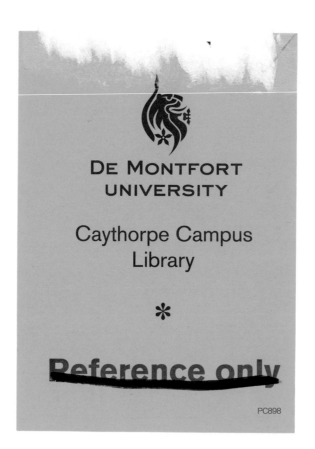

Biotechnology in Animal Feeds and Animal Feeding

Edited by
R. J. Wallace and A. Chesson

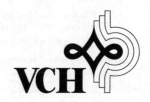

© VCH Verlagsgesellschaft mbH, D-69451 Weinheim (Federal Republic of Germany), 1995

Distribution:

VCH, P.O. Box 10 11 61, D-69451 Weinheim (Federal Republic of Germany)

Switzerland: VCH, P.O. Box, CH-4020 Basel (Switzerland)

United Kingdom and Ireland: VCH (UK) Ltd., 8 Wellington Court,
    Cambridge CB1 1HZ (England)

USA and Canada: VCH, 220 East 23rd Street, New York, NY 10010–4606 (USA)

Japan: VCH, Eikow Building, 10-9 Hongo 1-chome, Bunkyo-ku, Tokyo 113 (Japan)

ISBN 3-527-30065-1 (VCH, Weinheim)

Biotechnology in Animal Feeds and Animal Feeding

Edited by
R. John Wallace and Andrew Chesson

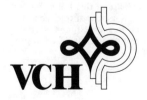

VCH

Weinheim · New York · Basel
Cambridge · Tokyo

Editors:
R. J. Wallace
A. Chesson
Nutrition Division
Rowett Research Institute
Bucksburn
Aberdeen AB2 9SB
Scotland, U.K.

This book was carefully produced. Nevertheless, authors, editors and publisher do not warrant the information contained therein to be free of errors. Readers are advised to keep in mind that statements, data, illustrations, procedural details or other items may inadvertently be inaccurate.

Published jointly by
VCH Verlagsgesellschaft mbH, Weinheim (Federal Republic of Germany)
VCH Publishers Inc., New York, NY (USA)

Editorial Director: Dr. Hans-Joachim Kraus
Production Manager: Dipl.-Wirt.-Ing. (FH) H.-J. Schmitt

Library of Congress Card No.: applied for

British Library Cataloguing-in-Publication Data:
A catalogue record for this book
is available from the British Library

Die Deutsche Bibliothek – CIP-Einheitsaufnahme:
Biotechnology in animal feeds and animal feeding / ed. by R.
John Wallace and Andrew Chesson. – Weinheim ; New York ;
Basel ; Cambridge ; Tokyo : VCH, 1995
ISBN 3-527-30065-1
NE: Wallace, R. John [Hrsg.]

© VCH Verlagsgesellschaft mbH, D-69451 Weinheim (Federal Republic of Germany), 1995

Printed on acid-free and chlorine-free paper

Printing: Druckhaus Diesbach, D-69469 Weinheim
Bookbinding: Großbuchbinderei J. Schäffer, D-67269 Grünstadt
Printed in the Federal Republic of Germany.

Preface

The problems faced by livestock producers and feed suppliers have probably never been greater. In most developed countries a static or falling demand for red meat coupled with downward pressure on prices exerted by the major retail buyers have meant that margins for the producer are ever smaller. In stark contrast, in many parts of the developing world the continuing shortage of feed of sufficient quality to allow even a modest production benefit means that animal products still contribute little to local food needs. Biotechnology offers hope for the amelioration of both of these extremes. In its more traditional guise of products from the fermentation industry, biotechnology already contributes much in the developed world to better diet formulation and to the provision of prophylactic agents that promote efficiency of feed conversion. This is set to continue and develop. Although the more traditional forms of biotechnology have had limited impact on livestock production in non-industrialised societies, recombinant DNA technology has the potential to extend the benefits of biotechnology and alleviate some of the many problems faced by livestock producers in these more deprived areas.

Biotechnology, and particularly genetic engineering, is viewed with concern by some. Public attitudes surveys still show that up to half of the national populations of countries of the European Union and the United States either are undecided about the merits of biotechnology or believe that biotechnology will adversely affect their lives. These concerns are reflected in legislation and, as a result, the statutes governing the introduction of products are more tightly drawn, more demanding in terms of proof of safety and more expensive to satisfy. The many vicissitudes surrounding the introduction of bovine and porcine somatotrophin well illustrates some of the present difficulties faced by manufacturers wishing to introduce engineered products. It is inevitable that public opinion will continue to influence the rate of development and introduction of new products. However public appreciation of biotechnology is not consistent. Applied to pollution control and bioremediation or to a reduction in the use of antibiotics, biotechnology is seen to offer solutions rather than problems. Consequently, products which have, or can be given a green image, or which do not directly impact on the human food supply are less likely to attract adverse attention. The registration of the enzyme phytase, one of the first products of genetic engineering introduced for use as a feed additive within the European Union, caused few problems. As a gene product it avoided the more stringent scrutiny applied to the release of genetically modified organisms and its intended use in reducing the need for added phosphorus in diets was seen by legislators to provide a solution to an acute environmental problem.

This book focuses on the application of biotechnology to animal feeds and feeding, deliberately avoiding the far more contentious issues surrounding the application of biotechnology to the animal itself. If this is a somewhat pragmatic stance, it reflects the editors views on which areas of current practice will develop and which areas of research are sufficiently well advanced to allow the early introduction of products. In this respect the book is intended to provide a guide to the possible and the practical in animal feeding. Despite this immediacy in the selection of topics for inclusion in this book, new possibilities have emerged during the time taken for its preparation and production. Two subjects of current interest to ruminant nutritionists are protected dietary peptides for use both as signal molecules and as a potential means of directed nutrition of the mammary gland, and the application of biotechnology to "by-pass" starch. Of more general interest is the potential use of oligosaccharides, particularly those of microbial origin, as agents able to stimulate a local and systemic immune response and the provision of minerals in organic form as more readily absorbed "bioplexes".

It is a mark of the vitality of the animal feed and animal production industries that developments move so rapidly from laboratory to field to become incorporated into the mainstream of production knowledge.

John Wallace
Andrew Chesson

Contributors

Susan B. Altenbach (71) USDA-ARS, Western Regional Research Center, 800 Buchanan Street, Albany, California 94710, USA.

Gilad Ashbell (33) Feed Conservation Laboratory, Agricultural Research Organisation, The Volcani Center, PO Box 6, Bet Dagan 50250, Israel.

Derek Balnave (295) Department of Animal Science, University of Sydney, Werombi Road, Camden, N.S.W. 2570, Australia.

Sharon A. Benz (28) Centre for Veterinary Medicine, Food and Drug Administration, Department of Health and Human Services, Rockville, Maryland 20857, USA.

Daniel Bercovici (93) Eurolysine, Siège Social, 16 Rue Ballu, 75009 Paris, France.

Keith K Bolsen (33) Department of Animal Sciences and Industry, Kansas State University, Manhattan, Kansas 66506, USA.

Daniel Demeyer (329) Department of Animal Production, University of Gent, Proefhoevestraat 10, B-9090 Melle, Belgium.

Trevor Doust (17) Veterinary Products Registration Section, National Registration Authority for Agricultural and Veterinary Chemicals, Box 240, Queen Victoria Terrace, Parkes, ACT 2600, Australia.

P. Anthony Fentem (279) Plant Biotechnology Section, Zeneca Seeds, Jealott's Hill Research Station, Bracknell, Berks RG12 6EY. UK.

Geoffry A. Foxon (279) Plant Biotechnology Section, Zeneca Seeds, Jealott's Hill Research Station, Bracknell, Berks RG12 6EY. UK.

Malcolm F. Fuller (93) Rowett Research Institute, Greenburn Road, Bucksburn, Aberdeen AB2 9SB, UK.

Masakazu Goto (26) Faculty of Bioresources, Mie University, 1515 Kamihama-cho, Tsu 514, Mie Prefecture, Japan.

Hadden Graham (295) Finnfeeds International Ltd., Market House, Ailesbury Court, High Street, Marlborough, Wiltshire SN8 1AA, UK.

Claire Halpin (279) Plant Biotechnology Section, Zeneca Seeds, Jealott's Hill Research Station, Bracknell, Berks RG12 6EY, UK.

Jean E. Hollebone (20) Biotechnology Strategies and Coordination Office, Management Strategies and Coordination Directorate, Agriculture and Agri-Food Canada, 930 Carling Avenue, Ottawa, Ontario K1A 0C5, Canada

Kate A. Jacques (247) Alltech Biotechnology Center, 3031 Catnip Hill Pike, Nicholasville, Kentucky 40356, USA.

Woodrow M. Knight (28) Centre for Veterinary Medicine, Food and Drug Administration, Department of Health and Human Services, Rockville, Maryland 20857, USA.

Ervin T. Kornegay (205) Department of Animal Sciences, College of Agriculture and Life Sciences, Virginia Polytechnic Institute and State University, Virginia 24061-0306, USA.

Pierre Monsan (233) Centre de Bioinéniere Gilbert Durand, INSA, Complexe

Scientifique de Rangueil, 31077 Toulouse, France.

T. G. Nagaraja (173) Department of Animal Sciences and Industry, Kansas State University, Manhattan, Kansas 66506, USA.

C. James Newbold (259) Rowett Research Institute, Greenburn Road, Bucksburn, Aberdeen AB2 9SB, UK.

Kyle E. Newman (247) Alltech Biotechnology Center, 3031 Catnip Hill Pike, Nicholasville, Kentucky 40356, USA.

Toshirou Nonomura (26) Commercial Feed Division, Livestock Industry Bureau, Ministry of Agriculture, Forestry and Fisheries, 1-2-1 Kasumigaseki, Chiyoda-ku, Tokyo 103, Japan.

Françoise Paul (233) BioEurope, BP 4196, 4 Impasse Didier-Daurat, 31031 Toulouse Cedex, France.

Frederick G. Perry (1) Rowett Research Services, Greenburn Road, Bucksburn, Aberdeen AB2 9SB, UK.

William D. Price (28) Centre for Veterinary Medicine, Food and Drug Administration, Department of Health and Human Services, Rockville, Maryland 20857, USA.

Anil Kumar Puniya (58) Division of Dairy Microbiology, National Dairy Research Institute, Karnal 132001, India.

Phillip T. Reeves (17) Veterinary Products Registration Section, National Registration Authority for Agricultural and Veterinary Chemicals, Box 240, Queen Victoria Terrace, Parkes, ACT 2600, Australia.

Gordon Rosen (143) 66 Bathgate Road, Wimbledon, London SW19 5PH, UK.

Charles G. Schwab (115) Department of Animal and Nutritional Sciences, University of New Hampshire, Durham, New Hampshire 03824-3542, USA.

Kishan Singh (58) Division of Dairy Microbiology, National Dairy Research Institute, Karnal 132001, India.

Stanislava Stavric (205) Bureau of Microbial Hazards, Food Directorate, Health and Welfare Canada, Sir Frederick G. Banting Research Centre, Ottawa, Ontario K1A OL2, Canada.

Judy Thompson (20) Plant Products Division, Plant Industry Directorate, Agriculture and Agri-Food Canada, 930 Carling Avenue, Ottawa, Ontario K1A 0C5, Canada.

Jeremy A. Townsend (71) Department of Biotechnology Research, Pioneer Hi-Bred International, Inc., 7300 N.W. 62nd Avenue, P.O. Box 38, Johnston, Iowa 50131 USA.

Marleen Vande Woestyne (311) Centre of Environmental Studies, Faculty of Agriculture and Applied Biological Sciences, University of Gent, Coupure Links 653, B-9000 Gent, Belgium.

Christian Van Nevel (329) Department of Animal Production, University of Gent, Proefhoevestraat 10, B-9090 Melle, Belgium.

Willy Verstraete (311) Centre of Environmental Studies, Faculty of Agriculture and Applied Biological Sciences, University of Gent, Coupure Links 653, B-9000 Gent, Belgium.

J. M. Wilkinson (33) Wye College, University of London, Wye, Ashford, Kent TN25 5AM, UK.

David R. Williams (22) Anitox Ltd., Anitox House, 80 Main Road, Earls Barton, Northamptonshire NN6 0HJ, UK.

Frantisek Zadrazil (55) Institut für Bodenbiologie, Bundesforschungsanstalt für Landwirtschaft, Bundesalle 50, D 38116 Braunschweig, Germany.

Contents

Preface

List of contributors

1 Biotechnology in animal feeds and animal feeding: an overview   1
F.G. Perry

2 Legislation and the legislative environment   17
P.T. Reeves and T. Doust (Australia), *J.E. Hollebone and J. Thompson* (Canada),
D.R. Williams (European Union), *T. Nonomura and M. Goto* (Japan),
W.M. Knight, S.A. Benz and W.D. Price (United States of America)

3 Silage additives   33
K.K. Bolsen, G. Ashbell and J.M. Wilkinson

4 Biological upgrading of feed and feed components   55
F. Zadrazil, A.K. Puniya and K. Singh

5 Transgenic plants with improved protein quality   71
S.B. Altenbach and J.A. Townsend

6 Industrial amino acids in nonruminant animal nutrition   93
D. Bercovici and M. F. Fuller

7 Protected proteins and amino acids for ruminants   115
C.G. Schwab

8 Antibacterials in poultry and pig nutrition   143
G.D. Rosen

9 Ionophores and antibiotics in ruminants   173
T.G. Nagaraja

10 Microbial probiotics for pigs and poultry   205
S. Stavric and E.T. Kornegay

11 Oligosaccharide feed additives   233
P.F. Monsan and F. Paul

12 Microbial feed additives for pre-ruminants   247
K.E. Newman and K.A. Jacques

13 Microbial feed additives for ruminants   259
C.J. Newbold

14 Transgenic plants with improved energy characteristics   279
C. Halpin, G.A. Foxon and P.A. Fentem

15 Dietary enzymes for increasing energy availability   295
H. Graham and D. Balnave

16 Biotechnology in the treatment of animal manure   311
M. Vande Woestyne and W. Verstraete

17 Feed additives and other interventions for decreasing methane emissions   329
C. Van Nevel and D. Demeyer

Index   351

1 Biotechnology in animal feeds and animal feeding: an overview

Frederick George Perry

Rowett Research Services, Bucksburn, Aberdeen AB2 9SB, UK

INTRODUCTION

Malnutrition affects about half a billion people throughout the world and a further 1.5 billion are undernourished or do not eat a properly balanced diet. Food shortages will become an ever increasing problem unless agricultural output can keep pace with population growth (Fig. 1). Animal products are crucial in this regard. They provide foods of high nutritive value, including milk, meat and eggs. In the case of ruminants in particular these products are formed from feedstuffs, such as forages and industrial by-products, that are not suitable for human consumption. Although biotechnology has been a component of the animal feed industry for many years it is essential that maximum use is made of the recent advances, notably in genetic engineering, to provide the increased production of animals and their products that will meet the needs of the human population in the coming decades.

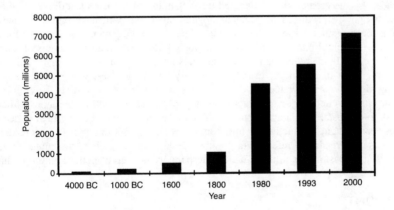

Figure 1. Growth of world population.

Improving the world supply of animal products generally means some form of intensification of animal production, although not all parts of the world are equally capable of adapting themselves to this challenge. There is no doubt that animal production in the Western World has improved over the last 30 years, in some cases quite dramatically (Table 1). Milk production per cow has improved in Europe by around 70%, most of this increase occurring in the last 10 years (Anon, 1992). Average milk yield per cow in Denmark and Netherlands, in 1991, was already in excess of 6200 kg per cow. Similar dramatic improvements have occurred in egg production. In pig meat production improvements have not been quite so dramatic, nonetheless increases approaching 50% have been achieved. Although the rate of improvement is showing signs of slowing down in the last decade, scope for improvement still exists in many countries. For example, in Greece, Spain and Portugal, milk yields are around

Table 1. Improvement in animal production over the last 30 years.

	Year			Improvement
	1960	1980	1990	
Milk production per cow (kg year^{-1})	3395	4400	6000	77%
Egg production per bird (year^{-1})	157	242	290	85%
Swine production				
Average daily weight gain (g)	450	600	630	40%
Feed efficiency (kg compound feed to yield 1 kg meat)	4.5	3.4	2.4	46%
Broilers				
Days to reach 2 kg liveweight	78	52	40	49%

3500 kg. While genetics and better management have contributed, improved nutrition of the cows, aided by the greater knowledge and understanding of the use of additives to the feed, many of which are produced by biotechnological processes, will have had a major role in achieving these results. Table 1 shows the effects of improvements in animal production under intensive conditions. It should be remembered, however, that large areas of the world have little or no choice other than to keep animals under extensive conditions. This usually means some form of roughage, often poor quality natural grasses, which are incapable of sustaining high levels of production. These feeds are never complete diets, lacking in trace elements, vitamins and major minerals such as phosphorus, as well as the animals being at some risk to a substantial parasitic burden. A well balanced, good quality feed is needed at all times for efficient production; a full stomach is simply not enough. For more detail of these issues, the reader is referred to Ørskov (1993), who describes the biotechnological constraints and possibilities in those nations desperately in need of better animal production.

FEED ADDITIVES

What are they?

Additives are now available in various forms ranging from direct-fed to slow release boluses which can substantially improve the efficiency of the diet, including low quality feeds, thereby improving animal production output for the local population. Biotechnology has been a significant contributor to the development of additives which help improve efficiency in both intensive and extensive forms of animal production. The range of additives used in the animal production industry is very broad, ranging from vitamins, trace minerals, growth promoters, disease preventing agents and auxiliary substances which, although not essential from the point of view of nutrition, have played a role in improving palatability, physical characteristics and preventing rancidity of the feed (Table 2).

Table 2. Classes of additives affecting efficiency of livestock production.

Supplements	Auxiliary substances	Disease preventing agents	Growth promoters
Vitamins	Antioxidants	Coccidiostats	Chemical
Trace elements	Flavours	Additives preventing	- ionophores
Amino acids	Emulsifiers	blackhead in	- antibiotics
Non-protein N	Free-flowing agents	turkeys	Biological
	Preservatives		- probiotics
	Pelleting additives		- enzymes
			- oligosaccharides

Consumer awareness

The addition of new additives to the list can take up to ten years or more, particularly with the exacting needs of toxicity testing and national and international registration requirements (Chapter 2). We can expect these regulations to increase, not only to protect the livestock and the farmer but also to impose safety standards which effectively ensure that food products from our animals are completely fit for human consumption. What the consumer wants from our end products will increasingly dictate our attitude to the way we feed our farm livestock.

Concern about the safety of the food we eat has increased, and will continue to increase, at least in the developed world. Food constitutes the inner environment of the human body and greater attention is now given to the involvement of our diet as a major factor in the development of a number of conditions affecting our health. This will undoubtedly lead to a call for animal products of different composition from those provided by the animal feed industry today. Biotechnological developments are beginning to address these issues. However, there will be problems of consumer acceptance. Some will say that such resultant products are far from natural, in much the same way some people distrust eggs from battery hens. We have yet to see the same distrust develop for stone ground flour from the modern genetically selected high yielding short straw varieties of wheat. This is a clear message to those involved in the biotechnological changes that affect the animal feed industry. Having satisfied the legislative, economic, toxicological and social requirements, they must ensure the consumer has confidence in the end product if they are to be successful in their mission.

At the present time we are used to seeing such headlines as "Biotech Comes of Age" and there is no doubt biotechnology already is having an impact on animal production, but it does bring its problems and dilemmas. For example, in Europe there are already substantial surpluses of some of the very products these biotechnology developments will assist with in greater production. Some, however, will result in lowered costs of production with no change in output and will thus become acceptable by making their contribution to better profitability of the industry.

THE DIET

Major feedstuffs

The majority of industrial animal feed formulations are composed of plant derived materials. Cereals and their by-products from various industries are the major components, followed by

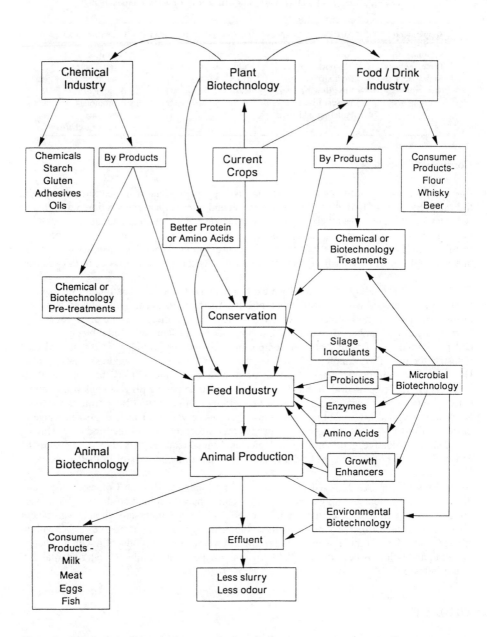

Figure 2. Contribution of biotechnology to animal production.

plant materials which are considered proteinaceous, such as legumes. Lesser components are animal by-products including meat and bone meal and fats such as tallow or lard. Additives such as vitamins, major and trace elements, synthetic amino acids, growth promoters and antibiotics generally complete the diet. More recently, enzymes and probiotics also feature as additives.

Depending on the animal production system, this formulated feed may be a complete diet as in the case of non-ruminants such as pigs and poultry and fish, or may be used as part of the diet to supplement locally grown and conserved forages for ruminating animals. This description forms the basis for a more detailed breakdown of the impact of biotechnology on the feed industry and animal production (Fig. 2).

By-products

Although this overview is concerned with the animal feed industry it has to be realised that many of its basic raw materials are by-products or waste products of other mature industries serving different consumer needs. Many of these by-products come from industries such as brewing, distilling and malting - starch conversion processes which in their own right have been subjected to developments in biotechnology and may be the carrier for that product into the feed industry. For example, by-products of the fermentation industry may contain within them the microbial residues upon which the process was based. These microbes themselves are likely to have been influenced by modern methods of biotechnology in order to improve the efficiency of the primary process.

Were it not for the use which the animal feed industry makes of by-products, they would create a major pollution problem. Fortunately, many of these raw materials lend themselves to upgrading either before the animal consumes them, or after consumption. Chemical and mechanical processes are often used before consumption, usually as part of the animal feed production process whereas biotechnological treatments, either as enzymes or microbes, are most often the choice after consumption.

Obviously all steps need to be taken to minimise pollution from the feed industry and farming community. Plant breeding techniques designed to produce better crops for livestock will have a major role to play. However, caution should be exercised in breeding plants for particular industrial uses. This must be a team effort, because these techniques will eventually lead to a by-product which will be targeted to the feed industry for its disposal. Plant breeders must ensure that there are no residual antinutritional components present, as well as keeping an eye on the volume produced: the industrialised feed industry can only cope with controlled volumes, otherwise the by-product of this effort will become a disposal problem.

Use of microorganisms

Microorganisms, long used for the preservation of food products, are playing an increasing role in the feed industry and gaining credibility both as inoculants for assisting in the preservation of forages such as grass or maize or as probiotics, where science is now bringing a better understanding to how these should be used in the animal.

Another interesting development has been the use of microbes to improve trace element supplementation. Some trace elements, such as selenium, have a narrow safety margin between nutritional requirement and toxicity. Selenium deficiency is on the increase, including in humans, as changes are brought about in the modern diet. The switch in the UK from less dependence on Canadian wheat compared to home grown wheat is currently being blamed for a significant fall in the daily intake of selenium to well below recommended levels for the population. To rectify this situation, selenium enriched yeast products are now a common sight on chemist's shelves as well as being used in the feed industry in bulk quantities. As scientists gain more knowledge of the role of minor trace elements we can expect to see more such products. Chromium and vanadium enriched yeasts are already in the pipeline.

APPLICATIONS OF BIOTECHNOLOGY

Improving the amino acid content of cereal grains

For poultry, pigs and fish fed conventional feed formulations, the essential amino acids lysine, methionine and threonine are usually present in limiting amounts unless the diet is supplemented with the synthetic version of these nutrients. However, considerable effort is being put into plant breeding to enhance the natural amino acid profile of the seeds (see Chapter 14).

Some success has already been achieved with conventional mutagenesis programmes. Wheat, maize, sorghum, milo and barley together with rice are the main cereal grains used in animal feeds, especially for non-ruminant animals. Each of these cereals has a drawback in their nutritional profile. For example it might be the tannin content of sorghum or the low protein content of rice. The protein component of the feed is probably the most critical part of the specification. Obviously as the nutritionist increases his understanding of what would be the ideal protein for the animal, in terms of its amino acid composition, then better use can be made of raw materials and better guidance can be given to the plant breeder.

As long ago as 1970, Munck *et al.* surveyed the world barley collection and identified one line named Hiproly which was high in protein and lysine content. Doll (1984) screened a large number of mutant barleys and identified several with enhanced lysine content. Miflin *et al* (1985) described future work aimed at identifying factors important in increasing gene expression not only for improving lysine but also the methionine and threonine content of barley. Although increases were achieved in terms of the free pool of amino acids they were not considered sufficient to satisfy nutritional requirements. None of the cultivars arising from this work has reached commercial production, largely due to other factors such as small grains or grain yield or poor disease resistance. In the current climate of cereal surpluses perhaps more attention should be given to acceptance of lower yields but better nutritional quality provided other factors are compatible with industry requirements.

Oats as a broiler feed

One recent example, obtained through conventional plant selection techniques, has achieved a cereal of a composition which is almost a complete diet in itself for broiler chickens. Oats is a cereal almost unknown as an ingredient in broiler feeds. The husk of the oat grain constitutes about 25% of the weight of the grain. The low metabolizable energy of oats excludes it from broiler diets but the protein content has always been regarded as being of high biological value with a constant amino acid composition over a wide range of protein content. A number of cultivars under the broad classification of "naked oats" have been developed. These cultivars have been found to have energy contents equal to maize as well as high protein contents. In addition the fat content is high and of the right fatty acid composition for poultry, thus making it with the addition of additives almost a complete diet in its own right. Table 3 illustrates one such experiment carried out with *Avena nuda* which clearly demonstrates its potential. On the negative side, harvesting remains a problem because the grain is easily shed from the crop, but advances in engineering including the use of stripper combine harvesters may help solve these difficulties.

Table 3. Performance of broilers fed different levels of naked oats (*Avena nuda* L).

Response Variable	Naked oats (% of feed)			
	0	20	40	69
	3 weeks			
Body weight (g)	545	567	563	493
FCR[1]	1.45	1.42	1.45	1.51
Feed (g bird^{-1} day^{-1})	35	36	36	32
	7 weeks			
Body weight (g)	1803	1865	1807	1744
FCR	1.93	1.88	1.87	1.92
Feed (g bird^{-1} day^{-1})	65	67	67	62
Dressing percentage	69.4	69.4	69.1	68.4

[1]FCR - Feed conversion ratio
From Maurice *et al.* (1985).

Other crops

In the long term, biotechnology researchers want to identify new uses for agricultural products, thus broadening the demand for the commodities farmers produce as their source of income. Already various EC countries are funding programmes looking at future non-food uses for crops. However, in the short term biotechnology can assist plant breeders develop a more stable performance of the traditional major crops, thereby reducing producer risks. Maize hybrids that contain a gene which confers resistance to specific herbicides are already being field tested. Hybrids of this type should mean that fewer herbicides will be used, which clearly has other environmental benefits.

These techniques, although highly relevant to cereal breeding, are now being applied to high-protein crops (Voelker and Davies, 1992). The target is often a product completely unrelated to the original crop and as such fits the role described in the last paragraph. It appears that it is only the imagination of scientists that is the most limiting factor of biotechnology applications for industry. Rapeseed is a good example of a crop included in normal farm production rotations in large areas of the world which has undergone considerable transformation. Gone are most of the nutritional problems associated with glucosinolates and high levels of erucic acid. However, wheels frequently turn full circle and there is now industrial interest in obtaining rapeseed crops with high levels of erucic acid. It must be remembered that the oil content of the rapeseed is only about a third of the seed. What happens to oil meal residue? Even if the antinutritional factors are kept under control the fact that the current animal feed industry cannot absorb massive volumes of such oil seed meals will add to this problem. Oil seed rape is currently in favour as a potential for production of "biodiesel". There is now plenty of evidence that rapeseed oil esters are perfectly satisfactory for a variety of circumstances in the fuel systems for the internal combustion engine, but every one tonne of oil for biodiesel produces an equivalent of two tonnes of rapeseed meal. Currently biodiesel is not economic but if this were to become the case then alternative uses will have to be found for the by-products.

Other crops such as peas, beans, soybean, alfalfa, clovers and grasses are all being subjected to modern biotechnology techniques on the laboratory scale. Some have been released for field testing. Some of the fears over the dangers of releasing genetically modified plants to the environment have been mollified by the results of the first comprehensive field trial in the UK of the invasiveness of a transgenic plant. Crawley *et al.* (1993) at Imperial College, London, have reported on a three-year trial which used two types of transgenic oilseed rape, a strain modified to tolerate the antibiotic kanamycin and another modified to tolerate the herbicide glufosinate. Each was planted out in four habitats in 3 different regions of UK along with an unmodified control. In the first year of the trial all of the plants had positive rates of increase. However this rate decreased for successive generations of plants which had grown from seeds shed by the prior generations, as the native plants began to recolonise the plots. In all test sites the hardiest strain was the unmodified control.

Soybean, because of its importance as one of the most widely grown crops, has received considerable attention from plant breeders. After oil extraction, the soybean meal is a major protein source for animal feeds but somewhat less than two thirds of its gross energy is available to the animal as metabolizable energy, mainly due to the presence of indigestible oligosaccharides. Scientists are now researching these aspects and seeds with reduced raffinose content and improved metabolizable energy content are now becoming available (Kerr, 1993).

While these results are encouraging, caution needs to be exercised in many ways. From the feed industry point of view it will be essential that by-products of this of exciting work are evaluated fully for effects on gut microorganisms and general body metabolism before they are acceptable as ingredients for inclusion in animal feeds.

DIETARY GROWTH ENHANCERS

There is no doubt that additives of a non-nutritional nature, based on biotechnology, have had a major input on growth and performance of livestock. It is often difficult to separate growth from better health and welfare. An animal which is in a good state of health, provided it is given adequate nutrition, will thrive. Products which influence these aspects include antibiotics, non-hormonal growth promoters, microbial products, including probiotics and enzymes and oligosaccharides.

Antibiotics as growth promoters

Although antibiotics have been used effectively for decades, particularly in a sub-therapeutic role, there is growing concern of consumers and the medical profession about their continued use as performance enhancers, especially from the point of view of build-up of resistance in the population. Zinc bacitracin and virginiamycin can be used without veterinary prescription and have been actively promoted as growth enhancers, making a significant contribution to animal production in the last two decades. However, being aware of the consumer concerns, the feed industry is actively pursuing alternatives with the aid of other biotechnology industries. Rosen (1991) summarised the use of antibacterials in disease control and performance enhancement, and highlighted the considerable variation in response using four well established products covering over 1200 trials. An update is presented in Chapter 8 of this volume.

Probiotics

Probiotics offer potential as natural products to fill the gap which would be left if the use of antibiotics were to be reduced. The proliferation of products described as probiotics has been enormous in recent times. A full account of progress to date is given in Chapter 10. Substantial funds are now being invested by government and companies to bring a better understanding to this area of considerable future importance to the feed industry. Both in Europe and North America, legislation is being introduced which will require probiotics to prove their efficacy in feeds if they are to continue to be marketed.

Recent evidence has clearly indicated the importance of selecting not only the correct organism, but the appropriate strain of that organism for the type of animal in which it is to be used, and the way in which the organism is cultured. Host specificity will take on increasing importance. For all the products to show a response in animal production following their feeding requires an increase in nutrient availability. Chesson (1991) described an excellent model of the effect of an increasing microbial load on the structure and metabolic activities of the upper digestive tract. Scientists involved in the development of existing or new probiotics should follow the logic of this model very closely.

Another area of interest related to probiotics is that of competitive exclusion, attempting to bring better control of pathogens entering the food chain from livestock production. Competitive exclusion has already become established in some parts of the world, notably Scandinavia, as a means of reducing salmonella and campylobacter contamination in poultry. However, current products, which are a diverse mixture of organisms originating from the caecal contents of adult poultry, are likely to find difficulties with widespread supermarket acceptance and impending legislation. Legislation will demand that the effective organisms are clearly identified in products of this nature (see Chapter 2). Further refinements of the concept of competitive exclusion together with a better knowledge of the substrates required to maintain the organism's viability in the gut environment will undoubtedly be developed in the near future.

In some parts of the world, climatic factors as well as the application of large amounts of nitrogen fertilizers are thought to be responsible for the build up of nitrates and nitrites in the stems and leaves of plants fed to ruminants. In the rumen, nitrates are converted to nitrites which are absorbed into the blood. Haemoglobin is then converted to methaemoglobin which results in a loss of oxygen transporting capacity of the blood and anoxia. Nitrite toxicity as it should be properly known leads to reduced performance, abortion and even death. Scientists at Oklahoma State University (Crummett *et al.*, 1992) have now identified from a collection of 154 cultures a particular strain of *Propionibacter* which, when fed to ruminants, is able to survive in the rumen and reduce nitrate and nitrite to nitrogen, thereby leading to a substantial improvement in the production losses associated with this problem.

Advances in recombinant DNA techniques and molecular biology have enabled considerable progress to be made in engineering rumen bacteria, and numerous genes encoding hydrolytic activities have been cloned in *Escherichia coli* (Hazlewood and Teather, 1988). The main objective is to increase fibre degradation by selecting the most efficient bacterial hydrolytic enzymes and introducing them into one or several dominant species of the rumen. Before this development reaches the commercial world, problems of gene stability within the host bacterium, ease of detection and control of the engineered bacteria will all have to be solved.

Enzymes

A small number of enzymes, probably less than 30 out of many millions in nature, are used on a large industrial scale. Of these, the majority are used in food and drink processing, detergents and textile industries. The animal feed industry is a relative newcomer in finding applications for industrial enzymes. Chesson (1987) and Hesselman (1989) reviewed the use of enzymes in poultry and pig rations, and listed numerous trials where the benefits of addition range from zero to 20% improvement in liveweight and feed conversion efficiency. This spread of results has given rise to confusion, but now a better understanding is being achieved as feed and enzyme producing companies invest in research specifically studying the role of enzymes in animal feeds. Table 4 summarizes the five main areas which have to be clearly understood before success can be achieved from the application of enzymes to feed.

Table 4. Criteria for successful application of enzymes to animal feeds.

Enzyme stability in the animal
Enzyme stability in the feed
Enzyme stability during and after processing
Interaction between the substrate and the enzyme
Ability of the animal to utilize the reaction product of the enzyme

Commercial enzymes with few exceptions are not yet designed specifically for the animal feed industry. Currently the largest application is in diets for non-ruminant animals that do not have the ability to digest cell wall components of the raw material. This has given rise to the addition of cell wall degrading enzymes which cause partial hydrolysis of the cell walls, releasing in some cases nutrients which would otherwise have been unavailable to the animal. The addition of β-glucanase enzymes to barley has now been widely adopted in Europe to allow this cereal to replace wheat in broiler feeds at considerable economic advantage and giving performance at least equal to that of wheat based formulations. However, more recent applications of xylanases to wheat-based formulations have generally shown that substantial economic performance benefits also can be obtained. A recent calculation by BP Nutrition (UK) suggested that the current addition of enzymes to poultry feeds is worth approximately

$40 million per annum to the UK broiler industry. There still remains a considerable challenge since many of the components of the other feed ingredients such as soya have yet to be made available as a nutrient to the animal.

Unfortunately, the level of success achieved with enzymes in poultry feeds has not been mirrored in pig feeds. As a result in the UK a substantial project funded by government and a group of companies has been initiated the Rowett Research Institute and the Flour Milling and Bread Research Association to address this issue. The future of enzymes looks exciting for the feed industry since the large industrial enzyme producers are now prepared to invest funds in developing enzyme applications for the feed industry. Sometimes the driving force may not be animal performance as we know it, but the reduction of effluent or pollution. Improving a feed digestibility from 85% to 90% does not sound too exciting but it reduces effluent by almost a third. In the areas of intensive livestock where manure output levies are imposed or threatened then this advance is attractive.

In some countries, components of the effluent are now coming under scrutiny. In the Netherlands, for example, pig and poultry farmers have to cut phosphorus waste by 30% by year 2000 from the 1986 levels or suffer severe cuts in livestock numbers. By 1995 farmers will be expected to maintain a mineral ledger to keep records of phosphorus arriving at the farm in form of fertilizer and feed. By 1995, farmers are expected to cut phosphorus from 175 kg ha^{-1} per year to 150 kg ha^{-1} and to achieve 65 kg ha^{-1} by year 2000. This will undoubtedly put significant emphasis on feed formulation to reduce the volume of phosphorus in manure, much of which comes from undigested phosphorus in the form of phytate, which is present in some of the plant raw materials used in the feed. This presented a clearly defined challenge capable of solution through an enzyme approach. Gist-brocades in the Netherlands have now cloned a phytase enzyme which scientifically is very successful but economics are still a little doubtful until the full impact of the pollution levy is imposed. Another group in the Netherlands has recently reported success in inserting of a phytase from *Aspergillus niger* into tobacco seeds (Pen *et al.*, 1993). Trials confirmed the efficacy of this development when seeds containing the phytase were fed to broiler chickens. Another product already developed is one containing a high level of α-galactosidase activity to promote the hydrolysis of oligosaccharides found in various legumes.

Enzymes have not generally been considered relevant for ruminants because of the role of the rumen microorganisms. However, there are now several indications that the additives of extract of *Aspergillus niger* or some strains of *Saccharomyces cerevisiae* may stimulate the numbers of cell wall degrading bacteria in the rumen, leading to an increase in the rate of fibre breakdown and an increased flow of microbial protein to the duodenum (Wallace and Newbold, 1992). Amylase has been shown to have small but significant benefits in some cases, where high cereal rations are used for fattening rations. More recently, work from Japan (Konno *et al.*, 1993) has found that an enzyme product obtained by culturing a basidiomycete, *Irpex lacteus*, has plant tissue digestion activity which, when the diet is also supplemented with amino acids, has a substantial benefit to ruminant production both in terms of milk production and composition as well as liveweight gain. It remains to be seen if these dramatic experimental results are repeated with the wide range of feeds found in farming practice.

Dietary oligosaccharides

Once known as "Neo Sugars", oligosaccharides are naturally present in many raw materials used in the animal feed industry. Many of the physiological effects of these dietary carbohydrates have been recognised to have human application, particularly in the Far East, notably Japan. In Japan, the significance and potential of these sugars has been highlighted by the renewed interest in the subject of glycobiology especially when linked to developments in analysis, purification and synthesis of these products. Table 5 lists some of the different types of products which are already commercially available, while Table 6 shows some of the potential applications for oligosaccharides. Chapter 11 deals with the topic in detail.

The recognition that cell surface carbohydrates have an important role as receptors for bacterial and viral pathogens, parasites, antibodies, food lectins and in normal cell processes has been the motivation behind recent interest in glycobiology. Also stimulating considerable current study is the effect mannose and manno-oligosaccharides may have in future to bring

Table 5. Some commercially available oligosaccharides.

Product	Production method
ß-Fructo-oligosaccharides	a) Transfructosylation of sucrose
	b) Hydrolysis of inulin
α-Galacto-oligosaccharides	Isolation from soybean whey
ß-Galacto-oligosaccharides	Transgalactosylation of lactose
Lactulos	Isomerisation of lactose
Isomalto-oligosaccharides	Transglucosylation of liquified starch
Maltotetraose	Enzymatic hydrolysis of starch
Xylo-oligosaccharides	Enzymatic hydrolysis of xylans
Chito-oligosaccharides	Enzymatic hydrolysis of chitin

some control to the animal feed chain, in reducing the incidence of *Salmonella* spp. in the food chain. Indeed mannose has already been shown to reduce salmonella colonization in young chickens. Commercial supplies of mannose or manno-oligosaccharides are not yet available.

Oligosaccharides bring a number of other advantages to the feed industry, such as their ability to withstand the high temperatures encountered in pelleting, their natural image from a product registration and consumer point of view, their stability to conditions in the intestinal tract, and their very low antigenicity. All of these factors favour their more widespread use in future.

CONSERVATION OF FEEDS

For generations, microorganisms have been used to conserve or ensile a variety of products, some of the earliest being the application of *Lactobacillus* cultures to preserve fish and animal offal for subsequent feeding to mink, foxes and fish. Similar cultures have been used for the manufacture of processed meat for the human market. More recently it has become increasingly common for farmers to ensile forage crops using biological additives. These commonly comprise enzymes designed to release sugars from the plant carbohydrates in order to promote the fermentation by naturally occurring organisms, or microbial inoculants which use endogenous sugars, again to promote the production of lactic acid by fermentation. In some instances, a combination of the two technologies has been used. Chapter 3 deals with silage additives in much more detail.

Because preserved forage forms such an important economic part of the livestock feeding regime, considerable effort has been made to improve our knowledge of the ensiling process and to develop products to aid a successful outcome. The vast range of organisms considered, together with the associated problems of viability, stability and safety, has lead to a proliferation of products, many of which have been patented because they relate to specific strains of an organism or specific processes for their production and stabilization, often combining other additives such as antioxidants (King, 1991).

If not properly ensiled, silages are prone to secondary fermentation by spoilage microorganisms, particularly if the acid concentration or pH is not sufficiently low to stabilize the silage. Such secondary fermentation is frequently characterized by the proliferation of *Clostridium* spp. which leads to reduced nutritional value and poor palatability of the feed caused by protein breakdown to ammonia and butyric acid. An interesting application in this area is the development of microbial additives containing bacteriophages (Day and Holton, 1988) specific to those *Clostridium* spp. most commonly found in silages in order to reduce or prevent the losses resulting from secondary fermentation. Claims have also been made for similar benefits in reducing butyric acid production in the rumen.

Table 6. Potential applications of oligosaccharides.

Substrate support in competitive exclusion treatment
Bifidogenic agent in animals (general)
Gut flora stabilization in young animals:
- piglets
- veal
- poultry
Gut flora stabilization during transport
E. coli suppression in rabbits
Component in competitive exclusion diets and premixes

Grass silage usually contains about 70% moisture and lends itself to biological pretreatment processes. For example silage quality is related to the quality of the forage which is harvested into the silo. Currently, grass for ensiling is cut at early stages of crop maturity in order to avoid the quality problems associated with lignification. However, there is now increasing attention being paid to harvesting the crop later to obtain higher bulk yields of dry matter per hectare and then using the silo as a reaction chamber to restore the nutritive value. With the development of enzymes, particularly those which have ligninolytic ability, studies are being made to establish if it is possible to degrade the lignin in the crop to gain access to the structural polysaccharide with which it is associated and at the same time not produce toxic phenolic compounds. If this approach can be made to work, the reduction in costs of harvesting, maybe two cuts of silage instead of the more usual three or four cuts, will pay substantial dividends to the farmer.

Although plant breeders have had considerable success in the past in producing new varieties of forage plants suited for particular purposes, whether it be for conservation or grazing, plant maturity still plays a significant role in determining nutritive value. In some ways, what determines nutritive value is elusive, since it is more than digestibility. Digestibility has a high heritability factor for a particular plant, but it changes throughout the life of the plant. Elucidation of the physicochemical features of forage digestion would go a long way to improving our understanding of nutritive value and could open the door for genetic manipulation to succeed. Nevertheless a number of seed companies are now working on producing forage plants which have lower lignin contents using biotechnology techniques in the broadest sense. It remains to be seen if these plants will stand up to harvesting conditions and the rigours of the climate in which they will be grown.

CONCLUSIONS

This overview has attempted to cover the implications of biotechnology in animal feed production without going into the detail provided in the following chapters of this book. There is no doubt that biotechnology is an accepted science in the feed industry, some aspects of which have been with us for many years. The advances being made by modern biotechnology techniques, although generally welcomed, have to be seen from the point of view that the animal feed industry is part of the food production chain. It will therefore be essential that all concerned with development affecting the animal feed industry keep the target customer in mind at all times if their work is to proceed to commercial practice.

REFERENCES

Anonymous. 1992. *EEC Dairy Facts and Figures.* Milk Marketing Board for England and Wales, Thames Ditton, Surrey.

Chesson, A. 1987. Supplementary enzymes to improve the utilization of pig and poultry diets. In *Recent Advances in Animal Nutrition* (W. Haresign and D.J.A. Cole, eds) pp. 71-90. Butterworths, London.

Chesson, A. 1991. Impact of biotechnology on livestock feeds and feeding. *Med. Fac. Landbouww., Rijksuniv. Gent* **56**, 1365-1391.

Crawley, M.J., Hails, R.S., Rees, M., Kohn, D. and Buxton, J. 1993. Ecology of transgenic oilseed rape in natural habitats. *Nature* **363**, 620-623.

Crummett, D., Hibberd, C. and Rehberger, T. 1992. *Oklahoma Beef Producer* 1-3.

Day, C.A. and Holton, B.W. 1988. Antimicrobial preparations. U.K. Patent Application GB 2206028A.

Doll, H. 1984. Nutritional aspects of cereal proteins and approaches to overcome their deficiencies. *Phil. Trans. Roy. Soc. Lond. B* **304**, 373-380.

Hazlewood, G.P. and Teather, R.M. 1988. The genetics of rumen bacteria. In *The Rumen Microbial Ecosystem* (P.N. Hobson, ed.) pp. 323-342. Elsevier, London.

Hesselman, K. 1989. *The use of enzymes in poultry diets.* Proceedings of the 7th European Symposium on Poultry Nutrition, Lloret del Mar. pp. 29-43. World Poultry Science Association.

Kerr, P.S. 1993. Soybean seeds with reduced raffinose saccharide content. World Patent Application WO 93 07742 A1.

King, A.B. 1991. Stabilized cultures of microorganisms. World Patent Application WO91 11509.

Konno, S., Matsuura, I. and Shirahata, K. 1993. Animal feed additive comprising enzyme and amino acid. UK Patent Application GB 2261877A.

Maurice, D.V., Jones, J.E., Hall, M.A., Castaldo, D.J., Whirenhunt, J.E. and McConnell, J.C. 1985. Chemical composition and nutritive value of naked oats (*Avena nuda* L.) in broiler diets. *Poultry Sci.* **64**, 529-535.

Miflin, B.J., Kreis, M., Bright, S.W.J. and Shewry, P.R. 1985. *Biotechnology and its Application to Agriculture.* SCI Monograph No. 32, pp. 71-78. Society of Chemical Industry, London.

Munck, L., Karlsson, K.E., Hagberg, A. and Eggum, B.O. 1970. Gene for improved nutritional value in barley seed protein. *Science* **168**, 985-987.

Ørskov, E.R. 1993. *Reality in Rural Development Aid.* Rowett Research Services Ltd., Aberdeen, UK.

Pen, J., Verwoerd, T., van Paridon, P.A., Beudeker, R.F., van den Elzen, P.J.M., Geerse, K., van der Klis, J., Versteegh, H.A.J., van Ooyen, A.J.J. and Hoekema, A. 1993. Phytase-containing transgenic seeds as a novel feed additive for improved phosphorus utilization. *Bio/technology* **11**, 811-813.

Rosen, G.D. 1991. Use of antibacterials in disease control and performance enhancement. In *Antibacterials and Bacteria*, pp. 1-30. Misset International, Doetinchem, Holland.

Voelker, T. and Davies, H. 1992. Plant medium chain thioesterases. World Patent Application WO 92 20236 A1.

Wallace, R.J. and Newbold, C.J. 1992. Probiotics for ruminants. In *Probiotics, the Scientific Basis* (R. Fuller, ed.) pp. 315-353. Chapman and Hall, London.

2 Legislation and the legislative environment

In this chapter the legislation governing the manufacture and use of the products of biotechnology in the feed industry as it applies to five regions of the world is described. The five regions chosen, Australia, Canada, the European Union, Japan and the United States, were selected because the existing trade is well regulated and because the systems of regulation developed in these countries have been adopted as models in many other parts of the world. However, this chapter should not be taken as a comprehensive guide to existing legislation. Amongst the countries of S-E Asia, for example, most tend to follow the example of the US Food and Drug Administration (FDA) or European Union, although Korea is somewhat influenced by the Japanese approach. However Malaysia, currently, has no registration requirements and Indonesia has developed its own unique system of control.

Of particular interest is the response of legislators to recombinant DNA technology since this will influence the rate at which genetically-manipulated organisms and their products will enter the marketplace. All five regions have dealt with, or are dealing with, requests to allow the use of products from genetically-modified organisms and the release of the organisms themselves. The response of the legislature in the selected areas to pressure for such release reflects, in part at least, the level of public concern about recombinant organisms and their gene products.

AUSTRALIA

Philip T. Reeves and Trevor Doust

Veterinary Products Section, National Registration Authority for Agricultural and Veterinary Chemicals, Parkes ACT 2600, Australia

Major changes to the Australian stock food regulations were approved in 1993 by the National Registration Authority for Agricultural and Veterinary Chemicals (NRA) in consultation with State regulatory authorities and industry. Under the revised arrangements, feed additives including therapeutics, parasiticides, growth promotants, performance enhancers, enzymes, microorganisms and vitamins, minerals and amino acids (where therapeutic, growth promotant or performance enhancing claims are made), as well as non-active ingredients of feeds are regulated by the Commonwealth under the Agricultural and Veterinary Chemicals Act, 1988. Medicated licks and blocks are also subject to Commonwealth registration which ensures that recommended medicament dosages result in acceptable efficacy. By contrast, medicated stock foods and medicated premixes no longer require registration *per se*. Nevertheless, dual Commonwealth and State control applies since the incorporated chemicals and their use levels are required to be registered by the Commonwealth, while ingredient standards and labelling of the end-use products are controlled at the State level. State regulations also apply to ingredient standards and labelling of feeds, non-medicated premixes, non-medicated licks and blocks, and vitamins, minerals and amino acids (where included at standard nutritional levels and where no specific label claims are made). None of these require to be registered by either the NRA or the State regulatory authorities.

The standard format of submissions for veterinary chemical product registrations in Australia is presented in the *Interim Requirements for the Registration of Agricultural and Veterinary Chemical Products* (the final edition of which is expected to be released in early 1995), and consists of the following Parts:

Part 1:   Submission Overview
Part 2:   Chemistry and Manufacture
Part 3:   Toxicology
Part 4:   Metabolism and Toxicokinetics
Part 5:   Residues
Part 6:   Occupational Health and Safety
Part 7:   Environmental Chemistry and Fate
Part 8:   Efficacy and Safety to Target Animals
Part 9:   Special Data
          9.1   Expert Panel on Antibiotics Approval
          9.2   Genetic Manipulation Advisory Committee Review
          9.3   Australian Quarantine and Inspection Service Approval
          9.4   Australian National Parks and Wildlife Service Permits

Because the standard format was considered inappropriate for enzyme- and microbial-based product submissions, new Guidelines for these product categories have been developed and draw heavily on the EU and Canadian Guidelines (*q.v.*)

The registration of enzyme- and microbial-based products generally requires preliminary evaluations by the Genetic Manipulation Advisory Committee (GMAC) and the Australian Quarantine and Inspection Service (AQIS) prior to submissions being lodged with the NRA. A separate application must be filed with GMAC when production strains involve recombinant DNA. An application to AQIS is mandatory when biologically-derived material is to be imported. Implicit in the issuance of an AQIS Import Permit is that the product conforms to the relevant specifications in terms of identity, purity and potency, and that the products are free from extraneous organisms, antibiotic activity or mycotoxin contaminants.

Submissions lodged with the NRA to register enzyme preparations are required to include general information on the identity of the end-use product and component enzymes, justification for product use(s), manufacturing details, and stability. The extent of the technical review undertaken for a particular ingredient reflects the adequacy of the information already on file and is structured around a two-tiered system. Under the first tier, the technical review is minimal for animal food additives that have GRAS status (prepared from microorganisms Generally Recognised As Safe) or have been evaluated by the National Food Authority (NFA), the Joint Expert Committee on Food Additives (JECFA) or the United States FDA, and approved as food enzymes. By comparison, the second tier involves more extensive reviews conducted on novel enzyme preparations which have not undergone previous assessment. Extensive reviews involve the Chemicals Safety Unit of the Department of Human Services and Health (CSU), Worksafe Australia (WSA), and the Commonwealth Environmental Protection Agency (CEPA) evaluating data on public health, occupational health and safety, and environmental issues, respectively. Important objectives of these assessments are to ensure that the production strain is non-pathogenic, potential hazards are identified, and measures to prevent risks and to protect workers during manufacture and handling are recommended.

Data in support of efficacy and safety to target animals are reviewed by experts within the State Departments of Agriculture. Extensive animal feeding trials are required to provide evidence that enzyme-based products are safe to target animals. Efficacy claims of enzyme preparations are categorised as generic (or non-specific) and specific. Claims such as "to increase the digestibility of certain feeds when fed to specific animals or subclasses of those animals" are allowed as generic claims. In this situation, the submitted information relates only to the identity and specifications of the ingredient(s) and end-use product, and justification of use in the target species. Local efficacy data are not required although efficacy data are needed to support justification of the product. By contrast, specific efficacy claims such as "improved feed conversion" or "specific productivity gains in target animals" must be substantiated by detailed efficacy studies and although overseas data might comprise the bulk of the data submitted, confirmatory local data are also required.

The submission requirements for microbial-based products include the identity of the end-use product, the identity and potency/activity of the component microorganisms, justification for use of the product, directions for use, and technical information related to stability and the manufacturing process. Other known uses of the microorganisms or the microbial preparation in human or animal foodstuffs, human or veterinary medicine, or industry, should also be included as this information may reduce the need to review certain submitted material. The technical review also is structured around a two-tiered system essentially identical to that described above for enzyme preparations.

The data requirements relating to efficacy and safety to target animals for microbial-based products are comparable to those for enzyme preparations. Briefly, safety to the target animals must be substantiated by clinical data generated from a single trial in which ten times the recommended dose is administered to the target species. Generic and specific claims are allowed for microbial products. A generic claim may be made when microbial preparations are administered to healthy or physiologically immature animals. Generic claims such as "for the maintenance of performance of healthy animals during normal animal husbandry practices such as shipping, dehorning, castration, weaning, ration changes, vaccination, debeaking etc." or "as an aid in the establishment of gastrointestinal microflora of physiologically immature animals" are not required to be substantiated by efficacy data. Detailed efficacy data are required to substantiate specific claims relating to animals with impaired physiology (for example, gastroenteritis or post-antibiotic therapy) or "for increased feed conversion efficiency and (or) productivity in healthy animals".

Non-active ingredients of feeds include antioxidants, pellet binding products, mould inhibitors, preservatives, colouring agents, anti-caking agents, deodorising agents and enzymes for which no therapeutic or performance enhancing label claims are made. Few of these ingredients are likely to be products of biotechnology. Under the revised arrangements, non-active feed ingredients destined to enter the food chain must be evaluated by the CSU via the NRA. Approved non-active ingredients are subsequently listed by the NRA and are exempted from registration. As an interim measure, those non-active ingredients currently included in feeds and premixes are considered approved, whereas new non-active ingredients need to be assessed for safety to the consumer. GMAC approval is required where recombinant technologies are involved in their manufacture, and AQIS approval where biologically-derived materials are imported.

In conclusion, biotechnology products which are intended for inclusion in animal feeds are evaluated by Australian regulatory authorities to the same standards as apply to conventional chemicals. However, the registration of genetically manipulated products by the NRA does require prior GMAC approval. While the establishment of a Genetic Manipulation Authority with legislative backing is imminent, it is presently unclear whether this body will be involved in the review process of feed additives.

Further information. Additional information on the Australian regulatory approach, or specific guidelines for chemical and biotechnological feed additives may be obtained from the Veterinary Registration Section, National Registration Authority for Agricultural and Veterinary Chemicals, PO Box 240, Queen Victoria Terrace, Parkes, ACT, Australia, 2600 (Tel + 616-272-3208, Fax + 616-272-4753).

CANADA

Jean E. Hollebone and Judy Thompson[1]

Biotechnology Strategies and Coordination Office, Management Strategies and Coordination Directorate, Agriculture and Agri-Food Canada, Nepean, Ontario K1A OY9, Canada, and [1]Plant Products Division, Plant Industry Directorate, Agriculture and Agri-Food Canada, Nepean, Ontario K1A OY9, Canada

The Canadian *Feeds Act* and Regulations govern feed and feed ingredients including those produced by biotechnology. Feeds are classified in eight broad categories including complete feeds, supplements, macro premixes, micro premixes, converter feeds, trace mineralised salts, mineral feeds, specialty feeds and single ingredient feeds. Bio-Feeds fall into the speciality feeds category which includes products such as forage additives, enzymes, flavouring agents and microbial products in non-viable or viable form (or the single ingredient feeds category if only one ingredient is involved).

Currently, there are no genetically engineered viable microorganisms (yeast or bacteria) commercially manufactured in Canada. However, there are a number of naturally occurring viable microbial products (probiotics) which are manufactured and registered for sale. As well, there are several products which have potential for modification through genetic engineering. These include:

- Fermentation products and other by-products, such as vitamins, amino acids, and flavours which are obtained through microbial fermentation. By-products from brewers, distillers and antibiotic production activities are also included. The resulting end products are highly purified and free of viable activity.
- Single cell (biomass) proteins, or microbial biomass proteins (MBP) which are the high protein cell mass remaining after microbial fermentation of a substrate.
- Microbial forage and grain inoculants used to conserve nutritional value of the feed.
- Viable microbial products designed to improve the performance of an animal or to modify specific physiological traits. This category includes live yeast and other fungi; bacteria; non-viable cultures of microorganisms and micro algae (MBP with a high potential for use in aquaculture).

Principles for the evaluation of genetically-engineered feed products

For evaluation purposes, products can be grouped into three classes based upon common risks that may be posed and assessed. These are:

- Chemical products of cell metabolism (amino acids and enzymes)
- Non-viable whole cells or part(s) of cells (e.g. from plant sources or single cell protein)
- Viable products (probiotics, yeast and forage inoculants).

Agriculture and Agri-Food Canada, in consultation with industry, is in the process of establishing criteria for product evaluations of bioengineered feeds. Some of the principles considered when evaluating the release of genetically engineered, viable microorganisms for risk are the nature of the microorganism; the intended use; and the nature of the environmental release site. Animal and human health and food safety aspects also must be considered if the product will ultimately be consumed by humans. The environmental fate of the product and toxicology of the organisms should also be reviewed, as well as the specific test site and the established experimental and safety protocols.

Because applications have not yet been received for genetically-engineered feed products, a general review of the present regulatory process is under way in order to integrate the new concerns of biotechnology into policy concerning the manufacturing of feed products. It is only with the advent of the first genetically-engineered product, however, that the proposed system can be adequately tested and adjusted. It is anticipated that the techniques of biotechnology used to produce feeds will, for the most part, involve recombinant DNA technologies. The first genetically engineered feed product is expected to be one developed to modify rumen function by enhancing fibre digestion.

Data requirements

Feeds are regulated by the Feeds Section of the Plant Products Division, Food Production and Inspection Branch, Agriculture and Agri-Food Canada. Under the current *Feeds Regulations*, most biofeeds would be registered as either a Specialty Feed or granted clearance as a Single Ingredient Feed. When possible, subcategories of the specialty feed designation with specific registration and evaluation requirements have been defined. These requirements outlined in trade memoranda are available to industry upon request. The data requirements for clearance of Single Ingredient Feeds are specified in T-3-141 and those pertaining to Specialty Feeds are set out in T-3-142. There are also specific Trade Memoranda for forage additive type products (T-3-122) and for viable microbial products (T-3-143). Although the level of information required varies depending on the specific product, the following is required regardless of the product.

1. Standard registration requirements including signing authority or Canadian agent (when the feed is imported) and a completed application form.
2. Five copies of the proposed label must accompany the application indicating the purpose of the product and appropriate guarantees, as per requirements set out in the *Feeds Regulations*.
3. A thorough description of the product is required, including:
   - A complete list of ingredients identified by generic name
   - The usefulness of the feed for its intended purpose
   - Scientific information supporting the claims of the product
   - A certificate of analysis and analytical methodology substantiating the guarantee

- Quality control procedures
- A product sample, if deemed necessary.

Toxicity and stability data should also be included when appropriate.

The type of information or scientific research data required will vary depending on the specific category of product. For example, requirements for the registration of a forage additive differ from those required for the registration of a viable microbial product (probiotic).

Feeds used for experimental purposes do not require permission for testing from the Plant Products Division. If such feeds are imported, however, details of the feed composition, the specific port of entry and the exact test location must be supplied before permission for importation can be granted.

Feeds in the Canadian Regulatory Framework

The Canadian approach to regulating biotechnology products is to build on current legislation and institutions. Hence, genetically engineered feeds will be regulated in the same way as conventional feeds. A similar approach has been taken for transgenic plants; they will continue to be regulated under the authority of the *Canadian Seeds Act*. Before a transgenic plant is approved for use as an animal feed it will be reviewed for livestock and environmental safety as well as nutritional utility by the Feed Section. In addition, before a transgenic plant is approved for use as an animal feed, it will be reviewed for human safety by the Department of Health and appropriate mixing and labelling requirements will be established.

Further information. Additional information on the Canadian regulatory approach, or specific guidelines for transgenic plants, biocontrol or pest control agents can be obtained from the Biotechnology Strategies and Coordination Office (Tel +1-613-952-8000, Fax +1-613-941-9421). For more information on animal feeds and feed additives, contact the Feeds Section, Plant Products Division, Agriculture and Agri-Food Canada (Tel +1-613-952-8000, Fax +1-613-992-5219).

EUROPEAN UNION

David R. Williams

Anitox Ltd., Earls Barton, Northants NN6 OHJ, UK

Comprehensive legislation is operative throughout the twelve member states of the European Union (EU) governing animal feedingstuffs. Most of the legislation is published as Commission Directives which are then adopted into the national legislation of each member state. In addition to the well known and long established products such as some vitamins, amino acids, yeast, brewery and distillery by-products etc., there are two new main categories of products deriving from biotechnology, namely enzymes and microorganism products which are covered by legislation introduced in December 1993. This forms part of the general framework of EU rules on animal nutrition and more particularly of the approval arrangements introduced by Council Directive 70/524 concerning additives in feedingstuffs.

The role of microorganisms and enzymes in feedingstuffs is, from a nutritional point of view, of the utmost importance, and the resulting economic advantages are far from negligible. These products, each according to its characteristics, improve the digestibility of nutrients present in feedingstuffs by facilitating their metabolism by the animal and, by stabilising the flora of the digestive system, they reduce the proliferation of pathogenic microorganisms. The latter quality helps considerably to reduce the mortality rate among young animals and improves homogeneity in animals at birth and later at the adult stage.

In terms of the environment, the positive effect on the capacity of animals to absorb certain nutrients (phosphorus, nitrogen, etc.) appears to be the way in which the quantity of phosphates or nitrates present in excreta is to be sharply reduced in the future. This latter aspect is of the greatest interest to the national authorities of those countries which are faced with the serious problems of pollution posed by the effluent in areas of intensive pig farming.

Purpose of the rules

In the absence of specific rules for the examination of this new generation of products, several Member States have allowed or temporarily permitted enzymes and microorganisms be used in animal feed. Other Member States have opposed the entry into free circulation of the products in question over the same period. The situation became critical owing to the distortions of competition which have progressively occurred in Member States at the level of both producers of enzymes and microorganisms and users (manufacturers of feedingstuffs and stock farmers). This state of affairs led some Member States to ask the Commission to regularise the situation. With a view to eliminating current distortions of competition progressively and achieving the level of harmonisation required by Community law relating to the authorisation of additives in feedingstuffs, it was proposed that:

- a status quo be established enabling Member States provisionally to permit the use of enzymes and microorganisms used or likely to be used on their territory pending a Community Decision in accordance with Directive 70/524/EEC;
- a timetable be adopted for the establishment of:
  - an inventory of all the products permitted in each Member State,
  - an identification note for the various products used
  - a dossier drawn up in accordance with Directive 87/153/EEC with a view to deciding at Community level on the authorisation to be given at national level
- rules on labelling be drawn up to which would apply to enzymes and microorganisms, and premixtures and feedingstuffs containing them.

The relevant Directives appeared in the Official Journal of the European Communities (OJ No. L334, 31.12.93 pp. 17 and 24) as Council Directives 93/113/EC and 93/114/EC.

The first step in the authorisation process is the drawing up of a list by each member state of products on the market, and the submission by companies of identification notes in support of their products. The format of the identification notes, which have to be completed and accepted by the authorities by 1st November 1994, is as follows:

1. Identity of the product
   - Trade name
   - Qualitative and quantitative composition (active substance(s), other components, impurities, and undesirable substances)

-    Name or business name and address or registered place of business of the manufacturer
-    Place of manufacture.
-    Name or business name and address or registered place of business of the person responsible for placing the product on the market, if he is not the manufacturer.

2.   Specifications concerning the active substance.
      For microorganisms:
-    Name and taxonomic description according to an international code of nomenclature
-    Name and place of culture collection where the strain is registered and deposited and the number of registration and deposit
-    State whether genetic manipulation has taken place.
-    The number of colony forming units (cfu g^{-1})
      For enzymes:
-    Name according to main enzymic activities and EC number (*Enzyme Nomenclature*, Academic Press, London, 1984)
-    State the biological origin. In the case of microbial origin, the relative information required for microorganisms above must be given
-    State whether the organism of origin has been genetically manipulated
-    Relevant activities with regard to appropriate types of chemically pure substances (expressed in activity units per g) e.g. μmole of product release per minute per gram of enzyme preparation.

Note: if the active substance is a mixture of active components, all the components must be described separately with an indication of their proportion in the mixture.

3.   Properties of the product
      Main effect:
-    Information concerning effectiveness.
-    Justification for the presence of each component if the substance is a mixture of active components.
      Other effects

4.   Product safety
-    Available information on safety.

5.   Conditions for the use of product
-    Uses provided for in animal nutrition (species or categories of animal, type of feedingstuffs, period of use, etc.)
-    Proposed dosage in premixes and feedingstuffs (appropriate units of biological activity such as cfu per gram of product for microorganisms or activity units per gram for enzyme preparations)
-    Other known uses of the active substances or the preparation (in foodstuffs, human or veterinary medicine, industry etc.)
-    Recommendations concerning product safety in relation to targeted species, the consumer and the environment
-    If necessary, measures for the prevention of risks and means of protection during manufacture and use.

6.   Technological information
-    Stability of the product with regard to atmospheric agents
-    Stability during the preparation of premixes and feedingstuffs

- Stability during the storage of premixes and feedingstuffs
- Description of the process of manufacture and methods used concerning the control of the quality of the product during its manufacture.

7.   Control
- Method(s) of analysis for determining the active component(s) in the product itself, in premixes and feedingstuffs.

8.   Attestation of the person responsible certifying the accuracy of the information given.

Long term authorisation

Once the Identification Notes have been submitted it will be necessary to begin work on the full product dossier, which must be submitted to the Commission and other Member States by 1st January 1996. There are formal guidelines on the information to be included in dossiers, detailed in the Annex to Directive 87/153. This Annex is in the process of being updated in order to take in the specific requirements of enzymes and microorganisms. The Commission also has recognised that the position of non-feed uses must be addressed when a further amendment of the feed additives directive (70/524/EEC) is discussed.

The Commission will publish the decision relating to all dossiers submitted up to 1st January 1996 before 1st January 1997.

Labelling

The directive applies to the use and marketing of enzymes, microorganisms and their preparations in animal nutrition, and there are specific labelling requirements for the products, premixes containing them and for compound feeds containing those products. The requirements for compound feeds are as follows and apply from 1st January 1995:

1.   Labels for compound feeds into which enzymes have been incorporated:
- The specific name of the active constituent(s) according to their enzymatic activity(ies) and the identification number according to the International Union of Biochemistry
- The activity units (activity units per kg or activity units per l) provided that such units are measurable by an official or scientifically valid method
- The expiry date of the guarantee or the storage life from the date of manufacture.

2.   Labels for compound feeds into which microorganisms have been incorporated:
- The identification of the strain(s) according to a recognised international code of nomenclature and the deposit number(s) of the strain(s)
- The number of colony forming units (cfu g^{-1}) provided that the number is measurable by an official or scientifically valid method
- The expiry date of the guarantee of the storage life from the date of manufacture
- Where appropriate, indication of any particular significant characteristics due to the manufacturing process.

The new legislation includes a number of other requirements especially when genetically modified organisms are involved. If the additive contains or consists of a genetically modified organism "A copy of any written consent from the competent authority to the deliberate release of the genetically modified organisms for research and development purposes provided for in Article 6 (4) of Directive 90/220/EEC, together with the results of the release(s) with respect to any risk to human health and the environment; together with the complete technical dossier supplying the information requested in Annexes II and III of Directive 90/220/EEC and the environmental risk assessment resulting from this information" must be provided.

It is estimated that several hundred enzyme and microorganism products are currently in use as animal feed additives, but many of them will be eliminated when the producers or suppliers fail to provide the extensive and detailed technical information on safety, quality and efficacy required for the dossiers.

Further information. Details of community legislation may be obtained from The Commission of the European Communities DG-VI, BII, 84-86 Rue de la Loi, 1049 Brussels, Belgium (Tel + 32-2-299-1111, Fax + 32-2-295-0130). Until full harmonisation of legislation throughout the community is achieved, specific and more or less restrictive rules may apply in the individual Member States.

JAPAN

Toshirou Nonomura and Masakazu Goto[1]

Commercial Feed Division, Livestock Industry Bureau, Ministry of Agriculture, Forestry and Fisheries, Chiyoda-ku, Tokyo 103, Japan, and [1]Faculty of Bioresources, Mie University, Tsu 514, Mie Prefecture, Japan

The Law concerning Safety Assurance and Quality Improvement of Feed has regulated the standards applied to the manufacture, use, preservation, labelling and components of feeds and feed additives since its introduction in 1953. It also established a system of inspection to ensure compliance. A major revision of the Law was introduced in 1975 and it has been steadily modified subsequently in order to achieve its objective: prevention of the production of harmful livestock products. In 1976, 44 types of feed additives were recognised under the law and registered by the Minister of Agriculture, Forestry and Fisheries. This has increased over the intervening period to the 132 types listed in 1994. In Japan, the designation of feed additives differs from that of medicinal substances used for prophylactic or therapeutic purposes. Medicinal substances are regulated by the Pharmaceutical Affairs Law. The former is based on generic specifications for each type of component, whereas medicinal substances are assessed on an individual basis.

Designation and specifications

Feed additives are grouped into three categories according to the purpose of their use. The first category, agents which do not directly contribute to the nutrition of the animal, includes antioxidants (3 types), mould inhibitors (3 types), binders (5 types), emulsifiers (5 types) and fermentation regulations (1 type). The second category of feed additives, amino acids (9 types), vitamins (31 types), minerals (34 types) and pigments (1 type), have a nutritional role in feed. Synthetic antibacterial agents (7 types), antibiotics (22 types), flavours (1 type), taste additive (1 type), and enzymes (9 types) form the third category and are used for promoting the more effective use of the nutritional components of a feed.

Criteria for each type of feed additive and feeds containing additives have been established to ensure public safety and to stabilise the production of livestock. Parameters designated for individual components include level of purity, titre and the maximum permitted concentration in specified feeds. The manufacture and use of antibacterial agents as growth promoters have been particularly cautiously treated. Regulations allow their use only for the designated animal and they are prohibited for lactating cows, breeding chickens and quails and calves until they are 6 months of age or older. A withdrawal period of seven days is required for pigs, chickens and quails to be killed for meat.

Antibacterial agents are grouped and no more than two from the same group are permitted to be used in the same feed. The groups are:

Group 1	Amprolium ethopabate, amprolium ethopabate sulphaquinoxaline, salinomycin sodium, decoquinate, nicarbazin, calcium halofuginone polystyrenesulfonate, monencin sodium, lasalocid sodium.
Group 2	Moranter citrate, destomycin A, hyglomycin B.
Group 3	Zinc bacitracin, avoparcin, alkyl trimethyl ammonium calcium oxytetracycline, efrotomycin, enramycin, kitasamycin, chlortetracycline, sedecamycin, thiopeptin, nosiheptide, virginiamycin, flavophospholipol, polinactin, tylosin phosphate.
Group 4	Alkyl trimethyl ammonium calcium oxytetracycline, chlortetracycline, bicozamycin, colistin sulfate, olaquindox.

In general, feed additives should be free from harmful substances and pathogenic microorganisms and the name and concentration of the active ingredient must be supplied. The date of manufacture (import), name and address of manufacturer (importer), and a statement of stability are also required. The necessary procedure to be followed for a new product allows the manufacturer (or importer) to experiment with the product under the experimental conditions stipulated by Ministerial Ordinance and then to apply for registration under 12 headings including the results of animal trials (efficiency, persistence, toxicity and effects on progeny). The data is then evaluated by the Agricultural Material Council and, finally registered by the Minister of Agriculture, Forestry and Fisheries.

Some agents, such as *Lactobacillus casei* used as a silage additive, have been legally used for other purposes including the production of human food. Where a bacterial species has been recognised to be safe for human foods, toxicity testing is required only exceptionally. In all other respects, the standards applied to the manufacture and use of bacteriostatic agents and the inspection thereof, established by Ministerial Ordinance introduced in 1992, are essentially those applied to other feeds and feed additives.

Examinations and assignment of manufacturing supervisor

The system of feed inspection introduced under the 1953 Law requires manufacturers or importers to operate to designated standards of manufacturing, preservation and use of feeds and feed additives. The six Fertiliser and Feed Inspection Stations of the Ministry of Agriculture, Forestry and Fisheries carry out inspections and regularly examine the components of all types of feeds and feed additives. For example, batch inspection for titre and toxicity of antibiotics manufactured in Japan appear to be carried out approximately once every two weeks.

The designation of a manufacturing supervisor, a requirement imposed by the Ministry on all manufacturers and farmers who produce and sell feeds and feed additives or who use feed additives in self-mixed feeds, has proved an effective mechanism for ensuring good manufacturing practice. Manufacturing supervisors are company employees who are held legally responsible for all activities at a particular site. They are not allowed to pass on these responsibilities to another. Generally they are qualified veterinarians or pharmacists, or have studied other relevant subjects (animal husbandry, fisheries or agricultural chemistry) at university, or have completed a Ministry training course and have had at least three years experience in the industry. There are currently about 800 manufacturers and 300 farmers who fall under the legislative framework of supervisor assignment.

New technical approaches in animal feeds

The application of molecular biology to the agricultural industry of Japan has been the subject of active experimentation. Since the first recombinant DNA experiments in 1976, more than 30,000 experiments have been completed under the guidelines for the genetic modification of organisms in contained laboratory system provided by the Ministry of Education or the Council of Science and Technology. Several processes for the production of agricultural products involving genetically modified organisms, including the production of amino acids, have been scaled-up using the open industrial-scale system provided by the Ministry of Agriculture, Forestry and Fisheries, although, currently, there are no commercial products. About 300 similar processes have been evaluated for practical use in the medicinal and industrial fields. Feeds and feed additives, produced from genetically engineered plants and microorganisms, will be regulated under the existing Law concerning Safety Assurance and Quality Improvement of Feed. No discrimination from conventional fermentation end products currently used for feed additives is envisaged. The standards with regard to manufacturing and use, the specifications applied to new bio-products, and the arrangements for inspection are the same as for the existing feeds and feed additives.

Further information Additional information concerning the Japanese regulatory approach to the agricultural use of genetically engineered plants and microorganisms, is available on application to the Biotechnology Division, Agriculture, Forestry and Fisheries Research Council Secretariat, 1-2-1 Kasumigaseki, Chiyoda-ku, Tokyo 100, (Tel + 03-3502-8111, Fax + 03-5511-8622). Information on feeds and feed additives may be obtained from the Commercial Feed Division, Livestock Industry Bureau, Ministry of Agriculture, Forestry and Fisheries, 1-2-1 Kasumigaseki, Chiyoda-ku, Tokyo 100, (Tel + 03-3501-3779, Fax + 03-3502-8766).

UNITED STATES OF AMERICA

Woodrow M. Knight, Sharon A. Benz and William D. Price

Centre for Veterinary Medicine, Food and Drug Administration, Department of Health and Human Services, 7500 Standish Place, Rockville, MD 20855, USA

The availability and use of products of biotechnology in the production of food for both man and animal is a reality. Because plants and plant products may find application in many different areas, including animal feed, they may be subject to federal oversight by different agencies in the United States. Presently, a number of agencies are involved in the regulation of biotechnology-derived products. Co-ordination of oversight by the different agencies and the pertinent federal statutes were discussed in a 1986 Federal Register publication (June 26, 1986; 51 FR 23302). In the developmental and experimental stage, the US Department of Agriculture's Animal and Plant Health Inspection Service (APHIS) is responsible for issuing field testing permits for genetically-modified plants under the Federal Plant Pest Act. The Environmental Protection Agency (EPA) is responsible for pesticides and toxic substances introduced into plants and sets tolerances for pesticide residues in food under the Toxic Substances Control Act (TSCA) and Federal Insecticide, Fungicide and Rodenticide Act (FIFRA). Governed by the Federal Food, Drug and Cosmetic Act (the Act), the Food and Drug Administration (FDA) has the regulatory authority and responsibility for ensuring the safety of food products from genetically modified plants under the adulterated food (section 402) and food additive (section 409) sections of the Act. Where possible, responsibility for review will lie with one agency. However, for certain products, it is anticipated that the lead agency will coordinate reviews with other agencies. For example, plants that have been modified to produce a pesticide or by-products from modified plants may also be used for animal feed purposes. Under these circumstances the EPA may request guidance from the FDA on the use of the plant in animal feed.

FDA has surveyed the scope of the nature of the biotechnological products that could enter the feed supply. These products fall under three definitions outlined in section 201 of the Act (food, food additive and drugs). Foods, such as corn and cottonseed, are not ordinarily pre-cleared by FDA, but are subject to regulation under section 402(a) of the Act. The Act gives FDA broad authority to initiate legal action against a food that is adulterated or misbranded within the meaning of the Act. Substances added to food are either food additives or generally recognized as safe (GRAS) by qualified experts. Both are pre-cleared by FDA unless the substance appears on the GRAS list established in 1976. The food additive definition broadly encompasses any substance that is added to food and, in 1986 and 1992, FDA published notices that indicated, in some cases, the genetic product from new plant varieties might fall within the scope of the food additive authority, and may require a food additive petition (FAP). It is also possible that genetic modification may result in a compound being produced by a plant such that the seller may be inclined to make a drug claim (cures or mitigates disease), in which case FDA may require a new animal drug application (NADA).

FDA recognizes that there are at least five different categories of feed products that may be derived using biotechnology:

- transgenic plants;
- fermentation products where genetically modified microorganisms are essential components of food;
- substances produced by genetically modified plants where the genetic modification is intended to colour food;
- food derived from animals that are subject to FDA's authority including seafood;
- ingredients produced by fermentation, such as enzymes, flavours, amino acids, thickeners, antioxidants, preservatives, colors and other substances.

Although there are no statutory provisions or regulations that address products of biotechnology specifically, FDA believes that it possesses extensive experience in the safety evaluation of products under its jurisdiction, and that feed ingredients derived from biotechnology can be regulated adequately within the framework of existing laws.

Because of limited resources and the many issues facing the FDA on a daily basis, regulatory discretion is used to avoid excessive expenditure of resources exploring issues which on face value represent minimal potential harm to the public. While there is truth in the idea that testing of the final product is the ultimate determination of safety, knowing the process used to develop the product is helpful in knowing the questions that should be asked to assure the product's safety. Thus FDA's approach to the regulation of genetically altered foods and food additives begins with an understanding of the process and procedure employed by the manufacturer.

FDA's policy toward testing and evaluating genetically modified plants was most recently outlined in the May 29, 1992, *Federal Register (57 FR 22984)*. This publication provides guidance for evaluating the safety and nutritional aspects of food derived from biotechnology that users of new technology should follow to assure that these foods are evaluated properly at all stages of production before their introduction to the food supply. It is organized according to issues that relate to the host plant that is being modified, the donor organism that is contributing the genetic information, new substances that are introduced into the food, or substances that have been modified. Decision trees and model questions in each of these areas are proposed that should be helpful to the sponsor in assessing the potential for the new food to cause harm to consumers. The document focuses on the traits and characteristics of the food and on what steps to take when certain changes are made to a conventional food.

Most genetic alterations of plants focus on productivity, and disease, herbicide, or pesticide resistance. In most cases, genetic modification will not likely result in significant changes in common food substances. Newly introduced or modified substances and changes in the level of common substances present in a food are core information to be considered in the safety assessment. Elevated levels of toxicants (e.g. glucosinates, alkaloids), or antinutritional factors (e.g. phytate, gossypol) would also be a safety concern.

The FDA has authority to require the establishment of food additive regulations regardless of the technique used to produce the food additive. A product that requires a food additive regulation (21 CFR 570) when added through conventional means would also be subject to a food additive regulation if it is the product of biotechnology. Thus a purified additive that is regulated as a food additive currently would be so regulated if it is produced at the same chemical purity via genetic manipulation of an organism. Here purity is an important statement because it is in the impurities associated with the manufacture of a natural substance using genetical engineering that is a primary concern. Impurities may arise from the microorganism fermentation materials and methods used to grow and harvest the enzyme. Demonstrating the safety of any impurities is the responsibility of the product breeder or manufacturer.

Direct-fed microorganisms (probiotics) are technically food additives and may require the publishing of a food additive regulation to provide for their safe use. Some forty microorganisms which present no safety concerns to the FDA are regulated in animal feed through an exercise of FDA's regulatory discretion. This list of organisms is published in the Official Publication of the Association of American Feed Control Officials. However, genetic modification of any organism on this list would cause the manufacturer to be required to submit information on the organism's safety and may eventually require the establishment of a food additive regulation for its use depending on the nature of the safety issues that develop.

The need for formal regulation and the nature of the required regulation of a food additive depends on the intended use and the labeling the manufacturer desires for the product. It is possible for the same product to be either a GRAS substance, a food additive, or a new animal drug. For example, if a GRAS substance is intended to have a new effect on animal feed when used, a food additive regulation may be required. When one labels that same substance to have an effect (health, production efficiency, etc.) on the animal, it will be regulated as a new animal drug. The regulation of identical forms of this substance would not differ regardless of whether it is derived from natural sources or from biotechnology. The labels for direct-fed microorganisms discussed in the above paragraph are permitted to state only that it is the source of the specific organism. Statements of benefits to animal health or productivity may cause these products to be considered new animals drugs. Products that have labeling that is either false or misleading are misbranded.

Future needs for regulating and labeling of products of biotechnology cannot be forecast. Based on responses to the "Statement of Policy: Foods Derived From New Plant Varieties", the public is interested in the labeling of genetically modified foods, and in the potential for development of allergies to food derived from genetically modified foods. The issues of premarket notification and the potential allergenicity of food derived from genetically engineered plants are not resolved and further discussions in these areas will occur. The influence of situations in other countries, particularly those involved in NAFTA and Europe, may influence our regulatory process as we attempt to achieve international harmonization in our food laws.

Further information. Additional information on the U.S. regulatory approach for animal feeds and feed additives can be obtained from the Division of Animal Feeds, Center for Veterinary Medicine (Tel. +1-301-594-1724, Fax +1-301-594-1812) and by reference to the documents cited below.

Code of Federal Regulations, Title 21, Parts 500-599. US Government Printing Office. Washington: 1993.

Federal Food Drug and Cosmetic Act, as Amended, and Related Laws. US Government Printing Office, Washington: 1990

Federal Register. Coordinated Framework for Regulation of Biotechnology; Announcement of Policy and Notice for Public Comment Vol. 51, pp. 23,3302 to 23,3313, June 26, 1986.

Federal Register. Statement of Policy: Foods Derived From New Plant Varieties; Notice. Vol. 47, pp. 22,984-23,005, May 29, 1992.

Kessler, D.A., Taylor, M.R.,. Maryanski, J.H., Flamm, E.L. and Kahl, L.S. 1992. The safety of foods developed by biotechnology. *Science* **256**, 1747-1749 and 1832.

3 Silage additives

Keith K. Bolsen, Gilad Ashbell[1] and J. M. Wilkinson[2]

Department of Animal Sciences and Industry, Kansas State University, Manhattan, KS 66506, USA; [1]Feed Conservation Laboratory, Agricultural Research Organization, The Volcani Center, Bet Dagan 50250, Israel; and [2]Wye College, University of London, Wye, Ashford, Kent TN25 5AM, UK

INTRODUCTION

Silage is the feedstuff produced by the fermentation of a crop, forage, or agricultural by-product of high moisture content, generally greater than 50%. Ensiling is the name given to the process, and the container (if used) is called a silo. Silage dates back to 1500-2000 B.C. However, the modern era did not begin until 1877, when a farmer in France, A. Goffart, published a book based upon his own experiences with corn silage.

Since the 1950s and 1960s, the amount of silage made in most industrialised countries (e.g. North America, Japan, Scandinavia and Europe) has increased steadily and often at the expense of hay (Wilkinson and Stark, 1992). Silage-making is much less weather-dependent than hay-making, and silage is more easily mechanized, is better suited to large-scale livestock production, and is adapted to a wider range of crops, such as corn (*Zea mays L.*), sorghums (*Sorghum bicolor (L.) Moench*), and winter or spring cereals (Bolsen, 1985).

Grass is the predominant silage crop in much of Europe. Although single species such as Italian ryegrass (*Lolium multiflorum*), perennial ryegrass (*Lolium perenne L.*), cocksfoot (*Dactylis glomerata L.*), timothy (*Phleum pratense L.*), and meadow fescue (*Festuca pratensis Huds.*) are the most common, mixed species of both grasses and legumes such as clovers (*Trifolium* spp.) are also ensiled. Corn and alfalfa (*Medicago sativa L.*) account for over 90% of the silage made in North America (Holland and Kezar, 1990), and over 50% of the silage in France and Germany is made from corn (Wilkinson and Stark, 1992).

A well-preserved silage of high nutritional value is achieved by harvesting the crop at the proper stage of maturity, which minimizes the activities of plant enzymes and undesirable, epiphytic microorganisms (i.e. those naturally present on the plant), and encourages the dominance of lactic acid bacteria (LAB) (McDonald, 1980). Additives have been used throughout the 20th century to improve silage preservation by ensuring that LAB dominate the fermentation phase. The silage additive industry has played a significant role in silage production, particularly in the past two or three decades. This is evidenced by the number of products being marketed.

In a comprehensive guide for silage additives available in the USA, Bolsen and Heidker (1985) included information on over 150 products and a more recent guide (Anon., 1992) described nearly 80 bacterial inoculants and about ten acid, enzyme and non-protein nitrogen (NPN) additives. A guide for silage products used in the UK contained over 100 additives, including 62 inoculants and 33 acid-based additives (Wilkinson, 1990). Spoelstra (1991) reported the results of a 1988 survey of silage additives marketed in the 12 countries of the

European Community. Of the 203 additives identified, 87 were inoculants and 83 were acid-based or salts of acids.

FACTORS AFFECTING SILAGE QUALITY

Silage preservation is influenced by numerous biological and technological factors (Fig. 1). Because many of these factors are interrelated, it is difficult to discuss their significance individually. However, the two dominant features to be considered for every silage are, firstly, the crop and its stage of maturity, and, secondly, the management and know-how imposed by the silage-maker.

The key "ensileability" criteria for a crop are: 1) dry matter (DM) content; 2) sugar content; and 3) buffering capacity (i.e. resistance to acidification). In these respects, corn is a nearly ideal crop, whereas alfalfa is at the other extreme and is the most difficult crop to preserve as silage. Grasses usually contain more water-soluble carbohydrates (WSC) and have less resistance to acidification than legumes.

CATEGORIES OF SILAGE ADDITIVES

In the early years of silage production, the reason for applying an additive was to prevent secondary fermentation and a butyric acid silage. As a result, the efficacy of the additive usually was judged by its effect on typical fermentation criteria, such as pH and concentrations of ammonia-nitrogen and lactic, acetic, and butyric acids (Spoelstra, 1991). This emphasis on fermentation was reflected in the traditional division of additives into categories of fermentation inhibitors, fermentation stimulants, and substrate or nutrient sources (Table 1) (Pitt, 1990; McDonald et al., 1991).

Fermentation inhibitors

In 1929 A. I. Virtanen, working in Finland, developed a method for rapid acidification of the crop with addition of mineral acids (hydrochloric and sulfuric) to a pH of about 3.5. This "AIV method" was used widely for decades by farmers in Scandinavia to ensile wet grasses. In the 1960s and 1970s, formic acid became the most widely used silage additive for low DM grasses and legumes throughout Western Europe. The addition of 2-4 l of 85% (w/w) formic acid per tonne of fresh crop reduces the pH of the forage from about 6.0 to 4.5-4.9 (Wilkinson, 1990). This has the effect of limiting the production of lactic acid during the fermentation phase, because less acid needs to be produced to lower the pH further to a stable level of approximately 4.0. The positive effects of formic acid on silage preservation and livestock performance have been extensively documented and reviewed (McDonald et al., 1991; Spoelstra, 1991). In many countries, formic acid is still the standard against which other additives usually are compared. The disadvantages of formic acid are its corrosive properties toward harvesting equipment, health risks to the user when not handled properly, and increased effluent production (Wilkinson, 1990). Sulfuric acid (45%, w/w) is also used in some European countries as a less expensive alternative to formic acid. In contrast to formic acid, sulfuric acid has no anti-microbial properties and merely acts as an acidifying agent (Woolford, 1984).

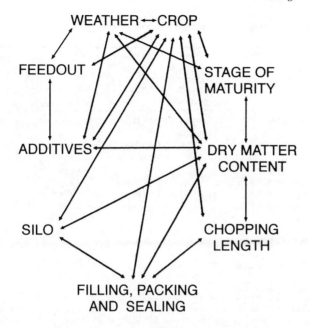

Figure 1. Factors affecting silage quality (interactions among factors are indicated by connecting lines).

Fermentation stimulants

In North America and several European countries where corn is an important silage crop, and alfalfa and grasses are more easily field-wilted to above 30 to 32% DM, LAB inoculants have become the most commonly used additives in the past 10 to 15 years (Bolsen and Heidker, 1985; Kung, 1992; Wilkinson and Stark, 1992; Muck, 1993). The bacteria in the commercial products include one or more of the following species: *Lactobacillus plantarum* or other *Lactobacillus* species, various *Pediococcus* species, and *Enterococcus faecium*. These strains of LAB have been isolated from silage crops or silages and were selected because they are homofermentative (i.e., ferment sugars predominantly to lactic acid), and they grow rapidly under a wide range of temperature and moisture conditions. Bacterial inoculants have inherent advantages over other additives, including low cost, safety in handling, a low application rate per tonne of chopped forage, and no residues or environmental problems. The ability of inoculants to improve the efficiency of the fermentation phase and thereby reduce DM losses in the ensiled material and increase its nutritional value depends upon two key factors. Firstly, enough WSC must be available for the production of sufficient lactic acid to achieve a stable pH in the silage (e.g. 4 - 4.5, depending on the initial DM content of the crop). Secondly, the LAB in the inoculant must retain a high viability from the time of manufacture to the time of use.

Enzyme products were introduced relatively recently as silage additives (Wilkinson, 1990; Muck and Bolsen, 1991). In the past, enzymes had sometimes been added to bacterial inoculants, but more recently products containing only enzymes have become available. These additives contain a variety of enzymes that degrade plant cell walls (cellulases,

Table 1. Categories of silage additives and additive ingredients[1].

Inhibitors[2]		Stimulants			Nutrient sources
Acids	Others	Bacterial inoculants[3]	Enzymes[4]	Substrate sources[5]	
Formic	Ammonia	Lactic acid bacteria	Amylases	Molasses	Ammonia
Propionic	Urea		Cellulases	Glucose	Urea
Acetic	Sodium chloride		Hemicellulases	Sucrose	Limestone
Lactic	Carbon dioxide		Pectinases	Dextrose	Other minerals
Caproic	Sodium nitrite		Proteases	Whey	
Sorbic	Sodium sulfate		Xylanases	Cereal grains	
Benzoic	Sodium sulfite			Beet pulp	
Acrylic	Sodium hydroxide			Citrus pulp	
Hydrochloric	Sulfur dioxide				
Sulfuric	Formaldehyde				
	Paraformaldehyde				

From Pitt (1990) and McDonald *et al.* (1991).
[1]Not all additives or ingredients used for silage are listed, not all listed are always effective, and not all listed are approved for use on ensiled material intended for livestock feed in all countries.
[2]Some inhibitors work aerobically, suppressing the growth of yeast, molds, and aerobic bacteria; others work anaerobically, restricting undesirable bacteria (e.g. clostridia and enterobacteria), plant enzymes, and possibly LAB.
[3]Most contain live cultures of LAB from the genera *Lactobacillus, Pediococcus, Enterococcus,* or *Streptococcus.*
[4]Most enzymes are microbial by-products having enzymic activity.
[5]Most ingredients also can be listed under nutrient sources.

hemicellulases, and pectinases) and/or starch-degrading amylases. In theory, additional sugars should become available for fermentation to lactic acid, and the partial hydrolysis of the cell wall could improve the rate and/or extent of digestion of the ensiled material.

Nutrient sources

Sources of NPN have been added to low-protein crops such as corn, forage sorghum, and mature winter or spring cereals primarily to increase the protein equivalent of the silage (Goodrich and Meiske, 1985). The main NPN products are urea, anhydrous ammonia and aqueous ammonia, and a few commercial additives also contain molasses, minerals, and acids. The justification for using NPN has been that it promotes a decreased protein degradation of the ensiled material, a prolonged aerobic stability during the feedout phase, and that the NPN is an economical nitrogen source. However, a major drawback to ammoniation of a crop is the potentially dangerous volatile and caustic properties of anhydrous ammonia, with the need for specialized application and safety equipment.

Molasses, which contains about one-half its weight as sucrose, is the most commonly used source of additional fermentable WSC, particularly for grasses and legumes that have less than 3% sugar on a fresh basis (Wilkinson, 1990). Cereal grains and their by-products also have been used, but to a lesser extent, to improve the fermentation quality of low DM forages. Because most LAB cannot ferment cereal starch, either amylase enzymes or substrates rich in amylases (e.g. malt) must be included (McDonald *et al.*, 1991). Citrus pulp, potatoes, chopped straw, and pelleted commercial products sometimes are added to wet crops with the objectives of reducing nutrient losses via effluent and improving fermentation efficiency.

THE FOUR PHASES OF SILAGE PRESERVATION

When making decisions about silage management techniques and additives, it is important to have a good understanding of the events that occur during silage preservation. The major processes involved can be divided into four phases: 1) aerobic; 2) fermentation; 3) stable; and 4) feedout. Each phase has distinctive characteristics that must be controlled in order to maintain silage quality throughout the periods of harvesting, silo filling, and silage storing and feeding.

Aerobic phase

When the chopped forage enters the silo, two important plant metabolic activities occur, namely respiration and proteolysis. Respiration is the complete breakdown of plant sugars to carbon dioxide and water, using oxygen and releasing heat. Simultaneously, plant proteases degrade proteins to primarily amino acids and ammonia and, to a lesser extent, peptides and amides (e.g. asparagine and glutamine) (McDonald *et al.*, 1991).

The loss of sugar during the aerobic phase is crucial from the standpoint of silage preservation. Sugars are the principal substrate that the LAB use to produce the acids which preserve the crop. Excessive heat production (i.e. temperatures above 42-44°C) can result in Maillard or browning reactions, which reduce the digestibility of both protein and fiber constituents. The main aerobic phase losses occur during exposure to air before a given layer of forage is covered by a sufficient quantity of additional forage to separate it from the atmosphere or before an impermeable cover (e.g. polyethylene sheeting) is applied.

Fermentation phase

Once anaerobic conditions are reached in the ensiled material, anaerobic microorganisms begin to grow. The LAB are the most important microflora, because forages are preserved by lactic acid. The other microorganisms, primarily members of the family *Enterobacteriaceae*, clostridial spores, and yeasts and molds, have negative impacts on silage quality. They compete with the LAB for fermentable carbohydrates, and many of their end products have no preservative action.

The enterobacteria have an optimum pH of 6-7, and most strains will not grow below pH 5.0. Consequently, the population of enterobacteria which is usually high in the pre-ensiled forage is active only during the first 24 h of ensiling (Lin *et al.*, 1992). Then their numbers decline rapidly, so they are not a factor after the first few days of the fermentation phase.

Growth of clostridial spores can have a pronounced effect on silage quality. Clostridia can cause secondary fermentation, which converts sugars and organic acids to butyric acid and results in significant losses of DM and digestible energy. Proteolytic clostridia ferment amino acids to a variety of products, including ammonia, amines, and volatile organic acids. Like the enterobacteria, clostridial spores are sensitive to low pH, and clostridia require wet conditions for active development. In general, clostridial growth is rare in crops ensiled with less than 65% moisture, because sufficient sugars are usually present to reduce the pH quickly to a level below 4.6-4.8, at which point clostridia will not grow. For wetter silages (70% moisture or more), reducing the pH to less than 4.6 either by the production of lactic acid or by direct acidification with the addition of acids or acid salts (see Section 3.5.4) is the only practical means of preventing the growth of these bacteria with today's technology.

The period of active fermentation lasts from 7-30 days. Forages ensiled wetter than 65% moisture ferment rapidly, whereas fermentation is quite slow when the moisture content is below 50%, such as in wilted haylages. For forages ensiled in the normal moisture range (55-75%), active fermentation is over within 7-21 days. At this point, fermentation of sugars by LAB has ceased, either because the low pH (below 4.0-4.2) stopped their growth or there was a lack of sugars for fermentation.

The populations of epiphytic microorganisms on forage crops are quite variable and are affected by forage species, stage of maturity, weather, mowing, field-wilting, and chopping (Fenton, 1987; Spoelstra and Hindle, 1989; Rooke, 1990). Numerous studies have shown that the chopping process tends to increase the microflora numbers compared with those on the standing crops, and the LAB population is most enhanced (Muck, 1989; Lin et al., 1992). This phenomenon was explained earlier as inoculation from the harvesting machine and microbial multiplication in the plant juices liberated during harvest. However, recent findings of Pahlow (1991) demonstrated that these large increases in microflora numbers were impossible to achieve by microbial proliferation and growth, because the time involved was too short, or by contamination from harvesting equipment, which could occur in the first load but not in later loads. A new "somnicell" hypothesis proposes that bacteria assume a viable but unculturable stage on the surface of intact plants (Pahlow and Müller, 1990). The chopping process activates the previously dormant population by releasing plant enzymes (e.g. catalase and superoxide dismutase) and manganese compounds.

The LAB ferment WSC to primarily lactic acid, but also produce some acetic acid, ethanol, carbon dioxide, and other minor products. This is a rather large group of bacteria, which includes species in six genera (Table 2). They are divided into two categories; the homofermentative LAB produce only lactic acid from fermenting glucose and other six-carbon sugars, whereas heterofermentative LAB produce acetic acid, ethanol, and carbon dioxide in addition to lactic acid (McDonald et al., 1991). Because lactic acid is a stronger acid than acetic and reduces the pH in the ensiled material faster, homofermentative LAB are preferred over heterofermentative species. In the fermentation phase, competition between strains of LAB determines how homofermentative the ensiling process will be.

Stable phase

Following the growth of LAB, the ensiled material enters the stable phase. If the silo is properly sealed and the pH has been reduced to a low level, little biological activity occurs in this phase. However, very slow rates of chemical breakdown of hemicellulose can occur, releasing some sugars. If active fermentation ceased because of a lack of WSC, the LAB might ferment the sugars released by hemicellulose breakdown, causing a further slow rate of pH decline.

Table 2. Lactic acid bacteria of importance in the ensiling process and their fermentation products.

Genus	Species	Glucose fermentation
Lactobacillus	*acidophilus* *casei* *coryniformis* *curvatus* *plantarum* *salivarius*	Homofermentative[1]
	brevis *buchneri* *fermentum* *viridescens*	Heterofermentative[2]
Pediococcus	*acidilactici* *cerevisiae* *pentosaceus*	Homofermentative
Enterococcus	*faecalis* *faecium*	Homofermentative
Lactococcus	*lactis*	Homofermentative
Streptococcus	*bovis*	Homofermentative
Leuconostoc	*mesenteroides*	Heterofermentative

From McDonald *et al.* (1991).
[1]Microorganisms that ferment sugars to predominantly lactic acid.
[2]Microorganisms that ferment sugars to a variety of organic acids, ethanol, and carbon dioxide.

Another major factor affecting silage quality during the stable phase is the permeability of the silo to air. Oxygen entering the silo is used by aerobic microorganisms (via microbial respiration), causing increases in yeast and mold populations, losses of silage DM, and heating of the ensiled mass. Pathogens such as *Listeria monocytogenes* have been found to proliferate in silages exposed to oxygen infiltration at low levels. The risk of *L. monocytogenes* is greatest in low DM silages and at high levels of oxygen ingress into the silo (Donald *et al.*, 1993).

The amount of aerobic loss in this phase is related not only to the permeability of the silo but also to the density of the silage. If the silage is left unsealed, substantial DM losses can occur at the exposed surface (Bolsen *et al.*, 1993). These losses can be reduced by covering the surface of the ensiled material with polyethylene sheeting, whether in vertical tower or horizontal bunker, trench, or stack silos (Dickerson *et al.*, 1992). Oxygen can pass through polyethylene, but at a very slow rate. Cracks in the silo wall or holes in the polyethylene seal obviously increase the rate at which oxygen can penetrate the silage mass.

Feedout phase

When the silo is opened, air usually has unrestricted access to the silage at the face. During this phase, the largest losses of DM and nutrients can occur because of aerobic microorganisms consuming sugars, fermentation products, (including lactic and acetic acids), and other soluble nutrients in the silage. These soluble components are respired to carbon dioxide and water, producing heat. Yeasts and molds are the most common microorganisms involved in the aerobic deterioration of the silage, but bacteria such as *Enterobacteriaceae* and *Bacillus* spp. also have been shown to be important in some circumstances (Woolford, 1984; Muck and Pitt, 1993). Besides the loss of highly digestible nutrients in the silage, some species of molds can produce mycotoxins and/or other toxic compounds that can affect livestock and human health.

The microbial activity in the feedout phase is the same as that occurring because of oxygen infiltration during the stable phase. The major difference is the amount of oxygen available to the microorganisms. At feedout, the microorganisms at the silage face have unlimited quantities of oxygen, allowing them to grow rapidly. Once yeasts or bacteria reach a population of 10^7-10^8 colony-forming units (cfu) g^{-1} of silage or molds reach 10^6-10^7 cfu g^{-1}, the silage will begin to heat, and digestible components, like sugars and fermentation products, will be lost quickly. The time required for heating to occur is dependent on several factors, including the numbers of aerobic microorganisms in the silage, the time the silage is exposed to oxygen prior to feeding, the silage fermentation characteristics, and ambient temperature.

Under farm conditions, feedout losses are largely a function of silage management practices. Few data are available to quantitate feedout losses in farm silos, but laboratory studies indicate that DM losses are about 1.5-3.0% per day for each 8-12°C rise in the silage temperature above ambient (Woolford, 1984). A fast filling rate and tight sealing of the silo minimize the buildup of aerobic microorganisms in the silage and maximize the production of fermentation products that inhibit their growth. Adequate packing of the ensiled material decreases the distance that oxygen can penetrate the silage face at feedout. Finally, feeding rate and silage density determine the length of time the silage is exposed to oxygen prior to feedout, and the shorter the exposure time, the less likely a silage is to heat during the feedout phase.

EFFICACY OF SILAGE ADDITIVES

Bacterial inoculants

The first known use of LAB cultures was with ensiled sugar beet pulp in France at the beginning of this century (Watson and Nash, 1960). Kuchler (1926) (as cited by Spoelstra, 1991) described an inoculant system developed in Germany, which included the growing of the bacteria on the farm. Many of these earlier attempts to inoculate silage crops were not successful because either the strains of LAB were not adapted to a silage environment or the bacterial cultures were not viable at the time of use (Spoelstra, 1991).

Whittenbury (1961) defined the criteria that a LAB should satisfy for use in silage, and additional characteristics were cited by Woolford (1984) and Lindgren (1984). Wieringa and

Beck (1964) reported that only one out of 81 strains of LAB isolated from silage was suitable for use as a silage inoculant. Woolford and Sawczyc (1984) screened 21 strains of LAB and found that none of them satisfied all criteria. *Lactobacillus plantarum* has been identified as one of the best suited LAB for inoculation of a silage crop, and single or multiple strains of this bacterium are included in virtually every commercial bacterial inoculant (Bolsen and Heidker, 1985; Wilkinson, 1990). Although *L. plantarum* satisfies most of the desired criteria, some strains are slow to produce lactic acid until the pH of the ensiled material falls below 5.0. Therefore, many commercial inoculants also contain species of *Pediococcus* and/or *Enterococcus*, which are active within the pH range of 5.0 to 6.5 and capable of dominating in the early stages of the fermentation phase (McDonald *et al.*, 1991).

Modern technology developed over the past three decades has greatly improved the commercial production of the bacterial cultures used in silage inoculants. An overview of the procedures was presented by Aimutis and Bolsen (1988), and a summary of the fermentation and stabilization techniques was reported by Risley (1992). After a specific microorganism has been isolated and selected, the commercial production of the bacteria involves growth (in a batch fermentor or bioreactor), recovery (filtration or centrifugation), and stabilization (freezing in liquid nitrogen, freeze-drying, or spray or fluidized-bed drying). Freezing in liquid nitrogen is the simplest procedure, but requires that the cell block be kept at low temperatures until it is used. Freeze-drying (lyophilization) takes this one step further, in that the water is removed as water vapor by putting the frozen cells under a vacuum and exposing them to controlled heating. The resulting freeze-dried cells are ground into a powder to be mixed with a variety of carriers. For both of these processes, several cryoprotectants are added to minimize cell death during the freezing period.

Perhaps no other area of silage management has received as much attention among both researchers and practitioners in the past decade as bacterial inoculants! It is beyond the scope of this chapter to cite all of the recently published scientific data. Summaries of several reviews will be presented, as well as results from selected studies to document the effect of inoculants on silage fermentation, preservation, and nutritive value.

Fermentation and preservation efficiency. Muck (1993) compiled data from over 250 studies conducted between 1985 and 1992 mostly with alfalfa, cool-season grasses, or corn in North America and Europe (Fig. 2). Inoculants significantly improved silage fermentation (e.g. decreasing pH and ammonia-nitrogen and increasing lactic-to-acetic acid ratio) in 65% of the studies. When the results were separated by crop, pH was lowered by the inoculants in 75% of the alfalfa, 77% of the grass, but only 40% of the corn studies. In an earlier review that included studies conducted between 1985 and 1990, Muck and Bolsen (1991) reported an improved fermentation efficiency in over 70% of the studies. At feedout, DM recovery was improved by the inoculants in 74% of the studies (25 out of 34), but aerobic stability was improved in only 42% of the studies (8 out of 19). The average increase in DM recovery in the studies that observed benefits from the inoculants was 2.5 percentage units. The authors stated that this was somewhat greater than would be expected from simply a more efficient fermentation phase alone, and that some improvement in aerobic stability during the feedout phase also must have occurred in many of the inoculated silages.

In the early 1980s, inoculants were being used to a limited extent in Europe, but results on farms were variable and scientific information was lacking on most aspects of bacterial inoculants (Castle, 1990). An international collaboration, EUROBAC, began in November,

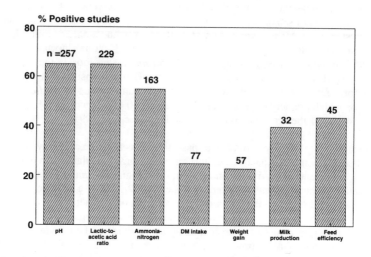

Figure 2. Proportion of studies in which inoculants significantly improved fermentation or livestock performance (the number of studies per measured response is shown above each bar). From Muck (1993).

1983, and joint studies on inoculants were conducted throughout Europe and Scandinavia. Results were obtained from 17 research institutes or universities in 11 countries, and data were available from 86 separate trials carried out both in the laboratory and on the farm. Classification of the grass silages based on DM content was: 1) direct-cut, <18%; 2) dry harvest conditions or "slightly wilted", 18-25%; 3) wilted, 25-35%; and 4) extensively wilted, >35%. It was the aim in these trials to compare the inoculant treatments to controls. The negative control was no additive and the positive control was the most widely used chemical additive, formic acid.

In a summary of the results, only the positive control was consistently effective in preserving the direct-cut silages (Zimmer, 1990). However, some results indicated that inoculants containing strains of the genera *Lactobacillus* and *Pediococcus* gave a more homolactic fermentation and a nearly 4% unit lower DM loss compared to the negative control, provided the grass had at least 1.5% WSC on a fresh basis. In the 18-25% DM silages, inoculants containing strains of *Lactobacillus* or *Lactobacillus* and *Pediococcus* were more effective than products that also contained a high proportion of *Streptococcus* (*Enterococcus*) *faecium*. Weather conditions during the wilting and harvesting periods produced a wide range in WSC content in the pre-ensiled grasses and a more variable response to the inoculants. In the rapidly wilted silages (25-35% DM), inoculants that contained *Lactobacillus* alone or in combination with *Pediococcus* markedly improved the fermentation process compared to the negative control, and they were as effective as formic acid. In the grasses ensiled above 35% DM (mean, 42.6%), the response to the inoculants was variable. When the grass was wilted quickly, inoculants gave a superior fermentation and a lower DM loss; however, if wilting was delayed by unfavorable weather and the WSC content was below 2% of the fresh crop, neither inoculants nor formic acid stabilized the preservation of the silages.

Grass suitable for inoculants contained a minimum of 1.5% WSC on a fresh basis and a DM content above 20-21%, but with either moderate or favorable wilting conditions to reach these values. Pooled data for the treatment groups according to these criteria are shown in Table 3. *Lactobacillus*-based inoculants gave silages of equal fermentation quality to the positive control (formic acid), but with significantly more lactic acid and a 1.1 percentage unit lower DM loss.

Table 3. Effect of formic acid and bacterial inoculant additives on the composition of grass silages with an initial DM content >18% and WSC content >1.5% of the fresh crop.

Treatment[1,2]	Pre-ensiled grass		Silage					
	DM (%)	WSC (%) fresh basis	pH	NH$_3$-N, (% of total N)	Acids (% of DM)			DM loss (%)
					lactic	acetic	butyric	
Control (63)	31.7	4.1	4.4	9.6	7.4	2.3	.4	7.4
Formic acid (29)	30.0	3.4	4.3	7.8	6.4	1.4	<.1	5.5
Lb or Lb + Pd (80)	32.0	3.5	4.2	8.1	9.1	1.4	.1	4.4
Str (31)	30.1	4.0	4.1	8.5	8.8	2.1	.4	8.1

From Zimmer (1990).
[1]Lb were inoculants that contained only *Lactobacillus*; Lb + Pd were inoculants that contained both *Lactobacillus* and *Pediococcus*, and Str were inoculants that contained a high proportion of *Streptococcus* (*Enterococcus*) *faecium*.
[2]The number of individual silages are given in parentheses.

During the EUROBAC Conference held in Uppsala, Sweden, in 1986, results of over 600 laboratory-scale experiments with silage inoculants were reported, and these were compiled by Spoelstra (1991). The data showed that inoculation of the majority of crops decreased pH values and ammonia-nitrogen concentrations and increased the lactic-to-acetic acid ratio by both increasing the lactic acid and decreasing the acetic acid contents of the silages. When averaged across all crop and ensiling conditions, *Lactobacillus*-based inoculants decreased DM losses by 2-3 percentage units.

From the EUROBAC results, the population of epiphytic LAB on the chopped forages was higher than expected, with counts below 10^3 cfu g^{-1} (fresh basis) being the exception (Pahlow, 1991). About 55% of the grasses were in the range of 10^4-10^5 LAB g^{-1} of crop. Since an average inoculation rate of 10^5 LAB g^{-1} was provided by the bacterial products, about one third of the forages had a LAB-flora count that was low enough to be increased by at least a factor of 10. For another 30% of the forages, the initial LAB population was doubled, but the remainder received significantly higher LAB populations only from products that provided 10^6 LAB g^{-1} of crop. Results showed that, in general, an inoculation factor (IF) of 2 was the minimum to achieve a positive effect on fermentation quality.

Bolsen *et al.* (1988) and Bolsen *et al.* (1990) determined the effect of bacterial inoculants on silage fermentation in a series of over 50 studies conducted from 1987-1989. The four principal crops used and their ranges in DM content were alfalfa (32-54%), wheat (30-42%), corn (32-38%), and forage sorghum (28-34%). Over 90% of the nearly 300 inoculated silages had a lower pH, higher lactic-to-acetic acid ratio, and lower ethanol and ammonia-nitrogen contents compared to control silages. IF was not a good predictor of the response to an inoculant, and applying more than 3 x 10^5 cfu of LAB per g of fresh crop did not provide additional benefit to fermentation quality. Fig. 3 shows the rate of fermentation for wheat harvested in the heading stage at 37% DM. Even though the chopped forage had 10^6 cfu of epiphytic LAB per g, all three inoculants produced lower pH and higher lactic acid values at 1, 2, 4, and 7 days postfilling. The data also suggested that strain selection for a particular bacterial inoculant was as important as the number of LAB it supplies per g of crop.

Pahlow (1990) indicated that a population of 10^6 LAB per g represents only a small fraction of the microflora that develop during the first two days of the ensiling process. Because few strains of epiphytic LAB have optimal properties for a silage environment, it was still worthwhile trying to establish a highly competitive strain or strains of silage-adapted LAB. Pitt and Leibensperger (1987), in a modelling approach, found that the effectiveness of bacterial inoculants increased with the number of LAB supplied, and they concluded that an IF greater than 1 was necessary. However, this was based on the assumption that the epiphytic and inoculant LAB had equal maximum growth rates. They also reported that an increased acid tolerance of the inoculant strains was more important than a homofermentative fermentation.

Nutritive value and animal performance. The number of studies with bacterial inoculants that have measured animal performance (e.g. liveweight gain, milk production, or feed efficiency) is much fewer than those that measured only fermentation and preservation criteria. In general, the effects of inoculated silages on beef or dairy cattle performance appear to be small, but consistently positive. In a review of data collected from 1985-1992, Muck (1993) reported that DM intake, daily gain, and milk production were increased in about 25, 25, and 40% of the studies when inoculated silages were compared to control silages (Fig. 2). Feed efficiency was improved in nearly 50% of the studies. When significant benefits from the bacterial inoculants were observed, DM intake, gain, milk production, and efficiency were increased on average by 11, 11, 5, and 9%, respectively.

Harrison (1989) compiled data published primarily in North America between 1982 and 1989 on the effects of inoculants, enzymes, or their combination on silage fermentation efficiency and dairy cattle performance. In 20 studies with predominantly alfalfa or grass silages, inoculants increased both actual and 4% fat-corrected milk by about 0.45 kg per cow per day. Cows fed inoculated silages also consumed more DM and had higher body weight gains. The greatest advantage for inoculated silages was obtained with wilted alfalfa and in studies that included at least 60% silage in the total ration on a DM basis.

Spoelstra (1991) summarized data published after 1985 with mainly low DM grass silages made under UK and Ireland conditions, as well as several dairy cattle studies using alfalfa silages in the USA. Overall, most inoculants were consistent in lowering pH, ammonia-nitrogen, and acetic acid compared to untreated, control silages. Lactic acid content was increased, on average, by the inoculants, but in 13 of 36 studies a decrease was observed. Feeding results showed that DM intake increased by an average of 3-4%, gain increased by 4%, and milk production increased by 3%; however, only about one-third of the increases in animal performance were statistically significant.

Bolsen *et al.* (1992a) summarized results from 26 studies conducted over a 14-year period at Kansas State University comparing fermentation efficiency, DM recovery, and beef cattle

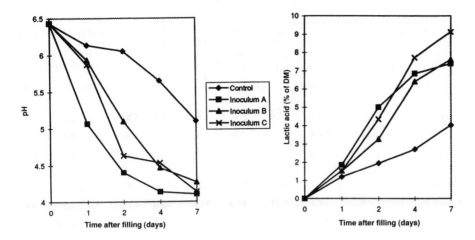

Figure 3. Effect of bacterial inoculants on pH decline and lactic acid production in wheat silages. The numbers of cfu of LAB supplied per g of forage were: inoculum A, 4.2 x 10^5; inoculum B, 3.1 x 10^5; inoculum C, 1.4 x 10^5. From Bolsen *et al.* (1988).

performance for inoculated or NPN-treated corn and forage sorghum silages. Treatment means for untreated, control silages and treated silages are shown in Table 4. The 19 inoculated corn silages had a 1.3 percentage unit higher DM recovery compared to untreated silages, and the inoculated silages supported a 1.8% more efficient gain and 1.8 kg increase in gain per tonne of crop ensiled. When the ten untreated and inoculated sorghum silages were compared, inoculants increased DM recovery, improved feed conversion, and produced 2.3 kg more gain per tonne of crop ensiled. In both crops, inoculants significantly decreased the acetic acid content of the silages and tended to decrease the ethanol content and increase the lactic-to-acetic acid ratio.

Overall, the magnitude of animal performance responses to inoculated silages are higher than might be expected from the shifts in fermentation products and the impact of increased DM recovery. One rather surprising finding from the recent reviews of Muck and Bolsen (1991), Spoelstra (1991), and Muck (1993) was that bacterial inoculants significantly increased both DM digestibility (in over 60% of the studies) and fiber digestibility (in over 35% of the studies). Why this should occur is not completely understood, because LAB are not known to degrade the cell wall or other components that are believed to limit digestibility in beef and dairy cattle. Muck (1993) speculated that the lower pH of inoculated silages causes additional acid hydrolysis of hemicellulose, which opened the cell wall fraction for more extensive and rapid digestion by rumen microorganisms.

Muck (1993) reported that animal performance benefits were linked closely to increases in digestibility in the 31 studies reviewed. Animal performance was improved in nearly 60%

Table 4. Summary of the effects of bacterial inoculants and NPN additions to corn and forage sorghum for silage fermentation, DM recovery, and cattle performance.

Crop and silage treatment	No. of silages	DM recovery[1]	Avg daily gain (kg)	Daily DM intake (kg)	DM per kg of gain (kg)	Gain per tonne of crop ensiled (kg)	pH	Products (% of DM)		
								Lactic acid	Acetic acid	Ethanol[2]
Corn										
Control	15	90.2	1.09	7.73	7.10	49.5	3.82	5.3	2.5	0.8
Inoculant	19	91.5	1.12	7.76	6.97	51.3	3.82	5.5	2.3	0.6
Probability level	---	0.01	NS	NS	0.11	0.01	NS	0.12	0.03	NS
Control	3	91.5	1.04	7.80	7.52	48.1	3.81	4.7	2.0	---
Anhydrous NH_3	3	89.4	1.01	7.96	7.84	45.0	4.19	6.1	2.5	---
Probability level	---	NS	0.16	NS	NS	0.07	0.01	0.01	0.12	---
Forage sorghum										
Control	10	83.1	0.75	5.96	8.32	35.3	3.94	5.1	2.6	1.4
Inoculant	10	85.2	0.76	5.85	7.98	37.6	3.93	5.2	2.1	1.2
Probability level	---	0.01	NS	0.20	0.04	0.01	NS	NS	0.02	NS
Control	3	87.7	0.61	5.41	9.52	37.3	3.91	5.1	2.0	---
Anhydrous NH_3 or urea[3]	3	82.6	0.49	5.13	10.58	30.3	4.63	6.1	3.6	---
Probability level	---	0.09	NS	NS	NS	0.24	0.10	NS	0.08	---

From Bolsen *et al.* (1992a)
[1]As a percent of the crop DM ensiled.
[2]Ethanol was not measured in studies conducted before 1984.
[3]One study with anhydrous NH_3 and two studies with urea.

of the studies (nine of 16) in which bacterial inoculants improved DM digestibility, and when digestibility was not affected by the inoculants, improved animal performance was observed in only 13% of the studies (two of 15).

The data reviewed indicate that bacterial inoculants are not always effective. The IF has been used to predict when an inoculant would be expected to give a significant improvement in animal performance for a particular silage crop. In studies at the U.S. Dairy Forage Research Center, increases in milk production from wilted alfalfa silages occurred only when the inoculant supplied at least ten times more LAB than the epiphytic, acid-tolerant LAB population on the forage (Satter *et al.*, 1991). Grass silage studies in Europe also confirm that an inoculant must provide a ten-fold increase in LAB to produce significant effects on animal performance (Spoelstra, 1991).   Corn usually has 10^5-10^6 epiphytic LAB per g, and commercial inoculants provide only an IF of 1 or less (Pahlow, 1991). However, data from farm-scale, inoculant studies often show increases in animal performance, and these benefits are not always explained by differences in fermentation efficiency (Bolsen *et al.*, 1992b; Honig and Daenicke, 1993). Gordon (1989) reported that DM intake and milk production were higher for cows fed inoculated ryegrass silage (10^6 cfu of *L. plantarum* g^{-1} of fresh crop) than for cows fed formic acid (85% w/w applied at 2.7 1 tonne^{-1} of fresh crop) or untreated silages. These improvements occurred despite similar fermentation characteristics for the three silages. Kung (1992) suggested that as yet unidentified constituents in the inoculated silages might be responsible for the nutritional benefits.

Enzymes

Forages contain the majority of their carbohydrate in the form of fibrous polymers of simple 6- and 5-carbon sugars. These polysaccharides (e.g. cellulose, hemicellulose, and starch) are not fermented to any significant extent by the epiphytic microflora on the ensiled crop (McDonald *et al.*, 1991). The concept of adding cell wall- or starch-degrading enzymes at harvest is attractive. If there is a shortage of fermentable substrate, more can be generated by the action of the enzyme preparation. In addition, by partially degrading the cell wall, cell contents should be rendered more accessible to the LAB population, which would increase the rate of fermentation. Many bacterial inoculant products also contain cellulases and hemicellulases, though rarely is their inclusion level or activity stated (Wilkinson, 1990), as an insurance against the crop having inadequate fermentable carbohydrate.

The consequences of adding an effective enzyme to forages would be to increase the extent of fermentation, producing silage with a lower final pH and a higher proportion of lactic and acetic acids by preventing secondary fermentation. Alternatively, if fermentation is restricted in higher DM crops by lack of available water, enzymes may increase the content of residual sugars in the silage. These sugars would then be expected to stimulate growth of the rumen microflora and thereby give an increased DM intake. A further benefit of adding enzymes could be that, by degrading the slowly digested fiber portion of the crop in the silo, the rate (and also extent) of digestion of the silage in the rumen may be increased, with consequent benefits to both DM intake and feed efficiency. On the negative side, excess sugars in the silage during the fermentation, storage, and feedout phases could encourage the growth of anaerobic yeasts, which would ferment the sugars to alcohol.

Little information exists on the activity of enzyme preparations, and few independent assays have been made of the activity of commercial products, possibly reflecting their recent introduction as major ingredients in silage additives. One such assay of a commercial preparation by Jacobs and McAllan (1990) showed that the predominant activity was hemicellulolytic, rather than cellulolytic. If 5-carbon sugars, such as xylose, are the predominant end-products of enzyme activity, then the bacteria to benefit most would be those that could ferment pentoses. Strictly homofermentative LAB are not able to ferment pentoses, though some genera that produce lactic acid, such as *Enterococcus* and *Pediococcus*, can do so (McDonald *et al.*, 1991). Therefore, it is desirable to have one or both of these genera as bacterial inoculants in additives containing cell wall-degrading enzymes. If the pentose sugars produced by the enzyme preparation are not fermented extensively by the bacterial population in the silo, then increased residual sugars should occur in the silage. This was confirmed by Henderson *et al.* (1991) with low DM grass silages.

McDonald *et al.* (1991) and Muck (1993) concluded that although enzyme additives in the majority of studies were able to increase the content of fermentable carbohydrate by hydrolysis of cell wall polysaccharides, their effects on digestibility and on animal performance have been disappointing. Thus, despite improvements in fermentation characteristics as measured by lower final pH, higher lactic-to-acetic acid ratio, and lower ammonia-nitrogen, higher DM intakes were achieved in less than 25% of the studies reviewed (Fig. 4). A similar low proportion of studies showed improvements in weight gain, milk production, and feed efficiency.

Muck (1993) noted that the reduction in cell wall (neutral detergent fiber) content following addition of enzymes to forages at ensiling was more consistent in grasses (80% of the studies) than in legumes (27% of the studies). This may simply reflect the fact that the commercial enzyme preparations tested were chosen for use with grasses and that the fiber content and structure of grasses and legumes differ. Stokes and Libby (1993) found that the inclusion of α-amylase, gluco-amylase, and pectinase in a commercial preparation (based on cellulase, cellobiase, and xylanase, and designated for use with grass) was more effective in reducing NDF content of alfalfa than grass silage. This suggests that pectinase, in particular, was effective in aiding enzyme access to the cellulose in the cell wall of alfalfa.

The lack of positive effects of enzyme additions to ensiled forages on DM intake might reflect an increased acidity of the treated silages. Failure to improve digestibility could be the result of solubilization of the same cell wall components that are digested relatively easily by the rumen microflora. In other words, the addition of the enzyme preparations did not increase the total content of rumen fermentable energy in the silage. Another possible reason for the relatively poor animal performance with enzyme-treated silages could lie in the observation that, with low DM crops, the addition of enzymes, with or without a bacterial inoculant, leads to increases in effluent loss (McAllan *et al.*, 1991). Because the constituents of effluent are derived principally from cell contents, which are virtually completely digestible, any increase in potential digestibility could be offset by increased nutrient losses in the effluent.

It could be argued that conversion of rumen fermentable polysaccharide to organic acids by solubilization and subsequent fermentation in the silo are not in the best interest of the rumen microflora, for which ATP-yielding substrates are at a premium. If this is the case, then a more logical point of addition of enzymes to silage would be at the time of feeding, rather than at the time of ensiling. In this way, the enzyme action would occur in the feed bunk rather than in the silo, with release of simple sugars for rapid fermentation by the rumen microbial population.

Nutrient sources

Nonprotein nitrogen. Earlier research with urea and anhydrous ammonia additions to corn and sorghum silages was reviewed by Ely (1978). Urea-treated silages gave small but consistent improvements in gain, milk production, and feed efficiency compared to silages that were supplemented with a similar amount of urea at feeding. Ammonia-treated silages provided benefits less frequently and had negative effects in several studies. The review did not include silage preservation results; however, retention of added nitrogen was 95% or higher for urea-treated silages but only 50-75% for ammonia treated silages. Adding ammonia immediately raises the pH of the crop to 8-9, and the combined effect of the ammonia and high pH reduces the yeast and mold populations and usually increases the

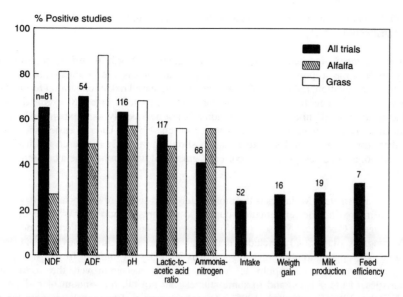

Figure 4. Studies conducted between 1985-1992 in which enzymes significantly improved fermentation or livestock performance (the number of studies per measured response is shown above each bar). From Muck (1993).

aerobic stability of the silage. Ammonia also decreases the number of LAB, and this delays the start of the fermentation phase. However, the amount of fermentation products (lactic and acetic acids) increases because of the much higher initial pH. Ammonia breaks some of the linkages between hemicellulose and other cell wall components, which should increase both rate and extent of digestion. The high initial pH also inactivates plant proteases, and this decreases the extent of protein degradation in the ensiled crop.

In a series of six studies conducted in farm-scale silos, Bolsen *et al.* (1992a) observed that anhydrous ammonia applied at 3.5-4.0 kg per tonne or urea at 5.0 kg per tonne increased the pH, lactic and acetic acid concentrations and DM losses in both corn and forage sorghum silages (Table 4). Performance of growing cattle was not improved by the NPN-treatments, but gain per tonne of crop ensiled was reduced by 3.1 and 7.0 kg in the corn and sorghum silages, respectively.

In a review of 39 studies reported since 1985, Muck (1993) found that NPN additives increased fermentation acids in approximately 60% of the silages, and in low DM crops (less than 30%) clostridial activity was a problem. In 12 of 21 studies, DM recovery was decreased in the NPN-treated silages and increased in only three studies. Aerobic stability was consistently improved in the NPN silages. Digestibility of the NPN silages (DM, NDF, or ADF) was increased in 16 of 19 studies, and most treated silages had a higher true protein content. These apparent improvements in nutritive value did not increase gain, milk production, or feed efficiency in most studies, especially in recent research with grass and legume silages. The author noted that the apparent paradoxes of improved bunk life with reduced DM recovery and improved digestibility with no benefit in animal performance need further clarification.

Anhydrous ammonia is used widely in a few regions of North America; however, it is unlikely to become a popular additive in the future unless the problems of handling, application, preservation, reduced DM intake, and the increased risk of clostridial fermentation are overcome. When economic analysis includes the increased silage DM loss and the cost of replacing the volatile nitrogen loss, ammonia is not necessarily an inexpensive source of supplemental protein for beef and dairy cattle (Bolsen, 1993). Urea is easier and safer to handle than ammonia, but unless future studies show significantly increased nutritive value for the traditional silage crops, such as corn and grasses, it will not become a commonly used additive.

Fermentable substrates. Molasses is the most widely used source of sugars and is particularly effective in improving the fermentation quality in wet grasses and low WSC legumes and tropical forages. Castle and Watson (1985) compared molasses and formic acid additions to low DM ryegrass silages and concluded that at 20-30 l per tonne, molasses was as effective as the acid. The application of high levels, such as 50-60 kg per tonne of fresh crop, of either cereal grains or sugar beet pulp to low DM crops has improved the fermentation characteristics of the silages, and in some studies, but not all, the amount of effluent was reduced (Done, 1988; Jones *et al.*, 1990). Thorough mixing of the substrates with the crop is particularly important because, if the adsorbents are added in layers in silos fitted with internal drains, effluent production might be increased (Wilkinson, 1990).

Acids and acid salts

In Europe and in many other areas where low DM grasses are important silage crops, formic acid is the standard against which most other silage additives have been tested. Formic acid not only restricts the growth of bacteria through its acidifying effect, it also has a selective antibacterial action, as does the weaker propionic acid (Woolford, 1975). In contrast, the mineral acids, sulfuric and hydrochloric, act solely by decreasing pH and they have no specific antimicrobial properties. Yeasts have been shown to be particularly tolerant of formic acid (McDonald *et al.*, 1991), and the aerobic stability of silages made with formic acid is often poor, partly because of the likely elevated yeast counts in the silage, and also because of the restricted fermentation, which leads to relatively higher contents of residual WSC in the silage.

Effects of formic acid on animal performance have been reviewed extensively (Waldo, 1978; Thomas and Thomas, 1985; McDonald *et al.*, 1991). The extent of the improvement in animal performance depends on the preservation quality of the untreated forage, with large benefits recorded when the untreated silage is badly preserved.

Salts of acids are used widely in Europe as safer alternatives to the acids themselves and efficacy is similar if similar rates of active ingredients are applied to the crop. Recently, the combined addition of bacterial inoculant and salts has been evaluated (Kalzendorf and Weissbach, 1993) with encouraging results. In ten studies with a wide range of crops, an added concentrated solution of sodium formate, in which freeze-dried LAB were dispersed, gave reduced fermentation losses, especially with forages that were difficult to ensile. Aerobic stability also was improved compared to silage with inoculant alone. The salt has little damaging effect on the LAB and develops its antibacterial action as the pH of the silage decreases. Because the LAB are relatively more acid-tolerant than the undesirable epiphytic microorganisms, they dominate the ensiling process.

CONCLUSIONS

In the second half of the 20th century, advances in silage technology, including high capacity, precision chop forage harvesters, improved silos, plastic sheeting, block and shear cutting silo unloaders, and the introduction of total or complete mixed ration equipment, have helped make silage the principal method of forage preservation. A better understanding of the biochemistry and microbiology of the ensiling processes has lead to the development of a wide range of additives which have increased the efficiency of silage preservation and nutritive value.

Although acids and acid salts still are used to ensile low DM forages in wet climatic conditions, bacterial inoculants have become the most widely used silage additives in the past five years. The major emphasis for use of commercial inoculants has been to ensure a rapid and efficient fermentation phase. However, in the future, these products must also contribute to other areas of silage management including the inhibition of clostridia, enterobacteria, and yeasts and molds and, perhaps, the production of polysaccharide-degrading enzymes. Aerobic deterioration continues to be a serious problem on many farms, especially in high DM silages. The introduction of competitive strains of propionic acid-producing bacteria which could assure aerobically stable silages during storage and feedout would improve most commercial additives.

Cell wall-degrading enzymes have potential to improve the ensileability of most crops and increase their nutritive value, but considerable work needs to be done before that potential is achieved in practice.

But most important is the development of new technologies that would allow the farmer to assess the chemical and microbial status of the silage crop on a given day, and then use the appropriate additive(s).

REFERENCES

Anonymous. 1992. Silage additives. In *1993 Direct-fed Microbial, Enzyme, and Forage Additive Compendium*, pp. 217-261. Miller Publishing Co, Minnetonka, Minnesota.

Aimutis, W.R. and Bolsen, K.K. 1988. Production of biological silage additives. In *Biological Silage Additives*, pp. 45-72. Chalcombe Publications, Canterbury, UK.

Bolsen, K.K. 1985. New technology in forage conservation-feeding systems. In *Proceedings of the XVth International Grassland Congress* pp. 82-88. Kyoto, Japan.

Bolsen, K.K. and Heidker, J.L. 1985. *Silage Additives USA*. Chalcombe Publications, Canterbury, UK.

Bolsen, K.K. 1993. Manejo del ensilaje (part II). In *México Holstein* vol. 24, pp.21-24. Hostein de México, Querétaro, Qro.

Bolsen, K.K., Laytimi, A., Hart, R., Nuzbach, L., Niroomand, F. and Leipold, L. 1988. Effect of commercial inoculants on fermentation of 1987 silage crops. In *Kansas Agric. Exp. Sta. Rpt Prog.*, vol. 539, pp. 137-153. Kansas State University, Manhattan.

Bolsen, K.K., Curtis, J.L., Lin, C.J. and Dickerson, J.T. 1990. Silage inoculants and indigenous microflora: with emphasis on alfalfa. In *Biotechnology in the Feed Industry* (T.P. Lyons, ed.) pp. 257-269. Alltech Technical Publications, Nicholasville, Kentucky.

Bolsen, K.K., Sonon, R.N., Dalke, B., Pope, R., Riley J.G. and Laytimi, A. 1992a. Evaluation of inoculant and NPN silage additives: a summary of 26 trials and 65 farm-scale silages. In *Kansas Agric. Exp. Sta. Rpt Prog.*, vol. 651, pp. 101-102. Kansas State University, Manhattan.

Bolsen, K.K., Tiemann, D.G., Sonon, R.N., Hart, R.A., Dalke, B., Dickerson, J.T., and Lin, C. 1992b. Evaluation of inoculant-treated corn silages. In *Kansas Agric. Exp. Sta. Rpt. Prog.*, vol. 651, pp. 103-106. Kansas State University, Manhattan.

Bolsen, K.K., Dickerson, J.T., Brent, B.E., Sonon, R.N., Jr., Dalke, B.S., Lin, C.J. and Boyer, J.E., Jr. 1993. Rate and extent of top spoilage in horizontal silos. *J. Dairy Sci.* **76**, 2940-2962.

Castle, M.E. 1990. Conclusions and future prospects. In *Proceedings of the EUROBAC Conference* (S. Lindgren and K.L. Pettersson, eds) pp. 184-188. Swedish University of Agricultural Sciences, Uppsala.

Castle, M.E. and Watson, J.N. 1985. Silage and milk production: studies with molasses and formic acid as additives for grass silage. *Grass and Forage Sci.* **40**, 85-92.

Dickerson, J.T., Ashbell, G., Bolsen, K.K., Brent, B.E., Pfaff, L. and Niwa, Y. 1992. Losses from top spoilage in horizontal silos in western Kansas. In *Kansas Agric Exp Sta Rpt. Prog,* vol. 651, pp. 131-134. Kansas State University, Manhattan.

Donald, S., Fenlon, D.R., and Seddon, B. 1993. The influence of oxygen tension on the growth of *Listeria monocytogenes* in grass silage. In *Silage Research 1993,* Proceedings of the 10th Silage Res. Conf., pp. 18-19. Dublin City University, Dublin, Ireland.

Done, D.L. 1988. The effect of absorbent additives on silage quality and on effluent production. In *Silage Effluent* (B.A. Stark and J.M. Wilkinson, eds) pp. 49-57. Chalcombe Publications, Canterbury, UK.

Ely, L.O. 1978. The use of added feedstuffs in silage production. In *Fermentation of Silage—A Review* (M.E. McCullough, ed.) pp. 233-280. Nat. Feed Ingred. Assoc, West Des Moines, Iowa.

Fenton, M.P. 1987. An investigation into the sources of lactic acid bacteria in grass silage. *J. Appl. Bacteriol.* **62**, 181-188.

Goodrich, R.D. and Meiske, J.C. 1985. Corn and sorghum silages. In *Forages* (M.E. Heath, R.F. Barnes, and D.S. Metcalf, eds) pp. 527-536. Iowa State University Press, Ames.

Gordon, F.J. 1989. An evaluation through lactating dairy cattle of a bacterial inoculant as an additive for grass silage. *Grass and Forage Sci.* **44**, 169-179.

Harrison, J.H. 1989. Use of silage additives and their effect on animal productivity. In *Proceedings of the Pacific Northwest Animal Nutrition Conference,* pp. 27-35. Boise, Idaho.

Henderson, A.R., Morgan, C.A., McGinn, R. and Kerr, W.D. 1991. The effect of sugars released by enzymolysis on the fermentation of low dry matter grass. In *Forage Conservation Towards 2000* (G. Pahlow and H. Honig, eds) pp. 301-304. Institute of Grassland Forage Research, Braunschweig, Germany.

Holland, C. and Kezar, W. 1990. *Pioneer Forage Manual: A Nutritional Guide.* Pioneer Hi-Bred International, Inc., Des Moines, Iowa.

Honig, H. and Daenicke, R. 1993. The effect of inoculation with lactic acid bacteria on the utilization of maize silage by bulls. In *Silage Research 1993*, Proceedings of the 10th Silage Research Conference, pp. 129-130. Dublin City University, Dublin, Ireland.

Jacobs, J.L. and McAllan, A.B. 1990. The effect of enzyme treatment on silage composition and increased degradability of ADF and NDF. In *Proceedings of the 9th Silage Conference,* pp. 86-87. Newcastle-upon-Tyne, UK.

Jones, D.I.H., Jones, R. and Moseley, G. 1990. Effect of incorporating rolled barley in autumn cut ryegrass silage on effluent production, silage fermentation and cattle performance. *J. Agric. Sci., Camb.,* **115**, 399-408.

Kalzendorf, C. and Weissbach, F. 1993. Studies on the effect of a combined application of inoculants and sodium formate. In *Silage Research 1993,* Proceedings of the 10th Silage Research Conference, pp. 89-90. Dublin City University, Dublin, Ireland.

Kung, L., Jr. 1992. Use of additives in silage fermentation. In *1993 Direct-fed Microbial, Enzyme, and Forage Additive Compendium,* pp. 31-35. Miller Publishing Co, Minnetonka, Minnesota.

Lin, C., Bolsen, K.K., Brent, B.E., Hart, R.A., Dickerson, J.T., Feyerherm, A.M. and Aimutis, W.R. 1992. Epiphytic microflora on alfalfa and whole-plant corn. *J. Dairy Sci.* **75**, 2484-93.

Lindgren, S. 1984. Silage inoculation. In *Proceedings of the 7th Silage Conf: Summary of Papers* (F.J. Gordon and E.F. Unsworth, eds) pp. 3-4. Queen's University, Belfast.

McAllan, A.B., Jacobs, J.L., and Merry, R.J. 1991. Factors influencing the amount and pattern of silage effluent production. In *Forage Conservation Towards 2000* (G. Pahlow and H. Honig, eds) pp. 368-370. Institute of Grassland Forage Research, Braunschweig, Germany.

McDonald, P. 1980. Silage fermentation. In *Occasional Symposium No 11,* pp. 161-174. British Grassland Society, Brighton, UK.

McDonald, P., Henderson, A.R., and Heron, S.J.E. 1991. *The Biochemistry of Silage,* 2nd ed, Chalcombe Publications, Canterbury, UK.

Muck, R.E. 1989. Initial bacterial numbers on lucerne prior to ensiling. *Grass and Forage Sci.* **44**, 19-25.

Muck, R.E. 1993. The role of silage additives in making high quality silage. In *Proceedings of the National Silage Producers Conference*, pp. 106-116. NREAS-67, Ithaca, NY.

Muck, R.E. and Bolsen, K.K. 1991. Silage preservation and silage additives. In *Hay and Silage Management in North America* (K.K. Bolsen, J.E. Baylor and M.E. McCullough, eds) pp. 105-125. National Feed Ingredients Association, West Des Moines, Iowa.

Muck, R.E. and Pitt, R.E. 1993. Progression of aerobic deterioration relative to the silo face. In *Silage Research 1993,* Proceedings of the 10th Silage Research Conference pp. 38-39. Dublin City University, Dublin, Ireland.

Pahlow, G. 1990. Microbiology of inoculants, crops, and silages. In *Proceedings of the EUROBAC Conference* (S. Lindgren and K.L. Pettersson, eds) pp. 13-22. Swedish University of Agricultural Sciences, Uppsala.

Pahlow, G. 1991. Role of microflora in forage conservation. In *Forage Conservation Towards 2000* (G. Pahlow and H. Honig, eds) pp. 26-36. Institute of Grassland Forage Research, Braunschweig, Germany.

Pahlow, G. and Müller, T. 1990. Determination of epiphytic microorganisms on grass as influenced by harvesting and sample preparation. In *Proceedings of the 9th Silage Conference,* pp. 23-24. Newcastle-upon-Tyne, UK.

Pitt, R.E. 1990. *Silage and hay preservation.* Cornell University Cooperative Extension Bulletin No NRAES-5, Ithaca, NY.

Pitt, R.E. and Leibensperger, R.Y. 1987. The effectiveness of silage inoculants: a systems approach. *Agricultural Systems* **25**, 27-49.

Risley, C. 1992. An overview of microbiology. In *1993 Direct-fed Microbial, Enzyme, and Forage Additive Compendium,* pp. 11-13. Miller Publishing Co, Minnetonka, Minnesota.

Rooke, J.A. 1990. The numbers of epiphytic bacteria on grass at ensilage on commercial farms. *J. Sci. Food Agric.* **51**, 525-533.

Satter, L.D., Muck, R.E., Jones, B.A., Ohiman, T.R., Woodford, J.A. and Wacek, C.M. 1991. Efficacy of bacterial inoculants for alfalfa silage. In *Forage Conservation Towards 2000* (G. Pahlow and H. Honig, eds) pp. 342-343. Institute of Grassland Forage Research, Braunschweig, Germany.

Spoelstra, S.F. 1991. Chemical and biological additives in forage conservation. In *Forage Conservation Towards 2000* (G. Pahlow and H. Honig, eds) pp. 48-70. Institute of Grassland Forage Research, Braunschweig, Germany.

Spoelstra, S.F. and Hindle, V.A. 1989. Influence of wilting on chemical and microbial parameters of grass relevant to ensiling. *Netherlands J. Agric. Sci.* **37**, 355-364.

Stokes, M.R. and Libby, T.L. 1993. Effects of two enzyme-inoculant silage additives and alfalfa content on fermentation and composition of mixed grass-legume silage. In *Silage Research 1993*, Proceedings of the 10th Silage Research Conference, pp. 93-94. Dublin City University, Dublin, Ireland.

Thomas, C. and Thomas, P.C. 1985. Factors affecting the nutritive value of grass silages. In *Recent Advances in Animal Nutrition* (W. Haresign and D.J.A. Cole, eds) pp. 223-256. Butterworths, London.

Waldo, D.R. 1978. Acid silage additives. In *Fermentation of Silage - A Review* (M.E. McCullough, ed.) pp. 120-179. National Feed Ingredients Association, West Des Moines, Iowa.

Watson, S.J. and Nash, M.J. 1960. *The Conservation of Grass and Forage Crops*. Oliver and Boyd, Edinburgh, Scotland.

Whittenbury, R. 1961. An investigation of lactic acid bacteria. Ph.D. Dissertation, University of Edinburgh, Edinburgh, Scotland.

Wieringa, G.W. and Beck, T. 1964. Untersuchungen über die Verwendung von Milchsäurebakterienkulturen bei der Gärfutterbereitung in Kleinbehältern. *Das Wirtschaftseigene Futter* **10**, 34-44.

Wilkinson, J.M. 1990. *Silage UK*, 6th ed. Chalcombe Publications, Canterbury, UK.

Wilkinson, J.M. and Stark, B.A. 1992. *Silage in Western Europe*. 2nd ed. Chalcombe Publications, Canterbury, UK.

Woolford, M.K. 1975. Microbiological screening of the straight chain fatty acids (C_2-C_{12}) as potential silage additives. *J. Sci. Food Agric.* **26**, 219-228.

Woolford, M.K. 1984. *The Silage Fermentation*. Marcel Dekker, New York.

Woolford, M.K and Sawczyc, M.K. 1984. An investigation into the effect of cultures of lactic acid bacteria on fermentation in silage. 1. Strain selection. *Grass and Forage Sci.* **39**, 139-148.

Zimmer, E. 1990. Evaluation of fermentation parameters from the silage experiments. In *Proceedings of the EUROBAC Conference* (S. Lindgren and K.L. Pettersson, eds) pp. 19-44. Swedish University of Agricultural Sciences, Uppsala.

Contribution number 94-154-B, Agricultural Experiment Station, Kansas State University, Manhattan 66506.

4 Biological upgrading of feed and feed components

Frantisek Zadrazil, Anil Kumar Puniya[1] and Kishan Singh[1]

Institut fur Bodenbiologie, Bundesforschungsanstalt fur Landwirtschaft, Bundesalle 50, D 38116 Braunschweig, Germany, and [1]Division of Dairy Microbiology, National Dairy Research Institute, Karnal - 132 001, India

INTRODUCTION

An inadequate supply of good quality feed is the main factor hindering the progress of animal production in many developing countries. Here, the system relies on fibrous crop-residues to bridge the gap between availability and need (Ibrahim and Schiere, 1987). Utilisation of fibrous crop residues by ruminants, even as a source of energy, is limited because the rumen microbial population does not possess ligninolytic activity. As a result, a large proportion of the potential energy in lignified crop residues remains unavailable; the lignin acts as a barrier to the utilisation of structural carbohydrate. The main short-comings of lignified feeds can be summarised as low digestibility, low protein content, poor palatability and bulkiness. If lignified crop residues are to be more widely used and the performance of animals on such feeds enhanced, their nutritional characteristics and palatability must be improved.

Solid state fermentation (SSF) systems have been used by humans for centuries, long before the underlying microbiological or biochemical events involved were understood. Traditionally, SSF is associated with the production of fermented foods in Asia (see Kahlon *et al.*, 1990), mould-ripened cheeses in Europe and composting; however, a number of industrial-scale SSF processes have been developed for the production of microbial protein for animal feed. These invariably make use of readily degradable substrates such as starch (Reade and Gregory, 1975; Skogma, 1976; Khor *et al.*, 1976), pre-treated cellulosic materials (Han, 1978: Moo-Young *et al.*, 1979; Singh *et al.*, 1989) or carbohydrate-rich wastes (Young and Scrimshaw, 1975: Han, 1978) as carbon source. An exception is the 'Pekilo' process developed in Finland, in which the fungus *Paecilomyces variatii* is grown on spent sulphite liquor (Romantschuk, 1975). The Finnish government has allowed the use of 'Pekilo protein' (55-60% protein, of which 87% is digestible) in animal feedstuffs. SSF has also been used to eliminate antinutritional compounds found in rapeseed meal (Bau *et al.*, 1994).

The amino acid composition of many plant proteins is less than ideal for animal production purposes. Protein content and the balance of amino acids can be enhanced by treatment with fungi. *Coprinus fimetarius*, a fungus able to tolerate high pH, has been used to capture the excess ammonia liberated during urea treatment of cereal straw (Singh *et al.*, 1989). The amino acid content of urea and *Coprinus*-treated wheat and rice straw was found to be five-fold greater than the straw recovered after urea treatment alone and the balance of amino acids was greatly improved (Table 1).

Use of SSF technology to improve the digestion of the fibre component of poorly digested lignified residues by ruminants has been relatively little studied although the concept is not new. Knoche *et al.* (1929) described *palo-podrido*, the highly digestible decayed wood of several hardwood trees, used for centuries as animal feed in southern Chile. Initial reports

Table 1. Amino acid content (µmol g^{-1}) of untreated, urea-treated and urea + *Coprinus fimetarius*-treated rice and wheat straws.

Amino acid	Wheat straw			Rice straw		
	Un-treated	Urea treated	Fungus treated	Un-treated	Urea treated	Fungus treated
Lys	0.56	2.17	9.73	0.81	1.08	7.24
His	0.88	0.26	1.34	0.25	0.19	1.09
Arg	0.34	1.26	103.53	0.28	0.51	2.12
Asp	3.78	21.98	89.59	7.22	3.37	89.97
Thr	1.51	5.98	57.42	2.34	9.57	46.42
Ser	1.75	9.98	128.95	3.39	6.00	40.30
Glu	5.99	24.65	171.98	7.38	19.53	170.00
Pro	2.70	4.99	21.01	2.80	2.40	15.95
Gly	3.41	14.88	113.71	7.47	15.78	85.51
Ala	0.68	4.06	22.17	2.68	4.99	33.75
Val	0.48	2.16	14.13	0.84	0.95	10.22
Met	0.24	2.25	20.60	0.68	1.52	22.91
Ile	0.84	5.04	30.30	0.91	2.53	30.33
Leu	0.47	2.07	17.11	1.07	1.68	13.94
Tyr	0.28	0.25	2.36	0.53	0.53	1.72
Phe	0.80	1.32	8.42	0.58	2.03	6.03
Total	24.71	102.80	812.35	39.23	72.66	577.30

From Singh *et al.* (1992)

suggested that the organisms responsible for formation of *palo-podrido* were yeasts (Kühlwein, 1963) but subsequently it was concluded that white-rot fungi were the causal agents (Zadrazil *et al.*, 1982)

In the natural environment many strains of fungi and bacteria are known to attack lignified plant residues although the exact mechanism is not always well understood. Few, however, are able to fully mineralise lignin fully to carbon dioxide and water and the majority simply modify the lignin macromolecule or further degrade lower molecular weight units released as a result of attack by other organisms. In general, strains of white-rot fungi are the most effective lignin degraders. They have the capacity to attack lignin polymers, open aromatic rings and cleave carbon-carbon and aryl-ether bonds, causing the formation of intermediate molecular weight polymers and the release of low molecular weight fragments. In contrast, brown-rot fungi are able to bring about limited change to the structure of lignin, such as demethylation of ring structures, and have, at best, only a limited capacity to effect a more substantial degradation. Soft rot fungi occupy an intermediate position and, in some moist environments, may be the dominant lignin-degrader. Many soil bacteria actively degrade mono- and dilignols with molecular weights up to 350 but lack the capacity to attack higher molecular weight structures. Only a few strains of bacteria, notably *Streptomyces* and *Nocardia* spp., have been shown to have any ability to degrade lignin and lignin derivatives.

The question of whether natural lignin is degraded in anaerobic environments is of some significance. Although early studies discounted the possibility that natural or synthetic lignins were decomposed anaerobically in anoxic soils and sediments (Hackett *et al*, 1977; Odier and Monties, 1983; Zeikus *et al*., 1982), laboratory investigations (Colberg and Young, 1982; Taylor, 1983) have suggested that molecular oxygen is not necessarily required for the cleavage of intermonomeric linkages or for ring opening. This view has been supported by studies made with radiolabelled synthetic lignins and lignin-carbohydrate complexes derived from grasses and hardwood which found that lignin could be degraded to carbon dioxide and methane in anoxic sediments over periods of weeks (Benner *et al*., 1984).

Treatment of lignified materials with ligninolytic microorganisms in laboratory SSF systems has been found to improve the nutritive value of some fibrous crop residues by increasing biomass protein and degrading the phenolic fraction at the expense of some energy from structural carbohydrate. This technology invariably has exploited white-rot fungi to improve the nutritive value of lignified by-products such as cereal straw, bagasse, rice husk and sawdust (Reid, 1989). Zadrazil (1985) tested approximately 200 strains of white-rot fungi for their effects on wheat straw and found increases in digestibility ranging from 15 to 32 units depending upon temperature and period of fermentation. Other studies aimed at estimating the changes in digestibility of fungal-treated substrates are summarised in Table 2. Spent straw from edible mushroom production (*Pleurotus* sp.) can also show improved digestibility when fed to ruminants (Zadrazil, 1977). Even when the process is optimised for straw treatment rather than fruiting body production, the added value provided by the mushroom crop considerably improves the economics of processing.

IMPROVED EXPLOITATION OF LIGNIFIED BY-PRODUCTS USING WHITE-ROT FUNGI

White-rot basidiomycetes differ considerably in the rates at which they decompose lignin and polysaccharides in woody tissues; some remove lignin preferentially while others attack both types of polymers at a similar rate. Based on this preference white-rot fungi can be divided into two groups (Zadrazil, 1985; Ljungdahl and Eriksson, 1985):

- simultaneous rot fungi, which degrade different wood components at same rates
- white mottled rot fungi (or white pocket fungi), which degrade lignin selectively, leaving considerable amounts of structural carbohydrate (Blanchatte, 1984).

Treatment with simultaneous rot fungi, such as *Polyporus versicolor*, at best produce no change in digestibility and often decrease the nutritive value of straws and other lignified by-products.

Selection of fungi for lignin degradation

The selection of an efficient culture is the key to the success of any biotechnological process. The type of substrate, method of processing and desired quality of fermented products should be the criteria for selection of a microbe. An ideal microorganism for SSF should have the following characteristics:

- high growth rate and the ability to grow in presence of the natural flora of the substrate (high saprophytic colonisation ability)
- selective ligninolytic activity

Table 2. Digestibility of lignocellulosic materials after solid state fermentation with fungi.

Substrate	Organism(s)	Duration of fermentation (days)	Change in digestibility (%)		Reference
			From	To	
Aspen wood	Polyporus berkeleyi	88	46	37	Kirk and Moore, 1972
	P. frondosus	64	46	71	
	Fomes ulmarius	77	46	64	
Barley straw	Coprinus cinereus	10	45	55	Burrows et al., 1979
	Peniophora gigantea	21	36	46	
Beech wood	Fomes lividus	14-21	5	26	Hartley et al., 1974
Pea straw	Ganoderma lucidum	21	40	48	Ibrahim and Pearce, 1980
Poplar shaving	Phanerochaete chrysosporium	28	30	62	Reade and MacQueen, 1983
Rape straw	Stropharia rugusoannulata	60	34	82	Zadrazil, 1980
	Pleurotus sp. florida	60	34	71	
	P. cornucopiae	60	34	62	
Sugarcane bagasse	P. gigantea	21	32	39	Ibrahim and Pearce, 1980
Wheat straw	Stropharia rugusoannulata	79	40	55-69	Zadrazil, 1977
	Lentinus edodes	60	40	77	Zadrazil and Brunnert, 1981
	Abortiporus bienis	26	40	79	Zadrazil and Brunnert, 1980
	Dichomitus squalens/Cyathus stercoreus	15-30	38	63-68	Agosin and Odier, 1985
	Pleurotus sajor-caju	40	15	46	Zadrazil et al., 1993
	Phanerochaete chrysosporium	30	28	43	Puniya et al., 1994
		10	41	46	Singh et al., 1993

- resistance to environmental stresses
- the minimum polysaccharidase required to sustain lignin degradation
- non-pathogenic and non-toxic to animals and humans
- ability to enhance digestibility and palatability of product
- genetically stable
- easy to prepare inoculum and convenient handling.

The ability of fungi to colonise crop residues depends on their competitive saprophytic ability under optimal conditions of culture during fermentation (Zadrazil, 1980, 1985). Efficient colonisation of non-sterile substrate is only possible if the culture possesses a higher saprophytic ability than the natural flora. Zadrazil and Peerally (1986) have described the quantitative differentiation of microbial activity and saprophytic colonisation in wheat straw during fermentation. The measurement of competitive saprophytic ability in terms of relative visible growth on solid substrate under defined culture conditions provides a practical method for selecting fungal cultures for SSF of fibrous crop-residues.

Maximum improvement of digestibility has been found to occur in the early stages of straw fermentation, which indicates that only a partial delignification is sufficient to produce a positive change in digestibility (Blanchatte, 1984). Degradation of lignin to water-soluble compounds is more important for enhancement of digestibility than is complete degradation to carbon dioxide. Low molecular weight phenolic compounds invariably are inhibitory to microorganisms including the cellulolytic bacteria found in rumen (Chesson *et al.*, 1982) but no obvious toxicity of phenolic compounds originating from lignin breakdown has been observed. Among the most promising white-rot fungi found for improving the degradability of wheat straw are strains of *Cyathus stercoreus* and *Dichomitus squalens* (Zadrazil and Brunnert, 1982), however both are characterised by a slow growth rate requiring the use of substrate in which the natural flora has been suppressed.

Several other white-rot fungi have been found useful for the treatment of wheat straw, notably *Pleurotus* spp., *Pycnoporus cinnabarinus, Phlebia radiata* and four other fungi belonging to this group (Hatakka *et al.*, 1989). In the best cases, the efficiency of biological pretreatment was comparable with that of alkali treatment. A higher proportion of glucose relative to the untreated straw was found in hydrolysates of some treated residues (Hatakka, 1983). This indicated that some fungi utilised xylan in preference to cellulose as a co-substrate for the degradation of lignin, which may be desirable when the pentose content of the residue is of lower nutritional value than the hexose content (Blanchatte *et al.*, 1985).

Genetic manipulation of ligninolytic microorganisms

Cellulase negative (cel⁻) mutants of white-rot fungi produced by conventional mutagenesis have shown a potential for the genetic improvement of ligninolytic fungi. Such mutants retain a capacity, albeit reduced, to modify lignin structure using energy from co-substrates other than cellulose which is not attacked. The first experiments to produce cel⁻ mutants were carried out by Eriksson and Goodell (1974) by UV light irradiation of spore suspensions of the white-rot fungus, *Polyporus adustus*. Several cel⁻ mutants also lacking mannase and xylanase were isolated, indicating that these enzymes are regulated coordinately in *P. adustus*.

Eriksson and his co-workers also isolated spontaneous acid induced cel⁻, xylanase positive and phenol-oxidase positive mutants of *Sporotrichum pulverulentum* (syn. *Phanerochaete chrysosporium*) and compared them with the parent strain (Eriksson *et al.*, 1983). However, these mutants had a low capacity for lignin degradation compared to wild types. Other cel⁻ mutants of *Phanerochaete chrysosporium* have been produced (Johnsrud and Eriksson, 1985) and compared for their ability to degrade lignin (Kirk *et al.*, 1986a,b). *P. chrysosporium* mutants obtained by traditional methods are pleiotrophic and have not allowed the roles of individual gene products to be established. Recombinant technology now has been applied extensively to the ligninolytic system of *P. chrysosporium* (Gold and Alic, 1993, for review) and gene families representing the major enzymes involved (laccase, lignin peroxidase and manganese-dependent lignin peroxidase) have been cloned. Gene disruption or deletion offers a means of obtaining mutants deficient only in specific isoenzymes. This will aid an understanding of the mechanism of lignin degradation and the regulatory system governing the expression of ligninolytic enzymes and, in the future, allow for the development of strains over-expressing key activities. Early attempts to circumvent the need for SSF by of use cell-free ligninolytic enzymes to delignify crop residues, made in the anticipation of cloned enzymes becoming available on a commercial scale, have proved singularly unsuccessful (Khazaal *et al.*, 1993).

FACTORS INFLUENCING THE FUNGAL UPGRADING OF LIGNIFIED RESIDUES

The fungus should grow optimally during SSF, to ensure maximum improvement in the nutritive value of crop-residues. Optimal conditions of moisture, pH, temperature, aeration and inoculum level need to be standardised to obtain a uniform fungal treated mass (Reid, 1989, for review).

Moisture content

In wet fibrous crop residues, moisture strongly influences the mass transfer rate of oxygen and carbon dioxide and the rate of heat dissipation with consequences for fungal growth, enzyme activity, the accessibility of the substrate and the rate of product formation. Water contents of 65-75% have been reported to be optimal for the growth of various fungi on solid substrates (Zadrazil and Brunnert, 1982; Babitskaya *et al.*, 1986). With water contents greater than 75%, the gas phase was found to be reduced and gas exchange increasingly impeded, creating anaerobic conditions within the substrate. At lower water contents, fungal growth was reduced because water tension was high and the degree of substrate swelling was low (Zadrazil and Brunnert, 1980). Abdullah *et al.* (1985) also noted that too little water inhibited fungal growth and led to early sporulation, whereas too much water caused leaching of nutrients and clogged interstitial spaces. This, in turn, reduced oxygen accessibility and favoured growth of contaminating bacteria.

Temperature and pH

Most lignin-degrading fungi grow best at temperatures between 20 and 30°C (Zadrazil, 1985). Higher temperatures have adverse effects on progress of fermentation and lead to less lignin degradation and a decreased digestibility of wheat straw (Zadrazil and Brunnert, 1982; Zadrazil, 1985). A temperature of 35°C was found by Parveen *et al.* (1983) to be optimum for SSF of wheat straw by *P. chrysosporium* (referred to as *S. pulverulantum*), while Abdullah *et al.* (1985) recorded 37°C as the optimum temperature for *Chaetomium cellulolyticum* growing on wheat straw. Good growth of *Coprinus fimaterius* was observed between 32 to 40°C (Flegel and Meevootisom, 1986).

Lignin degradation by most fungi occurs at acidic pH (Reid, 1985). However, alkali-tolerant fungi growing optimally between pH 7 to 9 have attracted interest in conjunction with the urea treatment of cereal straws (Meevootisom *et al.*, 1984; Singh *et al.*, 1990). The high pH generated by alkali treatment is sufficient to inhibit growth of most contaminating micro-organisms, so avoiding the need for expensive substrate pasteurisation while creating a niche for lignin degraders tolerant of alkaline conditions. Although *Coprinus* spp. have been the choice to date, some bacteria, including actinomycetes, also have been reported to attack lignin under neutral to alkaline pH conditions (Deschamps *et al.*, 1981; Pometto and Crawford, 1986).

Agitation and aeration

Lignin biodegradation occurs efficiently only under oxidative conditions. The ligninolytic activity of *Lentinus edodes* (Reid and Seifert, 1982), *Pleurotus sajor-caju* (Kamra and Zadrazil, 1986) and *Pleurotus ostreatus* were stimulated by oxygen, and agitation of liquid cultures generally has been found to enhance biodegradation (Reid *et al.*, 1985). However, very high rates of agitation or greater than ambient oxygen concentrations will inhibit ligninolytic activity (Leisola and Fiechter, 1985; Agosin *et al.*, 1986).

Mixing of solid substrate results in more uniform process conditions, improves the oxygen supply to microorganisms and removes gaseous metabolites from the void spaces of substrate. Mixing can prevent localised heating due to microbial heat evolution and may help to distribute additives uniformly in the fermenter. Mixing may be beneficial for continuous operation, automation and scale-up of processes (Weiland, 1988). On the other hand mixing influences the morphology of the microorganisms and may result in a change of metabolism. A lower product yield or failure of process also may occur if, during mixing, shear forces damage the growing tips of the hyphae (Markl and Bronnenmeyer, 1985).

Inoculum level and substrate density

Higher inoculum level of *P. chrysosporium* during SSF of natural birch lignin favoured biomass formation (Mudgett and Paradis, 1985). Density of packing of substrate is also an important factor (Zadrazil *et al.*, 1990a). Laukevics *et al.* (1985) examined some of the physical aspects of fungal growth in milled wheat straw, demonstrating that the interstitial space available for hyphae could have a limiting effect on biomass development.

DESIGN FOR A REACTOR FOR SOLID STATE FERMENTATION

The reactor used in Institute of Soil Biology, Braunschweig, is constructed of polyurethane foam sandwich panels covered with polyester board on both sides (Zadrazil *et al.*, 1990a,b). The filling height of substrate is approximately 2.0 m, the internal width is 2.3 m and the depth is 2.0 m, resulting in a net filling volume of 6.9 m^3, i.e. equivalent to 1.5 tonnes of straw or 3.0 tonnes of wood chip substrate. Two similarly insulated swing doors, situated at the front, occupy the full width of the reactor. Inside the reactor there is a raised slatted floor covered firstly with a gliding net and then with a drag net. The substrate is inoculated when moved between reactors (Fig. 1).

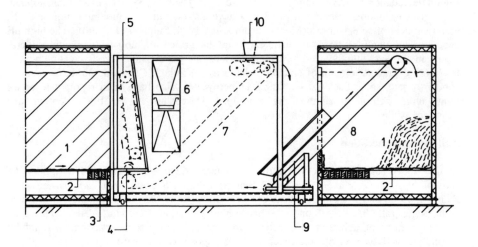

Figure 1. Horizontal cross section of SSF reactors showing transfer and inoculation of substrate. 1. SSF reactor; 2. Net for unloading the substrate; 3. Panels for aerating; 4. Equipment for unloading; 5. Equipment for fragmenting; 6. Equipment for filling; 7. Conveyor to bring substrate to spawning machinery; 8. Conveyor for filling the reactor; 9. Carrier for moving the conveyor; 10. Spawning machine.

Preconditioning and inoculation of substrate

The substrate is watered and transferred to the first reactor for thermal conditioning and inoculation. The substrate is transferred into the reactor using a specially designed machine (Fig. 1) which deposits it on the drag net. A removable front panel keeps the substrate from falling out of the container during filling. The temperature of substrate and gas phase is measured, recorded and controlled during the pretreatment stage which lasts for 48 to 140 h depending upon the type of substrate. The oxygen content of the gas phase during this process has an effect on the development of competitive microorganisms and carbon dioxide can be introduced to provide a degree of control. In the absence of added CO_2, the carbon dioxide content increases initially and then declines slowly while the opposite pattern is true for oxygen (Zadrazil *et al.*, 1990a).

The conditioned substrate is removed from the container by attaching the drag net to a winch. The substrate is loosened as it is pulled through a set of toothed bars before falling on to the elevator. During this step, the inoculum (grain spawn or liquid culture) applied at different rates (e.g. 50 l of liquid inoculum containing ~100 g mycelium dry matter, or 30-50 kg grain spawn) is added and mixed with 1000 kg of the conditioned cereal straw substrate. The inoculated substrate then is transferred to the second reactor. This transfer from one reactor into the other decreases the bulk density of the substrate and reduces the stream resistance of the gas phase by the substrate.

Control of SSF conditions

The most important problem of fungal growth in deep layers is the uniform control of temperature in the substrate and the removal of heat from the system. Heat exchange is achieved by the circulation of conditioned gas through the substrate and its isothermal state is maintained by altering the temperature, humidity and speed of gas movement (Weiland, 1988; Teifke and Bohnet, 1990; Schuchardt and Zadrazil, 1988). For the cultivation of *Pleurotus* spp. and other wood decaying fungi the gaseous phase is recycled. CO_2 and O_2 concentrations are monitored and the composition of the gas adjusted as appropriate (Schuchardt and Zadrazil, 1980, 1988). The system is illustrated here in Fig. 2 and 3, and described in detail elsewhere (Zadrazil *et al.*, 1990a,b).

The product

The final product differs from the starting material in water content and digestibility. One may assume that differences between the water contents of different layers have an influence on the digestibility of substrate. This phenomenon can be eliminated by better control of the gas phase. For example, the digestibility of substrate was increased after fermentation in the bioreactor by an average by 13.8 digestibility units (Zadrazil *et al.*, 1990b). The highest increase (18.7 units) was found in the layer near the substrate surface and the lowest (7.0 units) in the bottom layer. The observed increase in digestibility of cereal straw after fungal treatment on a large scale was comparable with results obtained by sodium hydroxide or ammonia treatment (see Sundstol and Owen, 1984).

The system described has also been used for production of edible fungi. Colonised substrate was transferred to a reactor for fructification. The yield of fruit bodies was satisfactory and was comparable to that obtained with other cultivation systems.

EVALUATION OF SSF PROCESSES

Biological approaches which utilise fungi for the bioconversion of lignified crop residues under optimised fermentation conditions have enabled the production of a feed with higher digestible organic matter and crude protein availability than the starting material. However, the successful introduction of processes of this type will also require that the fermented product meets the general requirements of economic production, safety, palatability and adequate dry matter intake by ruminants.

Toxicological evaluation

Guarding against toxicity must be a priority consideration in any biological treatment. This means that all the potential cultures must be tested chemically and biologically for acute and chronic toxicity. The fungus must not be pathogenic to the handlers or to the animals that will eventually consume the feed. There is a possibility that the microbe used will be allergenic when eaten, touched or breathed by the consumer especially when it produces spores (Flegel and Meevootisom, 1986). The biologically treated feeds involve a risk of

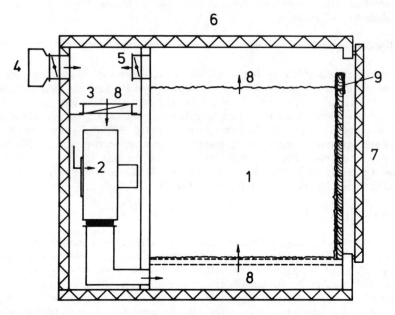

Figure 2. Vertical cross section of SSF reactor. 1. Substrate; 2. Fan for gas recycling; 3. Cooling and heating system; 4. Fresh air supply with anemometer; 5. Regulation of air movement; 6. Body of reactor; 7. Reactor door; 8. Direction of gas movement; 9. Net for substrate unloading.

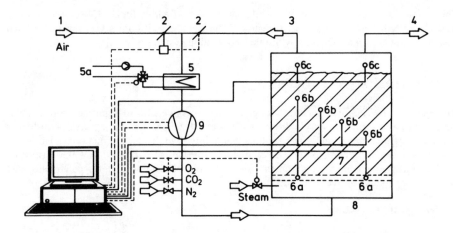

Figure 3. Scheme of control system of SSF reactor. 1. Fresh air supply; 2. Air damper; 3. Recirculation of gas phase; 4. Gas outlet; 5. Gas-cooling system: a - Liquid-cooling system; 6. Sensors for temperature control: a - Gas input, b - Temperature of substrate, c - Gas output; 7. Substrate; 8. Body of SSF reactor; 9. Fan.

toxicity at three different stages: toxin production by the strain itself during fermentation, toxin production by contaminating organisms under non-sterile conditions, and toxic metabolites produced as a result of lignin degradation.

Little toxicological testing of fungal strains likely to be used in SSF of lignified plant materials has been undertaken, an exception being Reddy (1985), who tested 21 different mould cultures to be used in SSF for aflatoxin production. Two-thermotolerant filamentous fungi used for single cell protein were evaluated by feeding their biomass to rats for 90 days (Kuo *et al.*, 1979). All the animals were found normal and healthy, except that transient alopecia was found for short duration in the initial period. Histopathological observations did not reveal any adverse effects on rats due to treatment.

Economic considerations

SSF is an attractive technology for upgrading agricultural residues because it more closely mimics the growth conditions encountered by fungi in their natural habit than liquid cultures. Generally, the reactor volume per unit substrate converted remains relatively small, since only small amounts of water must be added to the substrate. This results in lower capital and operating costs, and reduced space requirements. The reactor equipment is often simpler and requires less processing energy than corresponding liquid submerged fermentation (Weiland, 1988). The low moisture required to obtain maximum yield for the product with fungi excludes, in most instances, problems of bacterial contamination without the need for pasteurisation or sterilisation of the substrate.

Although capital costs may be small, especially for on-farm processes, the costs of pretreatment must be recovered by increased productivity gained by feeding treated residues. Inputs involved in upgrading of feed may include labour, transport and cost of the substrate used. Pretreatments involve additional costs of labour, chemicals and preparation of inoculum (Doyle *et al.*, 1986). Extra income can be in the form of increased animal productivity or in the combination of animal feed production and production of edible mushrooms. The cost-benefit analysis of a specific product depends on the availability of substrate, its alternate use, the availability of other food sources and the value of a more digestible feed within a specific farming system.

As digestibility increases with time in SSF, the economics are also affected by the duration of the process (Zadrazil and Brunnert, 1980, 1982). The increase in digestibility must be offset against a loss of organic matter. This also increases with time and argues for a shorter fermentation period. To obtain the maximum change in digestibility of substrates using white-rot fungi may take 4-5 weeks (Zadrazil *et al.*, 1990a,b). Because of dry matter losses it has been recommended that the fermentation period should be reduced to 1-2 weeks which maximises the total dry digestible matter rather than unit digestibility (Gupta, 1987).

Limitations

Despite the many advantages of SSF there are limitations which, to date, have prevented the exploitation of this technology on anything other than a modest scale. The main drawbacks are the difficulties in storing and handling solid substrates, especially for continuous operation, the difficult control of temperature and moisture in the fermenter and the lack of appropriate sensors for measuring environmental factors on-line during the course of fermentation.

Further disadvantages are the slow conversion rate due to the limitation on diffusion imposed by the substrate and the small added value accruing to the finished product (Weiland, 1988).

FUTURE RESEARCH NEEDS

At present there is a dichotomy in the development of SSF systems. SSF as a centralised activity has one set of needs which may include improved control measures and standardisation of the process. These activities are rarely appropriate for farm-scale operations, particularly in developing countries where the need is greatest and where access to expensive plant and control equipment presents problems. However, on the basis of earlier studies and experiences, the following needs common to both situations can be identified while recognising that the solutions may be very different:

- development of new designs and constructions of SSF reactors which ensure minimal differences in conditions in different layers of the substrate and which minimise energy inputs
- development of control systems to optimise air circulation in different parts of the reactor, to ensure constant air humidity and minimises water evaporation and movement within the substrate
- development of strategies for process control involving, where appropriate mathematical models of the SSF process
- elimination of contaminants and toxic substances
- genetic improvement of strains and isolation of thermotolerant strains suitable for use in the tropics
- cost-benefit studies in comparison with other processes available for the treatment of lignified plant residues.

Because of the ready availability of cereal grain and protein concentrates for animal production in industrialised countries, SSF technology may prove appropriate only in regions in which there is an absolute shortage of feed or where feed is prohibitively expensive for the majority of producers. There is evidence that SSF technology can be adapted to farm conditions and made relatively simple and economically viable. This technology does not replace the need for increased primary feed production, but could provide a useful supplement.

REFERENCES

Abdullah, A.L., Tangeraly, R.P. and Murphy, V.G. 1985. Optimization of solid substrate fermentation of wheat straw. *Biotechnol. Bioeng.* **27**, 20-27.
Agosin, E. and Odier, E. 1985. Solid-state fermentation, lignin degradation and resulting digestibility of wheat straw fermented by selected white-rot fungi. *Appl. Microbiol. Biotechnol.* **21**, 397-403.
Agosin, E., Tollier, M.T., Brillouet, J.M., Thirand, P. and Odier, E. 1986. Fungal pretreatment of wheat straw: effects on the biodegradability of cell walls, structural polysaccharides, lignin and phenolic acids by rumen micro-organisms. *J. Sci. Food Agric.* **37**, 97-106.
Babitskaya, V.G., Stakhev, I.V., Shcherba, V.V. and Vadetsky, B.Y. 1986. Bioconversion of lignocellulosic substrates by mycelial fungi in solid state culture. *Prikl. Biokhim. Mikrobiol.* **22**, 531-539.

Bau, H-M., Villaume, C., Lin, C.-F., Evrard, J., Quemener, B., Nicolas, J.-P. and Méjean, L. 1994. Effect of a solid-state fermentation using *Rhizopus oligosporus* sp. T-3 on elimination of antinutritional substances and modification of biochemical constituents of defatted rapeseed meal. *J. Sci. Food Agric.* **65**, 315-322.

Benner, R., MacCubbin, A.E. and Hodson, R.E. 1984. Anaerobic biodegradation of the lignin and polysaccharide components of lignocellulose and synthetic lignin by sediment microflora. *Appl. Environ. Microbiol.* **47**, 998-1004.

Blanchatte, R.A. 1984. Screening wood decayed by white rot fungi for preferential lignin degradation. *Appl. Environ. Microbiol.* **48**, 647-653.

Blanchatte, R.A., Otjen, L., Effland, M.J. and Eslyn, W.E. 1985. Changes in structural and chemical components of wood delignified by fungi. *Wood Sci. Technol.* **19**, 35-46.

Burrows, I., Seal, K.J. and Eggins, H.O.W. 1979. The biodegradation of barley straw by *Coprinus cinereus* for the production of ruminant feed. In *Straw Decay and its Effect on Disposal and Utilization* (Grossbred, E., ed.) pp. 147-154. John Wiley and Sons, Chichester, UK.

Chesson, A., Stewart, C.S. and Wallace, R.J. 1982. Influence of plant phenolic acids on growth and cellulolytic activity of rumen bacteria. *Appl. Environ. Microbiol.* **44**, 597-603.

Colberg, P.J. and Young, L.Y. 1982. Biodegradation of lignin-derived molecules under anaerobic conditions. *Can. J. Microbiol.* **28**, 886-889.

Deschamps, A.M., Gillie, J.P. and Lebeault, J.M. 1981. Direct delignification of untreated chips with cultures of bacteria. *Eur. J. Appl. Microbiol. Biotechnol.* **13**, 222-225.

Doyle, P.T., Devendra, C. and Pearce, G.R. 1986. *Rice Straw as a Feed for Ruminants.* Pub. Intl. Dev. Prog. of Australian Universities and Colleges Ltd., Canberra, Australia.

Eriksson, K.E. and Goodell, E.W. 1974. Pleiotrophic mutants of the wood-rotting fungus *Polyporus adjustus* lacking cellulase, mannase and xylanase. *Can. J. Microbiol.* **20**, 371-378.

Eriksson, K.E., Johnsrud, S.C. and Vallaneler, L. 1983. Degradation of lignin and lignin model compounds by the white-rot fungus *Sporotrichum pulverulentum. Arch. Microbiol.* **135**, 161-168.

Flegel, T.W. and Meevootisom, V. 1986. Biological treatment of straw for animal feed. In *Rice Straw and Related Feeds in Ruminant Rations* (M.N.M. Ibrahim and J.B. Schiere, eds) pp. 181-191. Straw Utilization Project Publication 2, Kandy, Sri Lanka.

Gold, M.H. and Alic, M. 1993. Molecular biology of the lignin-degrading Basidiomycete *Phanerochaete chrysosporium. Microbiol. Rev.* **57**, 605-622.

Gupta, B.N. 1987. Fungal treatment of cereal straws for ruminant feeding. In *Biological, Chemical and Physical Treatment of Crop-Residues for Use as Animal Feeds* (K. Singh, T.W. Flegal and J.B. Schiere, eds) pp. 26-36. ICAR, New Delhi, India.

Hackett, W.F., Connors, W.J., Kirk, T.K. and Zeikus, J.G. 1977. Microbial decomposition of synthetic ^{14}C labelled lignins in nature: lignin biodegradation in a variety of natural materials. *Appl. Environ. Microbiol.* **33**, 43-51.

Han, Y.W. 1978. Microbial utilisation of straw. *Adv. Appl. Microbiol.* **23**, 119-153.

Hartley, R.D., Jones, E.C., King, N.J. and Smith, G.A. 1974. Modified wood waste and straw as potential components of animal feeds. *J. Sci. Food Agric.* **25**, 433-437.

Hatakka, A.I. 1983. Pretreatment of wheat straw by white rot fungi for enzymic saccharification of cellulose. *Eur. J. Appl. Microbiol. Biotechnol.* **18**, 350-357.

Hatakka, A.I., Mohammadi, O.K. and Lundell, T.K. 1989. The potential of white rot fungi and their enzymes in the treatment of lignocellulosic feed. *Food Biotechnol.* **3**, 45-58.

Ibrahim, M.N.M. and Pearce, G.R. 1980. Effects of white rot fungi on the composition and *in vitro* digestibility of crop by-products. *Agric. Wastes* **2**, 199-205.

Ibrahim, M.N.M. and Schiere, J.B. 1987. Animal production possibilities using fibrous residues. In *Proc. 4th AAAP Anim. Sci. Congr.* pp. 74-77, New Zealand.

Johnsrud, S.C. and Eriksson, K.E. 1985. Cross-breeding of selected and mutated homokaryotic strains of *Phanerochaete chrysosporium* K-3: new cellulase deficient strains with increased ability to degrade lignin. *Appl. Microbiol. Biotechnol.* **21**, 320-327.

Kahlon, S.S., Kalra, K.L. and Grewal, H.S. 1990. Fungal single cell protein: current status. *Indian J. Microbiol.* **30**, 13-28.

Khazaal, K.A., Owen, E., Dodson, A.P., Palmer, J. and Harvey, P. 1993. Treatment of barley straw with ligninase: effect of activity and fate of the enzymes shortly after being added to straw. *Anim. Feed Sci. Technol.* **41**, 15-27.

Kamra, D.N. and Zadrazil, F. 1986. Influence of gaseous phase, light, and substrate pretreatment on fruit body formation, lignin degradation and *in vitro* digestion of wheat straw fermented with *Pleurotus* spp. *Agric. Wastes* **18**, 1-17.

Khor, G.L., Alexander, J.C., Santos-Nunej, J., Reade, A.E. and Gregory, K.F. 1976. Nutritional value of thermotolerant fungi grown on cassava. *Canadian Inst. Food Sci. Technol. J.* **9**, 139-143.

Kirk, T.K. and Moore, W.E. 1972. Removing lignin from wood with white-rot fungi and digestibility of resulting wood. *Wood Fiber* **4**, 72-79.

Kirk, T.K., Croan, S., Tien, M., Murtagh, K.E. and Farrell, R.L. 1986a. Production of multiple ligninases by *Phanerochaete chrysosporium*: effect of selected growth conditions and use of a mutant strain. *Enz. Microb. Technol.* **8**, 27-32.

Kirk, T.K., Tien, M., Johnsrud, S.C. and Eriksson, K.E. 1986b. Lignin degrading activity of *Phanerochaete chrysosporium* Burds.: comparison of cellulase-negative and other strains. *Enz. Microb. Technol.* **8**, 75-80.

Knoche, W., Cruz-Coke, E. and Pacotet, M. 1929. Der "palo podrido" auf Chiloe. Ein beitrag zur kenntnis der natürlichen umwandlung des holzes durch pilze in ein futtermittel. *Zentrab. Bakteriol. [Naturwiss]* **79**, 427-431.

Kühlwein, H. 1963. Zur kenntnis des "palo podrido", eines mikrobiell abjebauten holze aus südchile. *Zentrab. Bakteriol. [Naturwiss]* **116**, 294-299.

Kuo, C.Y., Alexander, J.C., Lumsden, J.H. and Thomson, R.C. 1979. Subchronic toxicity test for two thermotolerant filamentous fungi, used for single cell protein production. *Can. J. Comp. Med.* **43**, 50-58.

Laukevics, J.J., Apsite, A.F., Veisturs, U.S. and Tangerdy, R.P. 1985. Steric hindrance of growth of filamentous fungi in solid-substrate fermentation of wheat straw. *Biotechnol. Bioeng.* **27**, 1687-1691.

Leisola, M.S.A. and Fiechter, A. 1985. Ligninase production in agitated conditions by *Phanerochaete chrysosporium*. *FEMS Microbiol. Lett.* **29**, 33-36.

Ljungdahl, L.G. and Eriksson, K.E. 1985. Ecology of microbial cellulose degradation. *Adv. Microb. Ecol.* **8**, 237-299.

Markl, H. and Bronnenmeyer, R. 1985. Mechanical stress and microbial production. In *Biotechnology* Vol. 2 (H.J. Rehm and G. Reed, eds) pp. 369-394. VCH Verlagsgesellschaft, Weinheim, Germany.

Meevootisom, V., Flegel, T.W., Glinsukon, T., Sobhon, N. and Kiatpapan, S. 1984. Lytic fungi from Thailand for animal feed production. *J. Sci. Soc. Thailand* **10**, 147-178.

Moo-Young, M., Daugulis, A.J., Chahal, D.S. and MacDonald, D.C. 1979. The waterloo process for SCP production from waste biomass. *Process Biochem.* **14**, 38-40.

Mudgett, R.E. and Paradis, A.J. 1985. Solid state fermentation of natural birch lignin by *Phanerochaete chrysosporium*. *Enz. Microb. Technol.* **7**, 150-154.

Odier, E. and Monties, B. 1983. Absence of microbial mineralization of lignin in anaerobic enrichment cultures. *Appl. Environ. Microbiol.* **46**, 661-665.

Parveen, N., Kahlon, S.S., Sethi, R.D. and Chopra, A.K. 1983. Solid state fermentation of wheat straw into animal feed. *Indian J. Anim. Sci.* **53**, 1191-1194.

Pometto, I.I.I. and Crawford, D.L. 1986. Catabolic fate of *Streptomyces viridosporus* T7A-produced, acid precipitable polymeric lignin upon incubation with ligninolytic *Streptomyces* species and *Phanerochaete chrysosporium*. *Appl. Environ. Microbiol.* **51**, 171-179.

Puniya, A.K., Zadrazil, F. and Singh, K. 1994. Influence of gaseous phases on lignocellulose degradation by *Phanerochaete chrysosporium*. *Bioresource Technol.* **47**, 181-183.

Reade, A.E. and MacQueen, R.E. 1983. Investigation of white rot fungi for the conversion of poplar into a potential feedstuff for ruminants. *Can. J. Microbiol.* **29**, 457-463.

Reade, A.E. and Gregory, K.F. 1975. High temperature production of protein enriched feed from cassava by fungi. *Appl. Microbiol.* **30**, 897-904.

Reddy, P.P. 1985. Bioconversion of wheat straw and cellulosic substrates by molds under submerged and solid state fermentation. M.Sc. Thesis, Kurukshetra University, Kurukshetra, India.

Reid, I.D. 1985. Biological delignification of aspen wood by solid state fermentation with white rot fungus *Merulius tremellosus*. *Appl. Environ. Microbiol.* **50**, 133-139.

Reid, I.D. 1989. Solid state fermentation for biological delignification. *Enz. Microb. Technol.* **11**, 786-803.

Reid, I.D. and Seifert, K.A. 1982. Lignin degradation by *Phanerochaete chrysosporium* in hyperbaric oxygen. *Can. J. Bot.* **60**, 252-260.

Reid, I.D., Chao, E.E. and Dawson, P.S.S. 1985. Lignin degradation by *Phanerochaete chrysosporium* in agitated cultures. *Can. J. Microbiol.* **31**, 88-90.

Romantschuk, H. 1975. The pekile process: protein from spent sulphite liquor. In *Single Cell Protein II* (Tannenbaum, S.R. and Wang, D.I.C. eds) pp. 344-356. Cambridge Press, MIT, MA, US.

Schuchardt, F. and Zadrazil, F. 1980. Aufschluß von lignocellulose durch höhere pilze - entwicklung eines feststoff-fermenters. In *Energie durch Biotechnologie* (H. Dellweg, ed.) pp. 421-428. Berlin.

Schuchardt, F. and Zadrazil, F. 1988. A fermenter for solid state fermentation of straw by white-rot fungi. In *Treatment of Lignocellulosics with White Rot Fungi* (Zadrazil, F. and Reiniger, P., eds) pp. 77-89. Elsevier Applied Science, London, UK.

Singh, K., Rai, S.N., Singh, G.P. and Gupta, B.N. 1989. Solid state fermentation of urea-ammonia treated wheat straw and rice straw with *Coprinus fimetarius*. *Indian J. Microbiol.* **29**, 371-376.

Singh, K., Rai, S.N., Neelakantan, S. and Han, Y.W. 1990. Biochemical profiles of solid state fermentation of wheat straw with *Coprinus fimetarius*. *Indian J. Anim. Sci.* **60**, 984-990.

Singh, K., Singh, G.P. and Gupta, B.N. 1992. Biochemical studies of *Coprinus fimetarius* inoculated straws. *Indian J. Microbiol.* **32**, 473-477.

Singh, K., Singh, G.P. and Gupta, B.N. 1993. Effect of *Phanerochaete chrysosporium* inoculation on *in vitro* digestibility and chemical composition of wheat straw. *Indian J. Dairy Sci.* **46**, 177-179.

Skogma, H. 1976. Production of symba-yeast from potato wastes. In *Food from Waste* (K.J. Birch, K.G. Parker and J.T. Worgen, eds) pp. 167-176. Applied Science Publishers, London, UK.

Sundstol, F. and Owen, E. (eds) 1984. *Straw and Other Fibrous By-products*. Elsevier, Amsterdam, Netherlands.

Taylor, B.F. 1983. Aerobic and anaerobic catabolism of vanillic acid and some other methoxy-aromatic compounds by *Pseudomonas* sp. strain PN-1. *Appl. Environ. Microbiol.* **46**, 1286-1292.

Teifke, J. and Bohnet, M. 1990. Modelling of the physical process parameters of technical lignin degradation by *Pleurotus* spp. In *Advances in Biological Treatment of Lignocellulosic Materials* (M.P. Coughlan and M.T. Amaral Collaco, eds) pp. 71-83. Elsevier Applied Science, London, UK.

Weiland, P. 1988. Principles of solid state fermentation. In *Treatment of Lignocellulosics with White Rot Fungi*. (F. Zadrazil and P. Reiniger, eds) pp. 64-76. Elsevier Applied Science, London, UK.

Young, V.R. and Scrimshaw, N.S. 1975. Clinical studies on the nutritional value of SCP. In *Single Cell Protein II* (S.R. Tannenbaum, and D.I.C. Wang, eds) pp. 564-576. Cambridge Press, MIT, MA, US.

Zadrazil, F. 1977. The conversion of straw into feed by Basidiomycetes. *Eur. J. Appl. Microbiol.* **4**, 273-281.

Zadrazil, F. 1980. Conversion of different plant wastes into feed by basidiomycetes. *Eur. J. Appl. Microbiol. Biotechnol.* **9**, 243-248.

Zadrazil, F. 1985. Screening of fungi for lignin decomposition and conversion of straw into feed. *Angew. Botanik.* **59**, 433-452.

Zadrazil, F. and Brunnert, H. 1980. The influence of ammonium nitrate supplementation on degradation and *in vitro* digestibility of straw colonised by higher fungi. *Eur. J. Appl. Microbiol. Biotechnol.* **9**, 37-44.

Zadrazil, F. and Brunnert, H. 1981. Investigation of physical parameters important for the solid state fermentation of straw by white rot fungi. *Eur. J. Appl. Microbiol. Biotechnol.* **11**, 183-188.

Zadrazil, F. and Brunnert, H. 1982. Solid state fermentation of lignocellulose containing plant residues with *Sporotrichum pulverulentum* Nov. and *Dichomitus squalens* Karst. *Eur. J. Appl. Microbiol. Biotechnol.* **16**, 45-51.

Zadrazil, F., Diedrichs, M., Janssen, H., Schuchardt, F. and Park, J.S. 1990b. Large scale solid-state fermentation of cereal straw with *Pleurotus* spp. In *Advances in Biological Treatment of Lignocellulosic Materials* (M.P. Coughlan and M.T. Amaral Collaco, eds) pp. 43-58. Elsevier Applied Science, London, UK.

Zadrazil, F., Grinbergs, J. and Gonzalez, A. 1982. "Palo podrido" - decomposed wood which was used as a feed. *Eur. J. Appl. Microbiol. Biotechnol.* **15**, 167-171.

Zadrazil, F., Janssen, H., Diedrich, M. and Schuchdart, F. 1990a. Pilot-scale reactor for solid-state fermentation of lignocellulosics with higher fungi: production of feed, chemical feedstocks and substrates suitable for biofilters. In *Advances in Biological Treatment of Lignocellulosic Materials* (M.P. Coughlan and M.T. Amaral Collaco, eds) pp. 31-41. Elsevier Applied Science, London, UK.

Zadrazil, F. and Peerally, A. 1986. Effects of heat and microbial pretreatments of wheat straw substrate on the initial phase of solid state fermentation (SSF) by white rot fungi. *Biotechnol. Lett.* **30**, 103-109.

Zadrazil, F., Puniya, A.K. and Singh, K. 1993. Studies on effect of different gas compositions on degradation characteristics of crop-residues and resulting digestibility with *Pleurotus sajor-caju*. *Indian J. Microbiol.* **33**, 249-252.

Zeikus, J.G., Wellstein, A.L. and Kirk, T.K. 1982. Molecular basis for the biodegradative recalcitrance of lignin in anaerobic environments. *FEMS Microbiol. Lett.* **15**, 193-198.

5 Transgenic plants with improved protein quality

Susan B. Altenbach and Jeffrey A. Townsend[1]

USDA-ARS, Western Regional Research Center, 800 Buchanan Street, Albany, CA 94710, US, and [1]Department of Biotechnology Research, Pioneer Hi-Bred International, Inc., 7300 N.W. 62nd Avenue, PO Box 38, Johnston, IO 50131, US

INTRODUCTION

One of the goals of the animal feed industry is to provide feed formulations that allow for maximum growth of farm animals at the minimum cost. Because plant seeds, in particular corn and soybean, provide a concentrated source of protein, they provide the foundation of many animal feed formulations. Cereal seeds generally contain about 7-14% of their weight as protein and additionally are a good source of carbohydrates. Legume seeds are comprised of about 25-40% protein by weight and contribute the bulk of the protein to the feed. While plant seeds are an excellent source of protein in terms of quantity and availability, seed proteins from the major crop plants tend to be deficient in a number of essential amino acids that must be supplied in the diet to ensure maximum growth and development of non-ruminant livestock. Corn and other cereals are deficient in lysine and legume seeds are deficient in the sulfur-containing amino acids, methionine and cysteine. Part of these deficiencies is overcome by mixing seed meals from cereals and legumes, since cereals tend to have adequate levels of the sulfur amino acids while legumes provide a good supply of lysine. However, the entire requirement for these amino acids in intensively reared livestock cannot be met by mixing alone and most feeds for poultry are supplemented with additional methionine while lysine is added to the diets of both poultry and swine. The addition of amino acids to poultry and swine feeds adds significantly to the cost of production. For example, in the United States, these costs amount to approximately $120 million for methionine supplementation and $70 million for lysine supplementation annually.

The problem of protein quality in seed meals stems from the amino acid composition of the most abundant proteins accumulated in the seed. In the past, plant breeders have attempted to improve the complement of amino acids in plant seeds using traditional breeding methods. While these efforts have resulted in some success in the production of high lysine corn varieties, the increased lysine phenotype was found to be associated with undesirable agronomic characteristics and as a result these varieties have not been widely grown. Despite many years of breeding, soybean researchers have been unsuccessful in producing soybeans with improved levels of the sulfur-containing amino acids. The problem of seed protein quality is an area that is now being addressed by biotechnology and, without doubt, is one area in which plant molecular biology is likely to impact the animal feed industry in the near future. The nutritional quality of plant seeds might be improved by modifying the protein profiles of seeds and/or by altering the amino acid biosynthetic pathways of the plants. This chapter discusses molecular approaches for altering the amino acid composition of the seed with the aim of improving the quality of the protein in the seed meal.

THE TOOLS OF PLANT BIOTECHNOLOGY

In order to modify the protein profile of plant seeds, it is necessary to have adequate knowledge of the protein composition of the seed, the biosynthesis of the major protein constituents, the genes encoding those proteins and the regulation of those genes during seed development. It is also necessary to have a method for introducing new genes into the target crop plant. Because of the importance of plant seed proteins for both human and animal nutrition and the abundance of these proteins in the seeds, the seed storage proteins have been studied intensively and seed protein genes were among the first genes to be cloned from plants. Transformation technologies developed for tobacco and tomato in the early 1980s have recently been extended to major cereal and legume species. These developments in the field of plant molecular biology have set the stage for genetic engineering experiments aimed at altering protein quality.

Characterization of seed storage proteins

Plant seeds accumulate large quantities of a number of proteins that are deposited into compartments within the seed known as protein bodies where the proteins are stable during long periods of desiccation. Upon germination of the seed, the storage proteins are hydrolyzed and provide a source of reduced nitrogen for the developing seedling. It is the complement of these seed storage proteins that determines the amino acid composition of the seed.

The specific seed storage proteins vary among the different crop plants and are often classified on the basis of solubility using the scheme of Osborne (1924). In general, the predominant seed storage proteins from cereals such as corn, barley, and wheat are soluble in alcohol and referred to as prolamines. In corn, the major prolamines are referred to as zeins and comprise about 50-60% of the seed protein. The zeins contain high levels of proline and glutamine but essentially no lysine and are stored in the endosperm. In contrast, the major seed protein species of legumes and other dicotyledonous plants are soluble in either salt solutions or water and are referred to as globulins and albumins, respectively. These proteins are further distinguished by their sedimentation coefficients and classified as either 11S, 7S, or 2S species. In soybean, the 11S globulins are called glycinins and comprise about 40% of the total seed protein while the 7S globulins, called conglycinins, comprise another 40%. Soybean seeds also contain lectins and various small proteins some of which function as protease inhibitors in the seed. The major seed proteins from legumes generally accumulate in the cotyledons.

Biosynthesis and assembly of seed storage proteins

Because seed proteins must be transported to storage compartments within the seed, the proteins are usually synthesized as larger precursor polypeptides containing signal peptides that are cleaved co-translationally and direct the polypeptides into the endoplasmic reticulum. However, many seed proteins undergo additional post-translation modifications that may be very important in intracellular transport (Higgins, 1984; Utsumi, 1992 for reviews). These modifications are exemplified by comparing the biosynthesis and assembly of the 11S, 7S and 2S classes of seed proteins in dicotyledonous plants. After removal of signal peptides, 11S globulin precursors aggregate into trimers which are transported via the golgi to protein bodies. Within the protein bodies, a disulfide bridge is formed within the proprotein before the precursors undergo proteolytic cleavage into acidic and basic subunits. The protein species are further assembled into hexamers of 300 to 400 kDa. In contrast, after signal peptide cleavage, the 7S globulin precursors undergo glycosylation in the endoplasmic reticulum. The subunit precursors then assemble into trimers of 150 to 200 kDa and the oligosaccharides undergo further modification as the proteins pass through the golgi to protein bodies. The 2S albumins provide yet another distinct scheme of post-translational modification and are synthesized as precursors that undergo extensive proteolytic cleavage. In addition to the signal peptide, regions from both the amino- and the carboxyl-termini of the precursor as well an internal portion of the polypeptide are removed, resulting in monomers that consist of a large subunit and a small subunit linked by disulfide bonds.

Cloning of seed storage protein genes

Seeds generally accumulate a number of different isoforms of proteins within any given class and each isoform is encoded by a different member of a multi-gene family. For example, the family of 11S soybean glycinins has five members (Nielsen *et al.*, 1989) and the family of 7S soybean ß-conglycinins is believed to include at least 15 members (Harada *et al.*, 1989). The α-zein family from corn is even more complex and consists of about 75 genes which can be divided into four sub-families (Liu and Rubenstein, 1992). Individual members of a given gene family may be differentially regulated. For example, one family member may be expressed at maximum levels early in development, whereas a second family member may be expressed later. Some family members may be highly expressed while others are expressed only at low levels.

Seed storage protein genes have been cloned from many different plants (reviewed by Utsumi, 1992) and comparisons of nucleotide sequences obtained from different family members as well as from different species have revealed significant homologies. In addition, the availability of amino acid sequences derived from the nucleotide sequences has enabled the localization of sites of post-translational modifications and facilitated predictions about structures of seed proteins. Comparisons of cloned genes have also led to the identification of motifs in the upstream regulatory regions of genes that might play a role in tissue-specific, temporal or quantitative expression of the seed protein genes. Elements common among the prolamin genes are distinct from those found in either the 11S or the 7S globulin genes and there are numerous examples that indicate that regulatory regions from monocotyledonous plants such as cereals do not function particulary well in dicotyledonous plants such as legumes and other oilseeds. The cloned genes make available a collection of regulatory regions that might be used in the construction of chimeric genes for transgenic expression in specific plant species.

Transformation of important crop plants

Within the past ten years, methods for introducing DNA into plant cells from many of the important crops have been developed. Transformation procedures require a method of delivery of DNA into plant tissues and regeneration of entire fertile plants from those tissues. Target tissues may be protoplasts, callus cultures, embryogenic suspension cultures or explants from leaf or cotyledon tissue. One of two methods for DNA delivery is generally employed, either *Agrobacterium*-mediated transformation or particle bombardment.

In general, dicotyledonous plants are susceptible to a naturally occurring bacterium *Agrobacterium tumefaciens* that transfers bacterial genes to the chromosomes of wounded plant cells during the course of its natural infection thereby inducing the formation of tumors. DNA transfer involves genes located on a large plasmid called the Ti plasmid. In the early 1980s, the Ti plasmid was engineered so that the plasmid could carry desired DNA sequences into the plant instead of the bacterial genes that cause pathogenesis. The number of copies of the DNA that are inserted can be controlled somewhat by the concentration of the bacterial suspension that is used to inoculate the plants. Integrated DNA is stable in the transformed plants and is transmitted to the progeny via the seed. Tobacco was the first plant to be transformed reliably in the early 1980s (Zambryski *et al.*, 1983) and very soon became the model plant for analysis of transgenes. Transformation of the important legumes has proved more difficult because these plants are not good hosts for *Agrobacterium*. Transgenic soybean plants, however, have been produced using *Agrobacterium*-mediated transformation (Hinchee *et al.*, 1988).

The cereals have been particularly difficult to transform. However, in the last few years success has been reported with numerous grains including corn (Gordon-Kamm *et al.*, 1990) and barley (Wan and Lemaux, 1993). Monocotyledonous plants require a physical means of DNA delivery. The method that has met with the most success involves bombarding plant tissues with small gold or tungsten particles that have been coated with the DNA of interest. The projectiles wound plant cells and the DNA is incorporated into the genome of the plant by a mechanism that is not well understood. Under appropriate hormone and media regimes, the bombarded tissues are regenerated into whole plants which have been shown to be fertile and transmit the inserted DNA to the next generation. In most cases, this method delivers multiple copies of the target gene to the plant. Copies of the gene may be rearranged or only partly transferred. Although it is difficult to control the gene copy number, the DNA generally is inserted into a single location in the chromosome and segregates as a single genetic locus. Particle bombardment has also been used successfully for the transformation of soybean (McCabe *et al.*, 1988; Finer and McMullen, 1991).

MOLECULAR APPROACHES FOR ALTERING THE PROTEIN PROFILES OF SEEDS

The amino acid profile of the seed protein could be altered either by transferring genes encoding heterologous proteins rich in a desired amino acid to the target plant, or by modifying seed storage protein genes and then introducing the modified genes back into the plant. In order to have an appreciable effect on the amino acid content of the seed, the candidate protein must first contain proportions of the limiting amino acid that are significantly higher than the seed proteins of the target plant. Secondly, the gene encoding the protein must be expressed at high levels so that the protein represents a significant proportion of the total seed protein in the transgenic plant. The accumulation of either heterologous or modified proteins in seeds at high concentrations requires chimeric genes with regulatory regions that direct strong, seed-specific expression. The mRNA transcribed from the gene must be stable in the seeds and efficiently translated. Additionally, the proteins encoded by the genes must be correctly processed, transported and assembled in the transgenic plant.

Table 1. Approximate accumulation of proteins with different methionine contents required to achieve a 75% increase in seed protein methionine in transgenic soybean plants.

Methionine (%) in candidate protein	Accumulation (% of total seed protein)
3	50
5	25
10	10
20	5

Table 1 shows the approximate accumulation of proteins with different methionine contents that would be required to eliminate the need for methionine supplementation of poultry feeds in the United States. It is estimated that the methionine content of soybean seed protein would need to be increased by about 75% from a current level of 1.2% to about 2.1%. For simplicity, the values assume that the total amount of seed protein in the transgenic plant remains the same and that any endogenous protein species replaced by the expression of the introduced genes contain average levels of methionine.

Expression of heterologous proteins in transgenic seeds

The feasibility of expressing genes encoding heterologous proteins in plant seeds to correct for amino acid deficiencies, in particular methionine deficiencies, has been demonstrated in a number of different plant species. Most plant and animal proteins contain low levels of methionine (1-2%). A number of seed proteins have been identified in both monocotyledonous and dicotyledonous plants, however, which contain extremely high levels of the sulfur-containing amino acids (Table 2).

Of the candidate methionine-rich proteins, the 2S albumin from Brazil nut has been used in gene transfer experiments aimed at elevating seed methionine content. cDNA sequences encoding the 2S albumin from Brazil nut have been attached to a number of different regulatory regions and transformed into several different plant species. The chimeric gene that resulted in the highest levels of accumulation of the Brazil nut albumin in seeds from transgenic plants consisted of the regulatory regions of the phaseolin gene, a 7S seed storage protein from French bean, attached to the cDNA sequences encoding the 17 kDa precursor of the Brazil nut albumin (Altenbach *et al.*, 1989).

The feasibility of a gene transfer method for enhancing amino acid composition was first demonstrated in tobacco (Altenbach *et al.*, 1989), largely because of the availability of reliable transformation methods for this species. In tobacco transformed with the phaseolin-Brazil nut albumin chimeric gene, the Brazil nut protein encompassed as much as 8% of the total seed protein. The increased accumulation of the Brazil nut albumin was correlated with a 30% increase in the methionine content of the seed proteins. The 17 kDa precursor of the Brazil nut

Table 2. Seed proteins containing high levels of the sulfur amino acids.

Plant	Protein size (kDa)	Methionine (%)	Cysteine (%)	References
Corn	10	22.5	3.9	Kirihara *et al.*, 1988
Rice	10	20	10	Yamagata *et al.*, 1986
Brazil nut	12	19	8	Altenbach *et al.*, 1987
Sunflower	10	15.5	7.8	Lilley *et al.*, 1989; Kortt *et al.*, 1991
Soybean	10.8	12.1	2.5	George and de Lumen, 1991
Job's tears[1]	18.3	11.6	5.2	Leite *et al.*, 1991
Corn	15	11.3	4.4	Pedersen *et al.*, 1986
Cotton	?[2]	10	6.8	Galau *et al.*, 1992

[1]*Coix lachryma-jobi.*
[2]2S albumin, size not determined

albumin that was encoded by the chimeric gene was processed correctly in the transgenic seeds and the protein was hydrolyzed along with the endogenous tobacco seed proteins upon seed germination. Although the chimeric gene utilized the regulatory regions from a 7S gene, the Brazil nut protein accumulated early in the development of the tobacco seeds, during the time that the endogenous 2S proteins were accumulated (unpublished data). In tobacco, the 11S, 7S and 2S species encompass approximately 80, 10, and 10% of the total seed protein, respectively. Since neither the total protein content nor the quantity of the 2S protein fraction appeared to increase in the transgenic seeds, it was concluded that high levels of the Brazil protein were accumulated in tobacco seeds at the expense of some of the endogenous 2S seed proteins.

Large amounts of the Brazil nut albumin also were accumulated in transgenic seeds when the phaseolin-Brazil nut albumin chimeric gene was expressed in canola (rape) (Altenbach *et al.*, 1992). The Brazil nut methionine-rich protein comprised as much as 4% of the seed protein in this species and resulted in a 33% increase in seed protein methionine levels. As in tobacco, the precursor of the 2S albumin was processed correctly in the transgenic seeds and the protein was hydrolyzed upon germination. Canola seeds contain predominantly 11S and 2S protein species, in a ratio of about 60:40. Because canola seeds contain significant quantities of 2S proteins, it was difficult to determine whether the synthesis of the Brazil nut protein in the seeds influenced the accumulation of the endogenous 2S proteins. In canola, however, accumulation of the Brazil nut 2S albumin coincided with the accumulation of the 11S proteins rather than the 2S proteins.

Recent studies in which the chimeric phaseolin-Brazil nut albumin gene was inserted into soybean reveal that this gene is highly expressed in legume species (Townsend *et al.*, 1992a,b). Soybean contains predominantly 11S and 7S proteins. The accumulation of a protein species that co-migrated with the mature Brazil nut albumin on SDS-PAGE was easily detected in soybean and the Brazil nut albumin was estimated to encompass as much as 10% of the seed protein. The concentration of methionine in the transgenic seeds was increased significantly over control soybean seeds. However, the increase was not as high as expected (26% rather than the 80%

increase that would have been predicted). One reason may be that the synthesis of the methionine-rich albumin occurred at the expense of some of the soybean seed proteins. In particular, the accumulation of the Brazil nut protein in the transgenic seeds was accompanied by a decrease in a minor protein species of 10.8 kDa that is rich in methionine. There may be changes in other protein species as well.

The decrease in accumulation of an endogenous methionine-rich soybean protein in response to the expression of the chimeric phaseolin-Brazil nut albumin gene indicates that there may be competition between the synthesis of the heterologous and the endogenous protein species in transgenic soybean, similar to that observed previously among the 2S proteins in transgenic tobacco. One explanation would be that there are constraints on the amounts of this class of proteins that can be accumulated in the seed. Alternately, the inhibition of the accumulation of the soybean methionine-rich protein may be due to limitations on the sulfur pools available in the seeds. It has been known for some time that the synthesis of some seed proteins is influenced by the levels of sulfur available to the plant. In pea, the effects of sulfur deficiencies on seed protein synthesis are dramatic and can result in a 20% decrease in total seed protein, substantial decreases in the 11S and 2S protein species and a substantial increase in the amounts of the sulfur-poor 7S proteins present (Higgins, 1984). Experiments have shown that these changes result from dramatic changes in the concentration of the mRNA encoding the 11S and 7S proteins during seed development. mRNA for the 11S species are absent during sulfur-deficient periods while mRNA for the 7S proteins are stable throughout seed development. In soybean, sulfur deficiency has been associated with a 40% decrease in glycinins and a 3-fold increase in a ß-conglycinin subunit that contains no methionine (Gayler and Sykes, 1985). If the synthesis of the Brazil nut protein in large amounts in the seeds depletes existing sulfur pools, the expression of soybean genes regulated by sulfur might be affected. Quantitation of the different protein species accumulated in seeds of control and transgenic soybean plants should shed some light on this question. At the same time it might be interesting to determine whether the high transgenic expression of a 2S albumin containing average levels of methionine, such as the *Arabidopsis* 2S albumin, would have a similar effect on the accumulation of the endogenous soybean proteins.

Other attempts to express the Brazil nut methionine-rich protein in transgenic plants have met with limited success. Chimeric genes which utilized a promoter from a soybean lectin gene attached to a fusion protein in which a signal peptide from a soybean lectin gene was attached to the amino terminal processed peptide and downstream regions of the Brazil nut albumin precursor directed the accumulation of the methionine-rich protein in canola seeds at very low levels (< 0.05% of seed protein) (Guerche *et al.*, 1990). Other chimeric genes that have been tested consisted of a promoter from an *Arabidopsis* 2S albumin attached to fusion proteins that consisted of regions from the N-terminus of the *Arabidopsis* 2S albumin linked to sequences from the Brazil nut methionine-rich albumin. These chimeric genes resulted in the accumulation of the methionine-rich protein at concentrations estimated to be 0.05%, 0.1% and 0.3% of the total salt-soluble protein from tobacco, canola and *Arabidopsis* seeds respectively (de Clercq *et al.*, 1990). These results indicate that the choice of regulatory region as well as the choice of the coding sequence is critical for obtaining the high expression necessary to effect a change in the amino acid composition of seed proteins. Interestingly, the seeds from tobacco, canola,

Arabidopsis and soybean all contain the capacity for the extensive proteolytic processing of the 2S seed proteins.

Of the other methionine-rich proteins, there are reports of transgenic expression work in tobacco utilizing the 15 kDa zein protein from corn (Hoffman *et al.*, 1987). When the coding region of this alcohol-soluble protein was placed under the control of either dicot or viral regulatory regions, the zein was able to accumulate to concentrations as high as 1.6% of the total seed protein. The signal peptide was cleaved correctly from the precursors of the corn protein and the 15 kDa zein accumulated in the protein bodies of the tobacco seeds. However, the corn proteins were not degraded upon germination of the seed, potentially leading to problems with seedling viability if the proteins were accumulated in amounts sufficient to alter seed methionine concentration.

Seed storage proteins containing exceptionally high proportions of lysine have not been reported, although some 11S, 7S and 2S seed proteins from dicots do contain between 4 and 8% lysine. There are also reports of other plant proteins with significant lysine contents, most notably a chymotrypsin inhibitor from barley that contains 11.5% lysine (Williamson *et al.*, 1987) and several proteins believed to play roles in water stress with lysine contents around 13% (Hong *et al.*, 1988; Kurkela and Franck, 1990; Neven *et al.*, 1993). The seed-specific expression of genes encoding proteins that have specific functions in other plant tissues without having adverse effects on the plant would undoubtedly present even greater challenges than those encountered in expressing heterologous seed proteins.

Alteration of expression of endogenous seed protein genes

A variation on the approach of expressing heterologous proteins containing high proportions of a particular amino acid in transgenic seeds is to increase the expression of endogenous genes encoding proteins rich in the limiting amino acids. One advantage of this approach is that it is known that the protein can be processed, transported and assembled in the seed as well as hydrolyzed upon germination.

For soybean a good approach for improving the methionine content would be to increase the accumulation of the 10.8 kDa methionine-rich soybean protein identified by George and deLumen (1991). This protein encompasses about 0.6% of the total soybean seed protein and contains 12.1% methionine. In order to eliminate the need for methionine supplementation, this protein would need to contribute about 8% of the total seed protein. Based on work in transgenic tobacco and soybean with the phaseolin-Brazil nut albumin gene, this level of expression should be possible. The methionine content of corn seed proteins could also be increased in this manner by increasing the expression of genes containing either the 10 kDa methionine-rich zein (containing 22.5% methionine) or the 15 kDa zein (containing 11.3% methionine). Since corn contains adequate levels of methionine, elevating the methionine content would not improve its nutritional quality significantly when used as a sole protein source. However, the value would be increased if the corn were used as a part of a feed mixture with soybean.

It may be possible to increase the expression of members of gene families encoding proteins that are high in the desired amino acid and to decrease the expression of genes that encode proteins low in the desired amino acid, but this is a somewhat uncertain approach. For example, in soybean the glycinins contain approximately 1.8% methionine while the conglycinins contain much lower concentrations of methionine (approximately 0.6%). There is also variation in the methionine content of different glycinin subunits. The total methionine content of the seed might be increased somewhat if the ratio of glycinins to conglycinins could be altered. This might be accomplished by inserting additional genes in which strong promoters have been attached to coding regions for glycinin subunits with higher methionine levels. At the same time, the expression of the sulfur-poor conglycinins genes might be decreased using antisense technology. While modifying the expression of gene families could lead to an elevation in the overall methionine content of the seed, it is unlikely that this method alone could increase the levels of methionine sufficiently to eliminate the need for methionine supplementation of animal feeds. The approach is complicated by the fact that both the glycinins and the conglycinins are encoded by multiple genes. Additionally, it is not known whether subunits encoded by specific gene family members are required for correct protein assembly.

Alteration of coding regions of seed protein genes

If suitable proteins with high concentrations of a particular amino acid are not available, protein engineering techniques might be used to create genes encoding modified seed proteins with the desired composition. Multiple residues must be introduced into the target protein without effecting the folding of the protein, assembly into higher order structures, targeting to protein bodies, or degradation upon seed germination. Decisions regarding the regions of the protein to be modified can best be made when the three-dimensional structure of the candidate protein is known. Comparisons between sequences of seed proteins encoded by different members of a gene family and between homologous seed proteins in other plant species are also valuable in revealing potential sites for modification. Conserved domains may suggest that the region is important for protein accumulation while variable domains may be more likely to tolerate substitutions or additions of amino acid residues. In addition, studies of the *in vitro* assembly of protein subunits such as those made with soybean glycinin (Dickinson *et al.*, 1990) and conglycinin (Lelievre *et al.*, 1992) provide a complementary means of identifying regions likely to be critical in oligomer formation.

An 11S glycinin from soybean, a 7S phaseolin from French bean, a 2S albumin from *Arabidopsis* and an α-zein from corn have been the initial targets of protein engineering attempts to improve amino acid composition. The first experiments have focused on locating regions of these different proteins that might tolerate additional methionine or lysine residues, either as single amino acid substitutions or as part of larger insertions.

Hoffman *et al.* (1988) increased the number of methionine residues in phaseolin from three residues to nine residues by inserting a 45 bp section of DNA encoding a methionine-rich region of a zein protein into the phaseolin gene. Both the zein fragment and the region of phaseolin into which the insertion was made were believed to form α-helical structures. When a gene encoding this modified protein was expressed in tobacco seeds, only low levels of the modified protein accumulated despite the presence of the expected quantities of mRNA in the transgenic plants. Comparison between the expression of genes encoding normal phaseolin and the modified protein demonstrated that both proteins were synthesized at similar rates in the transgenic seeds and that both were glycosylated. However, the unaltered phaseolin accumulated in protein bodies in the tobacco seeds, while the modified protein could not be detected. It is clear, now that the three-dimensional structure of phaseolin has been determined at 0.3 nm resolution (Lawrence *et al.*, 1990), that the region modified was internal to the first helix-turn-helix motif of the protein and likely to be important in oligomer formation, explaining in part why this first attempt at protein engineering was unsuccessful. The availability of structural data for phaseolin should facilitate the identification of surface regions of the protein that may tolerate modifications better and thereby provide a better foundation for future engineering experiments.

Comparisons of the sequences of five glycinin genes were used to identify regions of the 11S soybean protein that might be modified. The analysis revealed three variable regions within the protein as well as a number of positions in which some glycinins contain methionines while others contain different hydrophobic residues (Argos *et al.*, 1985; Nielsen *et al*, 1989). One of the variable regions, a domain of about 80 amino acids at the carboxyl end of the acidic subunit of the protein, is particularly heterogeneous and has been termed the hypervariable region (HVR). Based on this information, Dickinson *et al.* (1990) made a series of deletions, insertions, and single amino acid substitutions throughout the glycinin protein. In some of the modified proteins, a portion of the HVR was replaced with domains between two and 20 amino acids in length that increased the methionine content of the resulting protein by as many as four residues. In an attempt to match the three dimensional structure of the inserted region with that of the surrounding glycinin protein, domains from a bacterial ferredoxin protein and a citrate synthase gene containing multiple methionine residues in turn regions were utilized. Other insertions in the HVR contained as many as five repetitions of an arginine-methionine sequence. *In vitro* transcription/translation products were produced from the modified coding sequences and the synthesized proteins were tested for their ability to assemble into oligomers similar in size to those found in soybean seeds. The assembly assays suggested that the hypervariable region in the carboxyl end of the protein could tolerate significant insertions without affecting the assembly of the protein subunits. However, changes in the amino terminal portion of the acidic subunit and changes in the basic subunit interfered with subunit interactions. Experiments in which modified coding sequences were expressed in transgenic tobacco plants under the direction of glycinin regulatory regions indicated that a number of modified subunits that were able to assemble in the *in vitro* assay were also able to accumulate in the seed although levels of accumulation were not reported (Scott *et al.*, 1991).

The 2S albumins from many plants, including *Arabidopsis*, canola, Brazil nut, sunflower and castor bean, are rich in cysteine (around 8%). The positions of cysteine residues in the various proteins are conserved, suggesting that disulfide bridges play an important role in the secondary structure and the stability of these proteins. Additionally, extensive post-translational proteolytic processing events involved in the biosynthesis of 2S proteins are similar in Brazil nut, canola and *Arabidopsis* (Ampe *et al.*, 1986; Ericson *et al.*, 1986; De Castro *et al.*, 1987; Sun *et al.*, 1987). While the overall structure of these proteins is likely to be similar, there is a good deal of variability in the primary sequences of these proteins as demonstrated by the fact that the Brazil nut albumin contains high concentrations of methionine (19%) and no lysine, while the *Arabidopsis* and canola 2S proteins contain low concentrations of methionine (about 2.5%) and significant quantities of lysine (around 7%). Sequence comparisons between 2S albumins from different species indicate that a region between the fourth and fifth cysteine residues of the large subunits of the proteins differs in both length and sequence and thus may not be critical to the structure of the protein (Krebbers *et al.*, 1986). Interestingly, the Brazil nut albumin stores almost half of its methionine in this variable region where methionine residues are clustered with arginine residues in two internal domains. The first evidence that the variable region of the 2S albumins might tolerate modifications came from the work of Vandekerckhove *et al.* (1989) in which the sequence for the five amino acid neuropeptide leu-enkephalin was engineered into a 2S albumin gene from *Arabidopsis* and expressed in both *Arabidopsis* and canola. De Clercq *et al.* (1990) extended this work, replacing a 69 base pair region of the coding sequence in the variable region of an *Arabidopsis* albumin with several different synthetic DNA fragments of 21, 54, and 72 nucleotides which were similar in sequence to that found in the Brazil nut albumin. The methionine content of the unmodified protein was thus elevated by either 4, 7 or 11 residues. These modified genes were expressed in tobacco, *Arabidopsis*, and canola plants at levels estimated by indirect methods to be 1-2% of the total seed protein.

In an attempt to investigate the effect of incorporating lysine residues into α-zeins from corn, Wallace *et al.* (1988) constructed a number of altered coding regions and examined the synthesis of the proteins in *Xenopus* oocytes. It had previously been demonstrated in *Xenopus* that zein mRNA could direct the synthesis and processing of zein proteins into membrane-enclosed structures similar to maize protein bodies. Five zein coding regions were constructed in which single codons for neutral amino acids in different positions of the protein were replaced with lysine codons. Four altered coding regions contained lysine substitutions for two amino acids and three coding regions contained insertions of either five or eight amino acids which included two lysine residues and one or two tryptophan residues. One additional coding region contained a large insertion encoding a 17 kDa protein from an animal virus. None of the modifications affected the translation, signal peptide cleavage or stability of the modified proteins in *Xenopus* oocytes and all of the modified proteins except the one containing the 17 kDa insertion were targeted to structures similar to maize protein bodies. While these experiments are encouraging, and suggest that zeins may be able to tolerate the insertion of lysine residues, the true test will be whether the modified zeins are stable in the seeds of transgenic plants. With this in mind, Ohtani *et al.* (1991) examined the expression of chimeric genes containing either the normal zein or zein coding sequences with single lysine substitutions under the direction of the phaseolin promoter in transgenic tobacco plants. Although the mRNA from both the normal zein and the modified zeins were present in the transgenic seeds in the expected amounts, accumulation of proteins in all cases was much lower than expected (<0.003% of the seed protein). Pulse-chase labeling experiments indicated that the newly synthesized zeins were unstable in the tobacco seeds and were rapidly degraded. The instability of these proteins in the tobacco seeds may be due to intrinsic differences between the seeds of corn and tobacco. Now that transformation methods are available for corn and other monocots, it will be interesting to examine the stability of these and other modified zeins in transgenic seeds from monocotyledonous plants.

Some of the early experiments bring to light complications in detecting and quantifying engineered proteins in transgenic seeds. Depending on how extensively a protein has been modified, antibodies directed against the protein may not react with the engineered version. Additionally, it may be very difficult to quantify the accumulation of a modified protein among the background of endogenous proteins in transgenic seeds, as was observed when the modified

2S albumin gene was introduced into *Arabidopsis*. Unfortunately, it is not a simple matter to detect a modified glycinin in soybean or an altered zein in corn.

Protein engineering approaches have not yet yielded transgenic plants in which the amino acid content of the seeds was altered. However, the initial experiments suggest that seed storage proteins have enough flexibility in their structures to tolerate insertions and amino acid substitutions in their primary sequences. Determining whether there is enough fluidity to create proteins with suitable methionine and/or lysine contents to solve the problem of amino acid deficiencies will be the focus of future work in this area.

MOLECULAR APPROACHES FOR MODIFYING AMINO ACID BIOSYNTHETIC PATHWAYS

Attempts to improve the quality of plant proteins used as food inevitably involve a consideration of the biosynthesis of amino acids. Improved diets could result from increases in free methionine or free lysine in plant seeds. However, since free amino acids generally represent only a small fraction (<5%) of the total in plant tissues, very large increases in the pools would be required to produce changes significant for the animal diet. Alternatively, overproduction of specific amino acids may enable proteins containing elevated levels of those same amino acids to accumulate in plant tissues.

Biosynthesis of the aspartate family of amino acids in plants

Lysine, methionine, threonine and isoleucine are members of a family of amino acids derived from aspartate (Fig. 1). In plants these amino acids are synthesized largely within the chloroplast. The biosynthetic pathway involved is very similar to one which operates in many bacterial species (Bryan, 1980). Feedback inhibition by the end products, lysine, S-adenosylmethionine, threonine and isoleucine, regulate the level of enzyme activity at key steps leading to their production, keeping free amino acids at constant and relatively low levels. Aspartate kinase (AK), the first enzyme in the pathway, phosphorylates aspartate to produce aspartyl phosphate. All of the end products of the pathway derive from the action of AK, but not all have been found to inhibit its activity. Native forms of AK have been identified which are inhibited by lysine or threonine or synergistically by combinations of lysine and S-adenosylmethionine. Mutant forms of AK have been identified which are less sensitive to feedback inhibition. The presence of such enzymes in plants has resulted in dramatic changes in the profile of free amino acids that are accumulated.

De-regulation of the aspartate family pathway by mutant forms of aspartate kinase

Green and Phillips (1974) designed a selective strategy for plant cell cultures where lysine plus threonine (LT) are used to inhibit normal growth. They found that growth inhibition results from lack of methionine and that growth is restored when methionine is added to LT medium. The strategy has been used to isolate AK mutants from corn (Hibberd and Green, 1982; Diedrick *et al.*, 1990), barley (Bright *et al.*, 1982), carrot (Cattoir-Reynearts *et al.*, 1983), and tobacco (Frankard *et al.*, 1991) desensitized to feedback inhibition. The inheritance pattern for these mutations was consistent with that of single dominant genes. Frankard *et al.* (1991) conducted extensive amino acid analysis on a tobacco plant which was homozygous for a mutant AK allele. Leaves from the plant (RTL70) had between a four and five fold increase in the total pool of free amino acids. Most of the increase was contributed by a massive (47-fold) increase in free threonine. Levels of the other aspartate-derived amino acids were also elevated compared to the wild type. Free isoleucine increased 12-fold and both free methionine and free lysine went up 5-fold. There was no change in the amount or quality of protein-bound amino acids. Seeds of RTL70 were changed even more dramatically than leaves and had nearly twenty times more free amino acid than the wild type. All free amino acid concentrations were increased, threonine by 70-fold and free lysine and isoleucine by 23 and 11-fold respectively. Free methionine was not detected in wild type seed but was 0.1% of total free amino acid in RTL70 seed. In seed, as in leaves, the quality of protein-bound amino acids remained unchanged, but, in contrast to RTL70 leaves, the seed of the mutant had a substantially higher protein content than the wild type suggesting that changes in amino acid biosynthesis may lead to increased protein accumulation in the seed. However, despite the dramatic changes in the free amino acid pools of RTL70 seed, only threonine, among the aspartate family amino acids, was increased as a percentage of the total (free plus bound) amino acids.

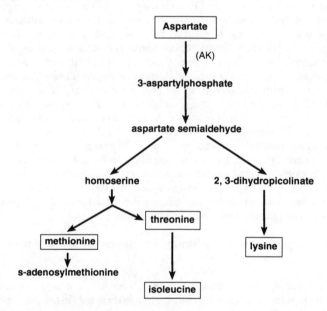

Figure 1. The asparate-family biosynthetic pathway. AK, Aspartate kinase; HDH, Homoserine dehydrogenase; DHPS, Dihydropicolinate synthase.

Shaul and Galili (1992a) have expressed a gene which codes for a mutant form of AK from *Escherichia coli*, the lysC gene, in transgenic tobacco plants. Bacterial AK was found to be even less sensitive to feedback inhibition than the mutant plant forms. The transgene approach allowed the authors to express the enzyme within the chloroplast, where presumably it would normally be located, or within the cytoplasm. While both types of plant had significant increases in free threonine, greater increases were achieved with chloroplast-specific expression. AK activity in several transgenics correlated well with their relative free threonine concentrations. Changes in the total pool of free amino acids were not reported but the observed free threonine increases in leaves were very similar to the work described above with the mutant plant enzyme. In these plants however, there was a smaller increase in free threonine in seed than in leaves. Possibly such differences result from the different expression patterns which the plant and chimeric genes must certainly have. They may as well result from abnormal seed development which caused partial sterility of these plants.

Shaul and Galili (1992a) and others have commented on deleterious effects which are presumed to result from overproduction of free amino acids. Among the altered phenotypes encountered are wrinkled, elongated, thickened or chlorotic leaves, slowed growth, delayed flowering and partial or complete sterility. Although it is difficult to be certain that these phenotypes are the consequence of greatly increased free amino acid pools, it does seem that some ill effects accompany large increases. Karchi *et al.* (1993) attempted to circumvent these problems by expressing the bacterial lysC gene specifically in seeds of transgenic tobacco. In their experiment, the lysC gene product was targeted to the chloroplast of developing seed by fusing the coding sequence to the pea rbcS-3A chloroplast transit peptide and the phaseolin promoter of French bean. Increased AK activity was detected in seed but not in leaves, roots or flowers of the transgenic plants. Several plants including those with the highest AK activities had phenotypes which were indistinguishable from the progenitor cultivar. The plants were fully fertile and produced seed with the same average weight and germination frequency as controls. Progeny of these plants that were homozygous for the transgene had a 17-fold increase in free threonine and a three-fold increase in free methionine (0.12% of total free amino acid). Quantitative and qualitative differences were detected in the protein-bound amino acids. The elevation in protein content was similar to that described above but in addition there was a significant increase in globulin-bound methionine which contributed to a total (free plus bound) methionine increase of nearly seven percent. The study showed that the aspartate family pathway is active in seed and that modification of the pathway can be conducted such that otherwise normal plants produce seed with elevated methionine content.

Deregulation of the aspartate family pathway by mutant forms of dihydropicolinate synthase

The third step in the aspartate family pathway is a branch point. Here aspartate semialdehyde is either condensed with pyruvate to form 2,3-dihydropicolinate in the first step specific to lysine biosynthesis or reduced to homoserine in the first step specific to methionine, threonine and isoleucine biosynthesis. Dihydropicolinate synthase (DHPS) catalyzes the condensation reaction toward lysine and homoserine dehydrogenase (HDH) catalyzes the reduction towards methionine, threonine and isoleucine. Both enzymes are regulated by end product feedback. Native forms of DHPS are sensitive to feedback inhibition by lysine but not by other pathway products. HDH is inhibited only by threonine but native forms have been identified which are threonine-insensitive as well. Many attempts have been made to identify DHPS mutants with the ultimate intention of overproducing lysine. Negrutiu *et al.* (1984) isolated a DHPS mutant from tobacco by selection of mutagenized protoplasts on a toxic analog of lysine, S-(2-aminoethyl) cysteine. DHPS activity was greatly increased in the mutant. AK activity was unchanged. Leaves from the mutant (RAEC-1) had a 30-fold increase in free lysine. Shaul and Galili (1992b) expressed in transgenic tobacco the dapA gene encoding a bacterial DHPS that is less sensitive to lysine inhibition than the mutant plant form. Free lysine was elevated 40-fold above normal in leaves of one such transgenic plant. The accumulation of free lysine was positively correlated with DHPS activity and with gene dose so that lysine accumulation could be tailored by generating transgenics with varied levels of gene expression. Expression of the gene in the cytoplasm did not result in increased lysine production, suggesting that DHPS, unlike AK, must be present within the chloroplast. As with the threonine overproducers, these lysine overproducers had abnormal phenotypes which increased in severity with the free lysine content of leaves.

Partitioning of amino acid biosynthesis between branches of the aspartate family pathway

The possibility now exists to deregulate the lysine biosynthetic pathway in plants completely by expressing genes coding for both desensitized AK and DHPS enzymes. The observations to date would suggest that this may represent the best possible approach for increasing the free lysine pool but that some control over the temporal and spatial expression of the genes will be required to obtain a normal plant phenotype. Characterization of such double mutants or double transformants may provide information about the partitioning of amino acid biosynthesis between pathway branches. HDH is implicated in such regulation. In carrot, HDH reversibly converts between a threonine-sensitive and a threonine-insensitive form (Matthews *et al.*, 1989). Understanding of the regulation is complicated by the knowledge that AK and HDH activities can reside on common proteins (Wilson *et al.*, 1991). To date, constitutively desensitized HDH mutants have not been identified, so further deregulation of this pathway branch has not been possible. An additional modification may be necessary before complete deregulation of the methionine biosynthetic pathway is achieved since homoserine kinase, the enzyme which immediately follows HDH in the pathway, is known to be feedback regulated by threonine, methionine, or S-adenosylmethionine (Bryan, 1990).

Aspartate itself has not been found to be a rate-limiting factor in the biosynthesis of amino acids. Thus far, its content has not been reduced in any deregulated plant. Several rate-limiting factors in the aspartate family pathway have been identified. Enhancements of AK activity have given increases in all the derived amino acid levels, with internal regulation seeming to favor the pathway branch which includes methionine. Enhancements of DHPS activity have driven overproduction of lysine by the alternate pathway branch. Overproduction of free amino acids in vegetative tissues is accompanied by negative effects on plant phenotype. Storage organs such as seed are more tolerant of increases in free amino acid pools and in seed the increases have resulted in gains in protein quantity and quality. However, these gains are not yet sufficient to impact the animal diet. Future attempts to increase the nutritional value of plants by deregulation of the aspartate family pathway may be complemented by the presence of lysine or methionine-rich storage proteins which could serve as sinks for the newly created amino acid pools.

CONSIDERATIONS OF MOLECULAR APPROACHES

Molecular approaches show great promise for improving the amino acid composition of feed ingredients. However, before products that will benefit the animal feed industry can emerge a number of important issues must be addressed. First of all, the alteration in amino acid content must not have a negative impact on the plant. Secondly, amino acids contained in the transgenic seed must be available to animals and the safety of products resulting from genetic engineering must be assessed for both humans and livestock. Finally, there will be challenges in marketing seeds containing enhanced amino acid contents.

Alteration of agronomic properties of the plant

There is a tremendous amount of variation in the complement of seed proteins in and between plant species with developmental, genetic and environmental influences all playing a role in determining the protein composition (Higgins, 1984, for review). Recent work suggests that the expression of heterologous seed protein genes can also influence the levels of certain endogenous proteins in the seed (Altenbach et al., 1989; Townsend et al., 1992a). It remains to be determined whether there are limits on the amounts of foreign proteins that can be accumulated in the seeds of transgenic plants or whether the form in which a seed stores its nitrogen is important as long as the seed maintains an adequate reserve for germination. Additionally, it is yet to be learned how the viability of a seedling might be affected if a heterologous or modified seed protein forming 10 or 20% of the total seed protein is resistant to proteolysis upon germination. While it is impossible to predict whether altering the protein profile of the seed might affect other characteristics of the plant, it is encouraging that transgenic tobacco, canola and soybean plants accumulating high levels of the Brazil nut albumin were indistinguishable from the control plants when grown under greenhouse conditions (Altenbach et al., 1989; 1992).

Whether a gene encodes a heterologous, endogenous, or engineered seed protein or an enzyme involved in amino acid biosynthesis, expression of the gene in transgenic plants must not compromise the agronomic properties of the plant. There must be no yield penalty associated with the transgenic plant or farmers will not grow the altered seed. Field trials in which the transgenic plants are grown side-by-side with control plants at a number of different test locations are critical for evaluating characteristics of the modified plants. Thus far, soybean plants accumulating the Brazil nut albumin have been tested in the field and the results show great promise. Transgenic soybean plants performed as well as control plants and there was no yield penalty associated with the accumulation of large quantities of the heterologous protein in the seed.

Availability of amino acids to livestock

Clearly, engineered seeds must contain increased levels of desired amino acids in a form that can be utilized by animals for growth and development without having toxic or antinutritional effects. When the candidate genes encode naturally-occurring seed proteins, preliminary animal feeding studies can be done relatively early in the research program. For example, early indications from rat feeding trials in which Brazil nut flour was used to supplement a navy bean based diet provided evidence that the methionine contained in the Brazil nut proteins was available to animals (Antunes and Markakis, 1977). Additionally, because the 2S albumin is a very abundant species and encompasses about 30% of the total seed protein in Brazil nut, the protein could be purified from seeds in quantities sufficient for use in feeding studies with Japanese quail. These studies indicated that the methionine contained in the Brazil nut albumin was available to the birds and that the addition of the protein to the feed did not have any deleterious effects (Tao *et al.*, 1987). The final test of product efficacy must be animal feeding trials comparing meal from transgenic seeds with meal from nontransformed seeds with and without amino acid supplementation. For transgenic soybean accumulating significant quantities of the Brazil nut albumin, these types of feeding trials are the next step in product development. In those cases where a protein has been modified, preliminary feeding trials are more difficult and can be done only if sufficient quantities of the engineered protein can be produced in microorganisms or other suitable expression systems. Again, feeding trials comparing meals from transgenic seed with the normal seed will be the definitive test of product usefulness.

Although the meals from transgenic seeds are intended for use as livestock feeds, safety of the transgenic plant to the farm animal is not the only concern. In many cases the seed meal is only a part of the equation. Oils extracted from transgenic soybean, corn, and other oilseeds may be used for human consumption. New proteins that are accumulated in the transgenic plants must be shown not to have harmful effects on humans. Of particular concern are proteins that might have allergenic properties since even small amounts of these proteins remaining as minor contaminants could induce strong reactions in sensitive individuals. The potential allergenicity of seed proteins from transgenic plants should be evaluated, especially those containing genes obtained from plants known to cause allergic responses such as wheat, legumes and nuts. The case of engineered proteins presents even greater challenges in that there is no *a priori* way to predict whether a protein that has been modified, in some cases, extensively, will have toxic, allergenic or antinutritional effects. This type of information is assessed best once the transgenic plant containing the modified protein is in hand.

Marketing issues

Currently, crops such as soybean and corn are commodities sold by quantity and not by seed properties. If plant varieties with nutritionally enhanced seeds are to be marketed, it will be necessary to distinguish the improved seeds from those that do not have this characteristic. This means that the new seeds will need to be segregated by farmers, elevator operators, seed processors, and feed formulators to preserve their identity. There has been some speculation that the added cost of segregating specialty seeds with improved amino acid contents might be prohibitive (Kidd, 1993). However, it should be noted that improved protein profiles are likely to be only one part of the specialty crop of the future. New soybean varieties are likely to emerge that produce specialty oils in addition to specialty proteins and new corn varieties may contain altered starches as well as altered proteins.

MODIFICATION OF OTHER FEED CROPS

Other grains and oilseeds such as barley, canola and sunflower are widely used in place of corn or soybean in feed formulations. Barley, like corn, is deficient in lysine. While canola and sunflower seed proteins have reasonably balanced amino acid compositions in terms of human nutritional requirements, the value of these seed meals for animal feed formulations would be increased by increasing the levels of lysine or methionine. Transformation of barley (Wan and Lemaux, 1993), canola (Radke *et al.*, 1988) and sunflower (Bidney et al., 1992) has been accomplished and transgenic canola seeds with elevated methionine contents discussed previously.

Although not addressed specifically in this chapter, forage crops have also been the target of genetic engineering efforts. Wool growth in sheep is limited by the availability of sulfur-containing amino acids. To increase these amino acids in a forage crop, Schroeder *et al.* (1991) expressed an ovalbumin gene from chicken in the leaves of lucerne. Ovalbumin was selected for this work because the protein is rumen resistant and has a balanced amino acid profile containing about 6.5% sulfur amino acids. The 2S methionine-rich albumin from sunflower has also been shown to be resistant to degradation by rumen bacteria and would be a good candidate protein for the improvement of forage crops (Spencer *et al.*, 1988). Different factors must be taken into consideration in order to achieve the accumulation of proteins in leaves and regulatory regions that lead to constitutive or leaf-specific expression must be used in the construction of chimeric genes. In initial gene transfer experiments expressing a chimeric ovalbumin gene in lucerne, ovalbumin represented only 0.005% of the total soluble leaf protein. These levels were far too low to have an effect on the amino acid content of the leaves.

Another approach for improving amino acid composition reported by Yang *et. al.* (1989) involved synthesizing a DNA sequence that would encode a protein composed of 80% essential amino acids. The synthetic gene was transferred to potato where the protein was detected at low levels (0.02 - 0.35% of the total tuber protein). This approach compounds problems inherent in engineering seed proteins. Parameters necessary for the stable accumulation of the protein in the target tissue must be addressed as well as potential negative effects on both the plant and the animal consumer.

CONCLUSIONS

The technology is available for improving the protein quality of crop plants of importance to the animal feed industry. Preliminary successes of a number of molecular approaches suggest that the technology should work either alone or in combination to produce plants with improved nutritional quality. In particular, there has been significant progress in increasing the methionine content of seed proteins. This work has been possible largely because of the availability of a number of naturally-occurring genes encoding methionine-rich seed storage proteins. The availability of regulatory regions from numerous genes from dicotyledonous plants and the ability to examine the expression of genes in transgenic systems over the past ten years have facilitated these efforts. The methionine content of soybean seeds has been increased appreciably by the expression of a gene encoding the methionine-rich Brazil nut albumin. However, in order to achieve the levels of methionine necessary to eliminate the need for supplementation of feeds, it may also be necessary to increase the expression of the 10.8 kDa methionine-rich soybean protein or to alter the free methionine pools in soybean if these prove to be limiting.

Protein engineering approaches are likely to be important in addressing the problem of lysine deficiencies of cereals. Critical to the success of this approach is the ability to delineate regions of seed proteins that will tolerate modifications without affecting the processing, targeting or assembly of the proteins. While attempts at engineering the 11S, 7S and 2S seed proteins from dicotyledonous plants have centered on increasing methionine content, these proteins might also be considered for engineering increased lysine since many of these proteins contain higher levels of lysine than are found in seed proteins of monocotyledonous plants. However, if such an approach is pursued, it will be important to evaluate the potential for proteins from dicotyledonous seeds to be transported, assembled and packaged in monocot seeds. In addition, it will be important to identify regulatory regions that will facilitate high gene expression of seed-specific in monocotyledonous plants such as corn. As in the case of methionine enhancement, such an approach might be complemented by a molecular approach for altering the pools of free lysine in the seed.

The ability to insert genes into economically important crop plants opens the door for molecular approaches aimed at overcoming amino acid deficiencies of plant seed proteins. While there is a need for more work that addresses the factors that regulate the expression of seed storage protein genes and the accumulation of different protein species in transgenic plants, it is likely that problems of inadequate levels of certain amino acids in seed proteins will be solved in the coming years using a combination of the approaches described in this chapter.

REFERENCES

Altenbach, S.B., Pearson, K.W., Meeker, G., Staraci, L.C. and Sun, S.S.M. 1989. Enhancement of the methionine content of seed proteins by the expression of a chimeric gene encoding a methionine-rich protein in transgenic plants. *Plant Mol. Biol.* **13**, 513-522.

Altenbach, S.B., Kuo, C-C., Staraci, L.C., Pearson, K.W., Wainwright, C., Georgescu, A. and Townsend, J. 1992. Accumulation of a Brazil nut albumin in seeds of transgenic canola results in enhanced levels of seed protein methionine. *Plant Mol. Biol.* **18**, 235-245.

Altenbach, S.B., Pearson, K.W., Leung, F.W. and Sun, S.S.M. 1987. Cloning and sequence analysis of a cDNA encoding a Brazil nut protein exceptionally rich in methionine. *Plant Mol. Biol.* **8**, 239-250.

Ampe, C., Van Damme, J., de Castro, L., Sampaio, M.J., Van Montagu, M. and Vandekerckhove, J. 1986. The amino acid sequence of the 2S sulphur-rich proteins from seeds of Brazil nut (*Bertholletia excelsa* H.B.K.). *Eur. J. Biochem.* **159**, 597-604.

Antunes, A.J. and Markakis, P. 1977. Protein supplementation of navy beans with brazil nuts. *J. Agric. Food Chem.* **25**, 1096-1098.

Argos, P., Narayana, S.V.L. and Nielsen, N.C. 1985. Structural similarity between legumin and vicilin storage proteins for legumes. *EMBO J.* **4**, 1111-1117.

Bidney, D.L., Seelonge, C.J. and Malone-Schaneberg, J.B. 1992. Transformed progeny can be recovered from chimeric plants regenerated from *Agrobacterium tumefaciens*-treated embryonic axes of sunflower. Proc. of the 13th International Sunflower Conference, Vol. 2, 1408-1412.

Bright, S.J.W., Miflin, B.J. and Rognes, S.E. 1982. Threonine accumulation in the seeds of a barley mutant with an altered aspartate kinase. *Biochem. Genet.* **20**, 229-243.

Bryan, J.K. 1990. Advances in the biochemistry of amino acid biosynthesis. In *The Biochemistry of Plants,* Vol. 16 (B.J. Miflin, ed.) pp. 161-195. Academic Press, New York, US.

Bryan, J.K. 1980. Synthesis of the aspartate family and branched-chain amino acids. In *The Biochemistry of Plants*, Vol. 5 (B.J. Miflin, ed.) pp. 403-452. Academic Press, New York, US.

Cattoir-Reynearts, A., Degryse, E., Verbruggen, I. and Jacobs, M. 1983. Selection and characterization of carrot embryoid cultures resistant to inhibition by lysine plus threonine. *Biochem. Physiol. Pflanzen.* **178**, 81-90.

De Clercq, A., Vandewiele, M., Van Damme, J., Guerche, P., Van Montagu, M., Vandekerckhove, J. and Krebbers, E. 1990. Stable accumulation of modified 2S albumin seed storage proteins with higher methionine content in trasgenic plants. *Plant Physiol.* **94**, 970-979.

De Castro, L.A.B., Lacerada, Z., Aramayo, R.A., Sampaio, M.J.A.M. and Gander, E.S. 1987. Evidence for a precursor molecule of Brazil nut 2S seed proteins from biosynthesis and cDNA analysis. *Mol. Gen. Genet.* **206**, 338-343.

Dickinson, C.D., Scott, M.P., Hussein, E.H.A., Argos, P. and Nielsen, N.C. 1990. Effect of structural modifications on the assembly of a glycinin subunit. *Plant Cell* **2**, 403-413.

Diedrick, T.J., Frisch R.A. and Gegenbach, B.G. 1990. Tissue culture isolation of a second mutant locus for increased threonine accumulation in maize. *Theor. Appl. Genet.* **79**, 209-215.

Ericson, M.L., Rodin, J., Lenman, M., Glimelius, K., Josefsson, L. and Rak, L. 1986. Structure of the rapeseed 1.7S storage protein, napin, and its precursor. *J. Biol. Chem.* **261**, 14576-14581.

Finer, J.J. and McMullen, M.D. 1991. Transformation of soybean via particle bombardment of embryogenic suspension culture tissue. *In Vitro Cell Dev. Biol.* **27**, 175-182.

Frankard, V., Ghislain, M., Negrutiu I. and Jacobs, M. 1991. High threonine producer mutant in *Nicotiana sylvestris* (Speg. and Comes). *Theor. Appl. Genet.* **82**, 273-282.

Galau, G.A., Wang, H. Y.-C. and Hughes, D.W. 1992. Cotton *Mat5*-A (C164) gene and *Mat5*-D cDNAs encoding methionine-rich 2S albumin storage proteins. *Plant Physiol.* **99**, 779-782.

Gayler, K.R. and Sykes, G.E. 1985. Effects of nutritional stress on the storage proteins of soybeans. *Plant Physiol.* **78**, 582-585.

George A.A. and de Lumen, B.O. 1991. A novel methionine-rich protein in soybean seed: identification, amino acid composition, and N-terminal sequence. *J. Agric. Food Chem.* **39**, 224-227.

Gordon-Kamm, W.J., Spencer, T.M., Manguno, M.L., Adams, T.R., Davies, R.J., Start, W.G., O'Brien, J.V., Chambers, S.A., Adams Jr., W.R., Willetts, N.G., Rice, T.B., Mackey, C.J., Krueger, R.W., Kausch, A.P. and Lemaux, P.G. 1990. Transformation of maize cells and regeneration of fertile transgenic plants. *Plant Cell* **2**, 603-618.

Green, C.E. and Phillips, R.L. 1974. Potential selection system for mutants with increased lysine, threonine and methionine in cereal crops. *Crop Sci.* **14**, 827-830.

Guerche, P., De Almeida, E.R.P., Schwarztein, M.A., Gander, E., Krebbers, E. and Pelletier, G. 1990. Expression of the 2S albumin from *Bertholletia excelsa* in *Brassica napus*. *Mol. Gen. Genet.* **221**, 306-314.

Harada, J.J., Barker, S.J. and Goldberg, R.B. 1989. Soybean β-conglycinin genes are clustered in several DNA regions and are regulated by transcriptional and posttranscriptional processes. *Plant Cell* **1**, 415-425.

Hibberd, K.A. and Green, C.E. 1982. Inheritance and expression of lysine plus threonine resistance selected in maize tissue culture. *Proc. Nat. Acad. Sci. USA* **79**, 559-563.

Higgins, T.J.V. 1984. Synthesis and regulation of major proteins in seeds. *Annu. Rev. Plant Physiol.* **15**, 191-221.

Hinchee, M.A.W., Conner-Ward, D.V., Newell, C.A., McDonnell, R.E., Sato, S.J., Gasser, S., Fischhoff, D.A., Re, D.B., Fraley, R.T., and Horsch, R.B. 1988. Production of transgenic soybean plants using *Agrobacterium*-mediated DNA transfer. *Bio/Technology* **6**, 915-922.

Hoffman, L.M., Donaldson, D.D., Bookland, R., Rashka, K. and Herman, E.M. 1987. Synthesis and protein body deposition of maize 15-kd zein in transgenic tobacco seeds. *EMBO J.* **6**, 3213-3221.

Hoffman, L.M., Donaldson, D.D. and Herman, E.M.   1988.   A modified storage protein is synthesized, processed, and degraded in the seeds of transgenic plants. *Plant Mol. Biol.* **11**, 717-729.

Hong, B., Uknes, S.J. and Ho, T-H.D.   1988. Cloning and characterization of a cDNA encoding a mRNA rapidly-induced by ABA in barley aleurone layers. *Plant Mol. Biol.* **11**, 495-506.

Karchi, H., Shaul, O. and Galili, G.   1993.   Seed-specific expression of a bacterial desensified aspartate kinase increases the production of seed threonine and methionine in transgenic tobacco. *The Plant Journal* **3**, 721-727.

Kidd, G.   1993.   Improved animal feed may be just "chicken feed". *Bio/Technology* **11**, 552.

Kirihara, J.A., Hunsperger, J.P., Mahoney, W.C., Messing, J.W.   1988.   Differential expression of a gene for a methionine-rich storage protein in maize. *Mol. Gen. Genet.* **211**, 359- 370.

Kurkela, S. and Franck, M.   1990.   Cloning and characterization of a cold- and ABA-inducible *Arabidopsis* gene. *Plant Mol. Biol.* **15**, 137-144.

Kortt, A.A., Caldwell, J.B., Lilley, G.G., Higgins, T.J.V.   1991.   Amino acid and cDNA sequences of a methionine-rich 2S protein from sunflower seed (*Helianthus anus* L.). *Eur. J. Biochem.* **195**, 329-334.

Krebbers, E., Herdies, L., De Clercq, A., Seurinck, J., Leemans, J., Van Damme, J., Segura, M., Gheysen, G., Van Montagu, M. and Vandekerckhove, J.   1988.   Determination of the processing sites of an *Arabidopsis* 2S albumin and characterization of the complete gene family. *Plant Physiol.* **87**, 859-866.

Lawrence, M.C., Suzuki, E., Varghese, J.N., Davis, P.C., Van Donkelaar, A., Tulloch, P.A. and Colman, P.M.   1990.   The three-dimensional structure of the seed storage protein phaseolin at 3Å resolution. *EMBO J.* **9**, 9-15.

Leite, A., Yunes, J.A., Turcinelli, S.R. and Arruda, P.   1991.   Cloning and characterization of a cDNA encoding a sulfur-rich coixin. *Plant Mol. Biol.* **18**, 171-174.

Lelievre, J-M., C.D. Dickinson and Dickinson, L.A., Nielsen, N.C.   1992.   Synthesis and assembly of soybean ß-conglycinin *in vitro*. *Plant Mol. Biol.* **18**, 259-274.

Lilley, G.G., Caldwell, J.B., Kortt, A.A., Higgins, T.J. and Spencer, D.   1989.   Isolation and primary structure for a novel methionine-rich protein from sunflower seeds (*Helianthus annus* L.).   In *Proceedings of the World Congress on Vegetable Protein Utilization in Human Foods and Animal Feedstuffs* (T.H. Applewhite, ed.) pp. 487-502.   American Oil Chemists Society, Champaign, IL, US.

Liu, C.-N. and Rubenstein, I.   1992.   Genomic organization of an alpha-zein gene cluster in maize. *Mol. Gen. Genet.* **231**, 304-312.

Matthews, B.F., Farrar, M.J. and Gray, A.C.   1989.   Purification and interconversion of homoserine dehydrogenase from *Daucus carota* cell suspension cultures. *Plant Physiol.* **91**, 1569-1574.

McCabe, D.E., Swain, W.F., Martinell, B.J. and Christou, P.   1988.   Stable transformation of soybean (*Glycine max*) by particle acceleration. *Bio/Technology* **6**, 923-926.

Negrutiu, I., Cattoir-Reynearts, A., Verbruggen, I. and Jacobs, M.   1984.   Lysine overproducer mutants with an altered dihydropicolinate synthase from protoplast culture of *Nicotiana sylvestris* (Spegazzini and Comes). *Theor. Appl. Genet.* **68**, 11-20.

Neven, L.G., Haskell, D.W., Hofig, A., Li, Q-B. and Guy, C.L.   1993.   Characterization of a spinach gene responsive to low temperature and water stress. *Plant Mol. Biol.* **21**, 291-305.

Nielsen, N.C., Dickinson, C.D., Cho, T.-J., Thanh, V.H., Scallon, B.J., Fischer, R.L., Sims, T.L., Drews, G.N. and Goldberg, R.B.   1989.   Characterization of the glycinin gene family in soybean. *Plant Cell* **1**, 313-328.

Ohtani, T., Galili, G., Wallace, J.C., Thompson, G.A. and Larkins, B.A.   1991.   Normal and lysine-containing zeins are unstable in transgenic tobacco seeds. *Plant Mol. Biol.* **16**, 117-128.

Osborne, T.B.   1924.   *The Vegetable Proteins*, 2nd ed., Longmans, London, UK.

Pedersen, K., Argos, P., Naravana, S.V.L. and Larkins, B.   1986.   Sequence analysis and characterization of a maize gene encoding a high sulfur zein protein of M_r 15,000. *J. Biol. Chem.* **261**, 6279-6284.

Radke, S.E., Andrews, B.M., Moloney, M.M., Crouch, M.L., Kridl, J.C. and Knauf, V.C. 1988. Transformation of *Brassica napus* L. using *Agrobacterium tumefaciens*: developmentally regulated expression of a reintroduced napin gene. *Theor. Appl. Genet.* **75**, 685-694.

Schroeder, H.E., Khan, M.R.I., Knibb, W.R., Spencer, D. and Higgins, T.J.V. 1991. Expression of a chicken ovalbumin gene in three lucerne cultivars. *Aust. J. Plant Physiol.* **18**, 495-505.

Scott, M.P., Lago, W.J.P., Nieslen, N.C. 1991. Molecular genetic control of protein composition and quality in soybean. In *Designing Value-added Soybeans for Markets of the Future* (R.F. Wilson, ed.) pp. 91-101. American Oil Chemists Society, Champaign, IL, US.

Shaul, O. and Galili, G. 1992a. Threonine overproduction in transgenic tobacco plants expressing a mutant desensitized aspartate kinase of *Escherichia coli*. *Plant Physiol.* **100**, 1157-1163.

Shaul, O and Galili, G. 1992b. Increased lysine synthesis in tobacco plants that express high levels of bacterial dihydrodipicolinate synthase in their chloroplasts. *Plant Journal* **2**, 203-209.

Spencer, D., Higgins, T.J.V., Freer, M., Dove, H. and Coombe, J. 1988. Monitoring the fate of dietary proteins in rumen fluid using gel electrophoresis. *Br. J. Nutr.* **60**, 241-247.

Sun, S.S.M., Altenbach, S.B. and Leung, F.W. 1987. Properties, biosynthesis and processing of a sulfur-rich protein in Brazil nut (*Bertholletia excelsa* H.B.K.). *Eur. J. Biochem.* **162**, 477-483.

Tao, S-H., Fox, M.R.S. Fry, B.E., Johnson, M.I., Lee, Y.H., Tomic, J.C. and Sun, S.M. 1987. Methionine bioavailability of a sulfur-rich protein from Brazil nuts. *Fed. Proc.* **46**, 891.

Townsend, J.A., Thomas, L.A., Kulisek, E.S., Daywalt, M.J., Winter, K.R.K. and Altenbach, S.B. 1992a. Improving the quality of seed proteins in soybean. In *Proc. 4th Biennial Conf. on Mol. and Cellular Biol. of the Soybean*. p.4, Iowa State University, Ames Iowa, US.

Townsend, J.A., Thomas, L.A., Kulisek, E.S., Daywalt, M.J., Winter, K.R.K., Grace, D.J., Crook, W.J., Schmidt, J.J., Corbin, T.C. and Altenbach, S.B. 1992b. Accumulation of a methionine-rich Brazil nut protein in seeds of transgenic soybean. *Agron. Abstr.*, **1**, 198.

Utsumi, S. 1992. Plant food protein engineering. *Adv. Food Nutr. Res.* **36**, 89-208.

Vandekerckhove, J., Van Damme, J., Van Lijsebettens, J., Botterman, J., De Block, M., Vandewiele, M., De Clercq, A., Leemans, J., Van Montagu, M. and Krebbers, E. 1989. Enkephalins produced in transgenic plants using modified 2S seed storage proteins. *Bio/Technology* **7**, 929-932.

Wallace, J.C., Galili, G., Kawata, E.E., Cuellar, R.E., Shotwell, M.A. and Larkins, B.A. 1988. Aggregation of lysine-containing zeins into protein bodies in *Xenopus* oocytes. *Science* **240**, 662-664.

Wan, Y. and Lemaux, P.G. 1993. Generation of large numbers of independently transformed, fertile barley plants. Plant Physiol. **104**, 37-48.

Williamson, M.S., Forde, J., Buxton, B. and Kreis, M. 1987. Nucleotide sequence of barley chymotrypsin inhibitor-2 (CI-2) and its expression in normal and high-lysine barley. *Eur. J. Biochem.* **165**, 99-106.

Wilson, B.J., Gray, A.C. and Matthews, B.F. 1991. Bifunctional protein in carrot contains both aspartokinase and homoserine dehydrogenase activities. *Plant Physiol.* **97**, 1323-1328.

Yamagata, H., Tamura, K., Tanaka, K., Kasai, Z. 1986. Cell-free synthesis of rice prolamin. *Plant Cell Physiol.* **27**, 1419-1422.

Yang, M.S., Espinoza, N.O., Nagpala, P.G. and Dodds, J.H., White, F.F., Schnorr, K.L., Jaynes, J.M. 1989. Expression of a synthetic gene for improved protein quality in transformed potato plants. *Plant Sci.* **64**, 99-111.

Zambryski, P., Joos, H., Genetello, C., Leemans, J., Von Montagu, M. and Schell, J. 1983. Ti plasmid vector for the introduction of DNA into plant cells without alteration of their normal regeneration capacity. *EMBO J.* **2**, 2143-2150.

6   Industrial amino acids in nonruminant animal nutrition

Daniel Bercovici[1] and Malcolm F. Fuller[2]

[1]*Eurolysine, Siège Social, 16 rue Ballu, 75009 Paris, France*
[2]*Rowett Research Institute, Buckburn, Aberdeen AB2 9SB, UK*

AMINO ACIDS

Amino acids are the building blocks of all the proteins found in nature, both plant and animal. About twenty amino acids are commonly found in natural proteins. The first to be discovered was glycine, which Braconnot isolated in 1820 from gelatin. The last was threonine, which Meyer and Rose isolated in 1936.

Chemical classification of amino acids

All α-amino acids consist of a carbon atom (the α-carbon or carbon-2) bonded to an amino (NH_2) group, a carboxyl (COOH) group, a hydrogen atom and a side chain (designated R) which is unique to that amino acid, as shown below.

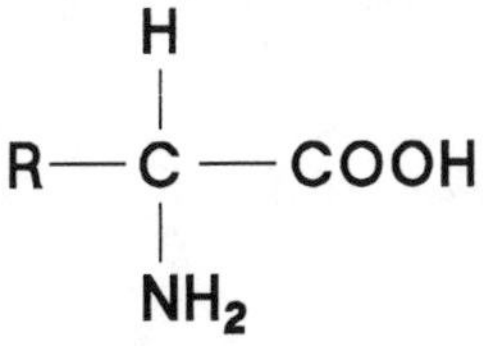

$$R - \underset{\underset{NH_2}{|}}{\overset{\overset{H}{|}}{C}} - COOH$$

Amino acids can be classified according to the chemical structure of the side chain (Table 1), which determines the physico-chemical characteristics of the amino acid.

Stereospecificity. All amino acids, except glycine, have optical activity due to the presence of at least one asymmetric carbon, which carries four different groups. Based on their stereospecificity amino acids are chemically defined as D- or L- isomers.

Although D-amino acids exist in nature (both free, in a number of plants and in complexes such as certain bacterial cell wall mucopolysaccharides, for instance), those found in most natural proteins are exclusively of the L-form. Most of the enzymes involved in the pathways of amino acid metabolism in living organisms selectively recognise the L-form. Amino acids obtained by chemical synthesis are racemic mixtures of the D- and L-enantiomorphs. However, the D-isomers of several amino acids can be utilised after conversion by an amino acid oxidase to the symmetrical oxo- form, followed by transamination. The bioavailability of the D-amino acids varies greatly from species to species and from one amino acid to another, depending on the efficiency of these conversions (Table 2).

Table 1.   Classification of amino acids and the structural formulae of their R-groups.

Classification	Amino acid	R-group
Aliphatic amino acids		
Neutral amino acids	Glycine (Gly)	H–
	Alanine (Ala)	CH_3-
Branched-chain amino acids	Valine (Val)	$(CH_3)_2-CH-$
	Leucine (Leu)	$(CH_3)_2-CH-CH_2-$
	Isoleucine (Ile)	$(CH_3)(C_2H_5)-CH-CH_2-$
Hydroxy amino acids	Serine (Ser)	$HO-CH_2-$
	Threonine (Thr)	$CH_3-CH.OH-$
Sulphur amino acids	Cysteine (Cys)	$HS-CH_2-$
	Methionine (Met)	$CH_3-S-(CH_2)_2-$
Acidic amino acids	Aspartic Acid (Asp)	$HOOC-CH_2-$
	Glutamic Acid (Glu)	$HOOC-(CH_2)_2-$
Amides	Asparagine (Asn)	$NH_2-CO-CH_2-$
	Glutamine (Gln)	$NH_2-CO-(CH_2)_2-$
Basic amino acids	Lysine (Lys)	$H_2N-(CH_2)_4-$
	Arginine (Arg)	$H_2N-C(=NH)-NH-(CH_2)_3-$
Aromatic amino acids		
Neutral amino acids	Phenylalanine (Phe)	
	Tyrosine (Tyr)	
Heterocyclic amino acids		
Neutral amino acids	Proline (Pro)*	
	Hydroxyproline (Hyp)*	
	Tryptophan (Trp)	
Basic amino acids	Histidine (His)	

* This is the complete amino acid, not just the R-group

Table 2. Relative bioavailability of amino acid isomers, analogues and precursors. Values are expressed as growth efficacy percentages (molar basis) of the L-isomer, which is assumed in all cases to represent 100% bioavailability.

Amino acid	Chick	Dog	Human	Pig
Lysine				
L-Lysine	100	–	–	100
D-Lysine	0	–	0	–
Threonine				
L-Threonine (2*S*, 3*S*)	100	–	–	100
D-Threonine (2*R*, 3*R*)	0	–	0	–
Tryptophan				
L-Tryptophan	100	–	–	100
D-Tryptophan	20	35	0	80
Methionine				
L-Methionine	100	–	–	100
D-Methionine	90	100	30	100
DL-Methionine	95	100	65	100
DL-OH-Methionine	80	–	–	100
Oxo-Methionine	90	–	–	–
L-Homocysteine	65	–	–	–
D-Homocysteine	7	–	–	–
Cyst(e)ine				
L-Cysteine	100	–	–	100
L-Cystine	100	–	–	100
D-Cystine	0	0	–	–
DL-Lanthionine	35	–	–	–
L-Homocysteine	100	–	–	–
D-Homocysteine	70	–	–	–
L-Methionine	100	–	–	100
Arginine				
L-Arginine	100	–	–	100
D-Arginine	0	–	–	–
L-Ornithine	0	0	–	0
L-Citrulline	90	90	–	90
Histidine				
L-Histidine	100	–	–	100
D-Histidine	10	–	–	–
Carnosine	100	–	–	–
Anserine	0	–	–	–
Balenine (ophidine)	0	–	–	–
Leucine				
L-Leucine	100	–	–	100
D-Leucine	100	–	–	–
Oxo-leucine	100	–	–	–
L-OH-leucine	100	–	–	–
D-OH-leucine	100	–	–	–

Table 2   *continued*

Amino acid	Chick	Dog	Human	Pig
Valine				
L-Valine	100	–	–	100
D-Valine	70	–	–	–
Oxo-valine	80	–	–	–
L-OH-valine	80	–	–	–
D-OH-valine	70	–	–	–
Isoleucine				
L-Isoleucine (2S, 3S)	100	–	–	100
D-Isoleucine (2R, 3R)	0	–	–	–
L-Alloisoleucine (2S, 3R)	0	–	–	–
D-Alloisoleucine (2R, 3S)	60	–	–	–
L-Oxo-isoleucine (3S)	85	–	–	–
D-Oxo-leucine (3R)	0	–	–	–
L-OH-isoleucine (2S, 3S)	85	–	–	–
D-OH-isoleucine (2R, 3R)	0	–	–	–
Phenylalanine				
L-Phenylalanine	100	–	–	100
D-Phenylalanine	75	–	–	–
Oxo-phenylalanine	85	–	–	–
L-OH-phenylalanine	70	–	–	–
D-OH-phenylalanine	0	–	–	–
Tyrosine				
L-Tyrosine	100	–	–	100
D-Tyrosine	100	–	–	100
L-Phenylalanine	100	–	–	100

From the data of Baker (1994).

Protein structure.   Proteins consist of a sequence of amino acids linked together through a peptide bond between the amino group of one and the carboxylic group of the next, as shown below.

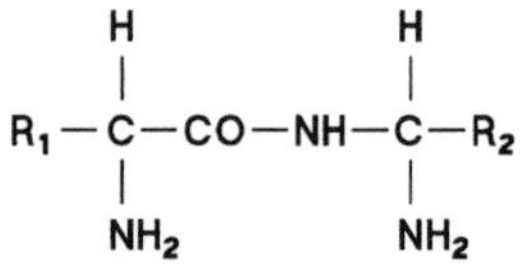

$$R_1 - \overset{\overset{\displaystyle H}{|}}{\underset{\underset{\displaystyle NH_2}{|}}{C}} - CO - NH - \overset{\overset{\displaystyle H}{|}}{\underset{\underset{\displaystyle NH_2}{|}}{C}} - R_2$$

Short chains of amino acids linked by these bonds are called peptides or oligopeptides.

Nutritional classification of amino acids

Amino acids are used for a great variety of functions in the body. These include their use as precursors for hormones, neurotransmitters, pigments and a variety of small molecules. However, by far the most important use, quantitatively, is for the synthesis of proteins. Proteins form the main structural and functional components of the animal body and the continuous provision of an adequate supply of all the twenty or so amino acids to the cells of the body is essential for their function. Protein synthesis requires the simultaneous presence of all constituent amino acids: the absence of any one restricts protein synthesis.

Some of these amino acids can be synthesised, by some or all of the cells of the body, from simpler constituents. These are the non-essential or dispensable amino acids. However, whereas plants and bacteria can synthesise the whole range of amino acids needed for protein synthesis, higher animals have lost the ability to synthesise certain of them and these must therefore be supplied preformed. These are the essential or indispensable amino acids. (The terms 'dispensable' and 'indispensable' are preferred because **all** the amino acids are essential for cellular function.)

Ruminant animals derive a large proportion of the amino acids they require by the digestion of microbial protein synthesised in the rumen. In contrast, the uptake of microbial amino acids in nonruminants, though not negligible, is of minor significance. However, as far as the requirements of the tissues are concerned, ruminants and nonruminant species behave in a similar way.

Essential amino acids. Amongst the twenty common amino acids found in proteins, nine are considered as absolutely indispensable in all higher animals. These are lysine, threonine, methionine, tryptophan, leucine, isoleucine, valine, histidine and phenylalanine. Certain other amino acids, although the pathways for their synthesis are present, may be synthesised at too low a rate to meet the animal's requirement. These amino acids then **behave** as indispensable amino acids. Some nutritionists prefer to consider these as indispensable amino acids **for that particular circumstance**. Thus, in mammals, but not in birds, arginine **can** be synthesised, but the rate of its synthesis may be too low to meet all the animal's requirements so that some must be provided in the diet if the animal is to grow (or otherwise produce protein) at its maximum rate. Glycine, proline and glutamine may also be incompletely dispensable in particular circumstances such as in very young birds and mammals.

Strictly speaking, lysine and threonine are the only two **amino acids** which are indispensable because all the others can be produced by transamination of the corresponding α-oxo acids; however, since these α-oxo acids cannot be synthesised, one or the other must be supplied in the diet.

NUTRITIONAL UTILISATION OF PROTEIN AND AMINO ACIDS: PHYSIOLOGICAL AND BIOCHEMICAL ASPECTS

Protein digestion

Individual free amino acids are released from the protein structure by chemical or enzymatic treatment. Digestion of food proteins is a complex process which involves four different steps:
1. mechanical breakdown of feeds
2. chemical action of hydrochloric acid in the stomach
3. enzymatic cleavage of complex molecules
4. microbial fermentation.

Proteolytic enzymes are active all along the digestive tract. Briefly, the processes involved in protein digestion can be described as follows. In the stomach, in the presence of HCl, gastric pepsins, with pH optima at 2.0 and 3.5, cleave intact proteins into long oligopeptides. On passing into the duodenum, pancreatic enzymes (trypsin, chymotrypsin, carboxypeptidases and elastase, which are secreted by the exocrine pancreas, selectively hydrolyse peptide bonds. Finally, intestinal peptidases cleave small peptides to yield a mixture of free amino acids, di-, and tri-peptides. These are transported from the lumen through the intestinal cell wall where other peptidases cleave the di- and tri-peptides to free amino acids which are transported into the blood stream. More complete descriptions of digestion in pigs and poultry may be found in Moran (1982), Low and Zebrowska (1989a,b) and Longland (1991). Some protein escapes digestion by this array of proteolytic activities either because it is inherently resistant to proteolysis or because it is enclosed within structures, especially plant cell walls, that are resistant to the host enzymes. Protein which thus escapes digestion may then be attacked by microbial enzymes. Because most of the microbial activity is concentrated in the large intestine, beyond the main sites of amino acid absorption, there is little or no nutritional benefit to be derived from this activity, the major end products of which are ammonia, which is absorbed, and microbial protein, which is passed in the faeces. In view of the difference between host enzymic digestion (mainly in the stomach and small intestine), yielding amino acids, and microbial fermentation (mainly in the large intestine), amino acid absorption is best assessed as the difference between the amino acids (both in protein and in the free form) in the diet and those which leave the ileum and enter the large intestine. Such measurements are commonly made by the collection of ileal digesta, either via a cannula or after slaughter. Measurements made in this way show no increase in ileal amino acid flow when diets are supplemented with free amino acids, indicating that these are fully absorbed, at least in the amounts used.

The extent of digestion of feed protein is influenced by several factors which can be grouped under three main headings:

- intrinsic protein digestibility of the raw material
  (protein structure, protection by plant cell structures, etc.)
- presence of antinutritional factors
- processing (especially with heating).

Because only amino acids that have been absorbed from the gastrointestinal tract can be used in metabolism, digestibility is an important attribute of feeds. Furthermore, because the free amino acids which are used to supplement diets are fully absorbable, the appropriate amount of an amino acid to be added can only be calculated accurately on the basis of the digestible amino acids in the feeds.

Amino acid metabolism

Amino acids are utilised for a great variety of functions in the body but one predominates over all others: that is protein synthesis. Even in an adult animal which is not growing or producing, protein is synthesised continuously but equally is being continuously broken down. This process of protein turnover continues throughout life: during growth the rate of whole-body protein synthesis exceeds the rate of breakdown and there is body protein accretion but as maturity is approached the difference between the rates disappears and the normally fed adult is, with minor fluctuations, in protein equilibrium. In this state the requirement for amino acids is to replace those lost through various routes, both by excretion and in metabolism. The need to replace these obligatory losses constitutes the maintenance requirements. In addition to these, any productive process creates an increased requirement for amino acids: this need is closely related to the amount and composition of the products formed, which may be body tissues in growing or gestating animals, milk proteins in the case of lactation or egg protein in the case of the laying hen. The animal's total amino acid requirements are the sum of those needed for maintenance and those needed for production.

Amino acid imbalance. The excesses of certain amino acids may lead to reduced utilisation of the limiting amino acid and thence of the diet as a whole. These amino acid imbalances are of particular importance in cases of amino acids which share common enzyme or transport system in their metabolism and which therefore compete. The most important cases are the interactions amongst the branched-chain amino acids and that between lysine and arginine. Because all three branched chain amino acids are oxidised via one enzyme complex (the branched-chain oxo-acid dehydrogenase complex) and control the activity of the enzyme, a dietary excess of one (especially leucine) increases the oxidation of the others. The antagonism between lysine and arginine is especially important in poultry, for which arginine is indispensable. In pigs, it appears to be of significance only in the neonate. These effects are reviewed by D'Mello (1994a). The primary response of animals to dietary amino acid imbalance is a reduction in food intake and most of the growth depressing effects are consequences of that. However, excess leucine reduces the utilisation of valine and isoleucine in pigs even when food intake is equalised (Langer and Fuller, 1994).

Amino acid requirements

The amino acid requirements of any individual vary during its life according to a number of genetic and environmental factors. The requirements also vary according to the function of the animal, i.e. whether it is growing, pregnant, lactating, laying eggs, etc.

Table 3. Indicative amino acid requirements (g kg^{-1} diet) of pigs (NRC, 1988) and chickens (NRC, 1994) in various categories.

	Growing pigs (kg)			Lactating sows	Broiler (weeks)			Laying hens[1]
	10-20	20-50	50-110		0-3	3-6	6-8	
Threonine	5.6	4.8	4.0	4.3	8.0	7.4	6.8	4.3
Glycine + serine	–	–	–	–	12.5	11.4	9.7	–
Valine	–	–	–	–	9.0	8.2	7.0	6.4
Methionine + cyst(e)ine	4.8	4.1	3.4	3.6	9.0	7.2	6.0	5.3
Methionine					5.0	3.8	3.2	2.7
Isoleucine	5.3	4.6	3.8	3.9	8.0	7.3	6.2	5.9
Leucine	7.0	6.0	5.0	4.8	12.0	10.9	9.3	7.5
Phenylalanine + tyrosine	7.7	6.6	5.5	7.0	13.4	12.2	10.4	7.5
Phenylalanine					7.2	6.5	5.6	4.3
Lysine	9.5	7.5	6.0	6.0	11.0	10.0	8.5	6.3
Histidine	2.5	2.2	1.8	2.5	3.5	3.2	2.7	1.5
Arginine	4.0	2.5	1.0	4.0	12.5	11.0	10.0	6.4
Tryptophan	1.4	1.2	1.0	1.2	2.0	1.8	1.6	1.5

[1]White egg layers

A synopsis of the amino acid requirements of pigs and poultry is given in Table 3. Requirement is expressed as the minimum daily supply or dietary concentration to achieve maximal growth or optimal performance. More complete information is given in D'Mello (1994b).

Limiting amino acids. When the dietary supply of any one amino acid is not sufficient to fulfil the animal's requirement, this amino acid is said to be limiting. Amino acid limitation relates to the difference between the amino acid composition of feeds and the ability of those feeds to satisfy all the animal's requirements. The amino acid in greatest deficit in the feed **relative** to the animal's requirement is said to be first limiting, the one in the next greatest deficit second limiting and so on. Lysine, threonine, tryptophan and methionine are frequently limiting for pigs and poultry when given diets based on commonly used feeds. Cereals, for example, which represent a major fraction of animal feeds in developed countries, are poor in these essential amino acids. To meet the animal's requirements they must be supplemented either with protein concentrates such as soya bean meal and fish meal which are rich in essential amino acids or with free amino acids. The use of free industrial amino acids allows the requirements for all amino acids to be satisfied with less total protein in the diet than is possible using protein concentrates which tend to result in large surpluses of some non-limiting amino acids. An example of this is shown in Table 4. Supplementation with industrial amino acids, by providing specific complementation of the amino acid pattern of the chosen feedstuffs, allows the final diet to conform closely to the animal's requirements.

Table 4.   An example of formulation of alternative diets, based on digestible amino acids, to meet the target amino acid specification.

	Diet A		Diet B	
Wheat (g kg^{-1})	620		865	
Soya bean meal (g kg^{-1})	250		65	
Maize gluten meal (g kg^{-1})	100		40	
L-Lysine.HCl (g kg^{-1})	0		5.30	
L-Threonine (g kg^{-1})	0		2.15	
		% of requirement		% of requirement
Crude protein (N x 6.25)	255		166	
Digestible crude protein (N x 6.25)	209		137	
Digestible lysine (g kg^{-1})	8.44	100	8.44	100
Digestible threonine (g kg^{-1})	6.55	107	6.11	100
Digestible methionine + cysteine (g kg^{-1})	7.98	150	5.54	104
Digestible tryptophan (g kg^{-1})	2.79	179	1.67	107
Digestible valine (g kg^{-1})	11.62	183	6.65	105
Digestible isoleucine (g kg^{-1})	8.40	170	5.06	103

However, it is usual that, in the course of meeting the animal's requirement for the most limiting amino acid, a number of others will be present in excess. This is seen in the examples given in Table 4. Although, as described above, excesses of some amino acids may affect the utilisation of others, the most general consequence of amino acid excess is simply poorer utilisation of the protein as a whole. Because amino acids in excess of those quantities needed to balance the most limiting cannot be utilised for protein synthesis they are necessarily degraded. Figure 1 shows this schematically, using four amino acids as examples.

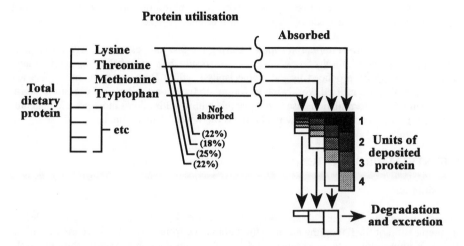

Figure 1. Schematic of amino acid utilisation for growth. Dietary amino acids are digested to varying extents; the absorbed amino acids are utilised in units of 'ideal protein' required for deposition; the excesses are degraded and excreted. Supplementation with additional lysine would allow these to be utilised. For simplicity, maintenance requirements are ignored.

Ideal protein. A pattern of amino acids which exactly conforms to the pattern of the animal's requirements is called 'ideal protein'. This can be provided by a mixture of proteins or of proteins and free amino acids. In an ideal protein all indispensable amino acids and the sum of the dispensable amino acids are equally limiting. The concept has two important applications:

- it allows the requirements for all amino acids to be expressed in terms of a single quantity
- it provides a reference pattern against which actual proteins can be evaluated.

By including digestibility (measured at the terminal ileum) the concept is refined to describe both the animal's amino acid requirements and the amino acid composition of an ideal protein in terms of the quantities actually absorbed. The use of Digestible Ideal Protein as a means of both summarising dietary amino acid provision and describing a maximally utilisable protein, greatly simplifies the expression of both.

Diets used in practice very rarely conform to the pattern of ideal protein. The expense of ensuring an exact conformity is usually greater than the benefit. Instead, rather more protein, which conforms less closely to the ideal, is given. It is the product of protein concentration and protein quality which determines the protein value of the diet. Protein quality can be evaluated numerically by comparison with the ideal pattern. This is called the 'Chemical Score', a term devised by Block and Mitchell (1946), although they originally used egg protein as their reference pattern rather than the experimentally derived pattern of ideal protein which is now available. Stated simply, the Chemical Score is the lowest of the values obtained by expressing the content of each amino acid in an actual protein as a proportion (or percentage) of what the same amount of ideal protein would contain. Thus it allows direct comparison of protein value between proteins with different limiting amino acids: indeed, such comparisons can only be made by the use of a reference pattern.

Practical applications in animal nutrition. During the last ten years, extensive research on the amino acid digestibility of raw materials has resulted in the establishment of reliable databases (e.g. those produced by the Netherlands Feeding Bureau, Heartland Lysine and Degussa), which are utilised worldwide to formulate feeds on the basis of digestible amino acids. Amino acid formulation based on digestible amino acids allows more precise matching of the amino acids supplied by raw materials to the needs of the animal.

INDUSTRIAL PRODUCTION OF AMINO ACIDS

Introduction

Amino acid production was first described at the beginning of this century (Ikeda, 1908) for the preparation of the flavouring agent sodium glutamate from seaweed. Since then the usage of monosodium glutamate as a human food ingredient has developed rapidly throughout the world. Today it is produced by fermentation technology. Industrial amino acids produced by biotechnology are identical to amino acids found in the proteins of plants and animals. Like all other living organisms, microorganisms produce L-amino acids.

During the last 20 years, usage of amino acids as ingredients in pig and poultry diets has developed worldwide. There are both economic and technical reasons for this:
- substitution of plant and animal protein sources
- optimisation of dietary amino acid supply to the animal
- reduction of dietary protein levels.

Three methods are used to produce amino acids:
- isolation from protein hydrolysates
- chemical synthesis
- fermentation technology.

Products

Four pure amino acids are available for the feed industry. Three of them, L-lysine, L-threonine and L-tryptophan, are produced through biotechnologies, by fermentation of substrates derived from crop plants, such as sugar beet molasses or corn starch hydrolysates, using specialised microorganisms. Industrial amino acids produced by micro-organisms are identical to those found in vegetables and animals, providing to the feed industry fully available nutritional supplements.

Lysine was first produced on an industrial scale in the 1960s as the animal feeding industry began to consider the importance of this amino acid in feed formulation. At this time lysine was produced by chemical synthesis but this later proved uneconomic in the face of competition from the developing biotechnological industries. L-Lysine is primarily used in animal feeds to supplement plant protein sources many of which have low concentrations of lysine. Pure industrial L-lysine is marketed essentially as a monohydrochloride salt which is a crystalline powder. Impure L-lysine products are also available (Table 5).

The production of methionine by chemical synthesis began in the 1950s. Today both methionine and its hydroxy- analogue are still produced by this method rather than by biotechnology. There are several advantages of chemical rather than biotechnological synthesis. Firstly, the complexity of the methionine biosynthetic pathway is an obstacle to obtaining methionine overproducing microorganisms. Secondly, chemical methods involve economical intermediate reagents permitting the production of DL-methionine at low cost.The third reason, probably the most important, is that animals have the ability to convert the D-isomer of methionine into the L-form, which is the only form appropriate for body protein synthesis. In pigs and poultry, the D- and L- forms of methionine are utilised almost equally well (see Table 2).

Thus methionine produced by chemical synthesis, which is a racemic mixture, has very little disadvantage from this point of view in comparison to naturally occurring methionine. Because the methionine (+ cystine) requirements of poultry are relatively higher than those of pigs, methionine usage is especially important in the poultry feed industry.

Moreover, a competitive product, DL-2-hydroxy-4-methyl-mercaptobutyric acid, which is a methionine analogue, has entered the feed market during the last ten years, and is generally produced in a liquid form. This molecule does not carry any amino function but is converted to methionine by oxidation and transamination. Industrial availability of the liquid form of methionine hydroxy- analogue is one of the factors in its commercial success.

L-Threonine and L-tryptophan are marketed as technically pure crystalline amino acids. During the 1980s large scale production of L-threonine was developed, using fermentation technology. This stimulated its usage in feeds for nonruminants, especially pigs. Production of DL-tryptophan through bioconversion has now been replaced by fermentation technology, which is more competitive. Its use in animal feeding is limited by the total amount produced.

Feed grade amino acid production is today a worldwide industrial activity. The largest production is of methionine with more than 200,000 tons annually, followed by L-lysine, L-threonine and L-tryptophan. In addition to pure amino acids, several amino acid-based products are utilised in the feed industry, as for example concentrated liquid products, methionine complexes and analogues. Utilisation of such products is regulated in Europe by the Directive 82/471, which lists the registered products (Table 5).

Production technologies

L-Lysine, L-threonine and L-tryptophan are produced by fermentation of sugars from raw materials such as beet or cane molasses and cereal starch hydrolysates by specialised microorganisms.

Biosynthesis of amino acids in microorganisms is normally regulated to meet the organism's needs, but metabolic distortions can result in the overproduction of particular amino acids.

Table 5.   Amino acid products registered for feed usage in Europe.

Product name	Composition	Species
3. AMINO ACIDS AND THEIR SALTS		
3.1.Methionine		
3.1.1. DL-Methionine, technically pure	DL-Methionine: min. 98%	All animal species
3.1.2. Dihydrated calcium salt of N-hydroxymethyl-DL-methionine, technically pure	DL-Methionine: min. 67% Formaldehyde: max 14%, Ca: min. 9%	Ruminants from the beginning of lactation
3.1.3. Methionine-zinc, technically pure	DL-Methionine: min. 80%, Zn: max 18.5%	same as 3.1.2
3.1.4. Concentrated liquid sodium DL-methionine technically pure	DL-Methionine: min. 40% Na: min. 6.2%	All animal species
3.1.5. DL-Methionine, technically pure protected with a co-polymer.	DL-Methionine: min. 65% Vinyl-pyridine/styrene copolymer: max. 3%.	Dairy cows
3.2. Lysine		
3.2.1. L-Lysine, technically pure	L-Lysine: min. 98%	All animal species
3.2.2. Concentrated liquid L-lysine (base)	L-Lysine: min. 50%	same as 3.2.1
3.2.3. L-Lysine monohydrochloride, technically pure	L-Lysine: min. 78%	same as 3.2.1
3.2.4. Concentrated liquid L-lysine monohydrochloride	L-Lysine: min. 22.4%	same as 3.2.1
3.2.5. L-Lysine sulphate produced by fermentation with *Corynebacterium glutamicum*	L-Lysine: min. 40%	same as 3.2.1
3.2.6. L-Lysine phosphate and its by-products produced by fermentation with *Brevibacterium lactofermentum* NRRLB-11470	L-Lysine: min. 35% Phosphorus: min. 4.3%	Poultry, pigs
3.2.7. Protected mixture with co-polymer of: a) L-Lysine monohydrochloride, technically pure b) DL-Methionine, technically pure	L-Lysine + DL-Methionine: min. 50% (of which DL-methionine: min. 15%) Vinyl-pyridine/styrene co-polymer: max. 3%	Dairy cows
3.3. Threonine		
3.3.1. L-Threonine, technically pure	L-Threonine: min. 98%	All animalspecies
3.4. Tryptophan		
3.4.1. L-Tryptophan, technically pure	L-Tryptophan: min. 98%	All animalspecies
3.4.2. DL-Tryptophan, technically pure	DL-Tryptophan: min. 98%	same as 3.4.1
IV. ANALOGUES OF AMINO ACIDS		
4.1 Methionine analogues		
4.1.1. DL-2-Hydroxy-4-methyl mercaptobutyric acid	Total acids: min. 85% Monomer acid: min. 65%	All animal species except ruminants
4.1.2. Calcium salt of DL-2-hydroxy-4-methyl-mercaptobutyric acid.	Monomer acid: min. 83% Calcium: min. 12%	same as 4.1.1

Adapted from European Directive 82/471/EC

Efficient L-lysine producers are found among glutamic-acid-producing auxotroph mutants of *Corynebacterium* and *Brevibacterium*. High-lysine-producing strains are also found among organisms resistant to the lysine antimetabolite S-(3-aminoethyl)-L-cysteine. In addition to the conventional mutation techniques used to obtain such strains, recombinant DNA technologies have been introduced more recently. Overproduction is obtained by increasing the number of genes which encode the key enzyme(s) for the biosynthesis of an amino acid. Recombinant DNA technologies have introduced new species of microorganisms in industrial processes, such as *Escherichia coli*. Such technologies have been developed to produce L-threonine.

Extraction of amino acids from natural materials of plant and animal origin involves protein hydrolysis followed by separation of the individual amino acids. For example, L-cystine and L-tyrosine are commonly obtained industrially by extraction. As both amino acids are poorly soluble they can be separated from a water soluble fraction after hydrolysis of a protein such as feather meal, which is rich in both amino acids.

For more information, a fully documented review has been published by Aida *et al.* (1986).

ROLE OF INDUSTRIAL AMINO ACIDS IN ANIMAL NUTRITION

Introduction

During the last 30 years, the development of industrial production of feed grade amino acids accompanied the modernisation of animal production. Intensification of pig and poultry production resulted in increased economic pressure to optimise feed conversion ratio, a key parameter of the profitability of animal production. This can be achieved by optimising the dietary supply of the limiting amino acid. Genetic improvement of animals increased their daily protein deposition, rate of egg production, etc and consequently increased their dietary amino acid requirements. Although all nutrients can be found in agricultural raw materials, the adequate supply of amino acids required by advanced animal nutrition is difficult to achieve when only vegetable and animal protein sources are available. Energy-rich sources such as cereals contain poor levels of essential amino acids. Therefore, L-lysine, L-threonine, L-methionine and L-tryptophan are the most common limiting amino acids of farm animal diets, as described above.

Incorporation of amino acids in animal feeds is motivated by several aims:
- to optimise animal production performances
- to improve protein nutrition through better amino acid balance
- to guarantee the amino acid composition of feeds
- to decrease crude protein levels
- to increase formulation flexibility
- to reduce feed cost.

Some of the most important improvements in animal nutrition are linked to the usage of industrial amino acids (Table 6).

Table 6.   Nutritional improvements related to industrial amino acid usage.

Improvement	Consequences
Diversification of raw material sources for the feed industry	Improved use of energy-rich cereal substitutes and protein sources (vegetable, animal by-products)
Increased supply of dietary amino acids	Better knowledge of requirements; improvement of animal genetics
Optimisation of feed conversion ratio	Better raw materials quality; ideal protein balance
Development of feedstuff evaluation system	Net energy system; digestible amino acids
Reduction of dietary crude protein levels	Flexibility in raw material selection Reduction of N-pollution

For references, see Gatel and Grosjean (1992), Baker *et al.* (1993), Latimier *et al.* (1993), Valaja *et al.* (1993) and Noblet *et al.* (1994).

Optimisation of animal production: use of L-threonine

The threonine requirement of growing pigs has been extensively studied during the last ten years. Analysis of published scientific information shows that optimal threonine supply to the animal is equivalent to 65-70% of dietary lysine content. Threonine requirement tends to increase according to the weight of the animal (Table 7).

Table 7.   Threonine requirement of growing pigs

Reference	Weight (kg)	Lysine (% of diet)	Threonine/Lysine (%)
Cole and Bong (1989)	10-25	1.00	67
Gatel and Fekete (1989)	10-28	1.18	69
Wang and Fuller (1989)	20	–	72
Esteve (1990)	9-15	1.15	65-68
Lenis and van Diepen (1990)	45-105	0.87	67
Schutte *et al.* (1990)	9-25	1.15	67
	9-23	1.25	71
	10-30	1.26	>65
	20-40	1.05	68
Chung and Baker (1992)	10	–	65
Sève *et al.* (1993)*	25-50	0.77	69
Average			**68**

* Expressed as digestible content

European pig feed surveys during the late 1980s showed that the optimum threonine to lysine ratio in pig feeds varied between 55 and 60%. Figure 2 shows an example of the effect of increasing the threonine:lysine ratio in piglets from 54% up to 65%. The response was a 5% body weight gain increase and almost 0.1 point reduction of food conversion ratio in piglets fed at different levels of threonine between 9 and 27 kg. The availability of industrial L-threonine allows the threonine:lysine ratio to be increased leading to better utilisation of raw materials and improved pig performance.

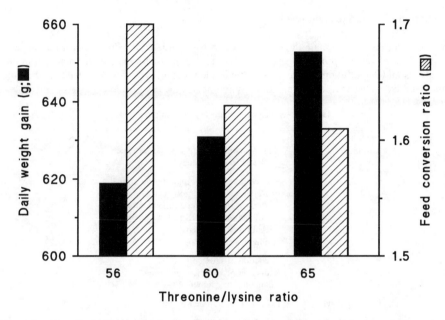

Figure 2. The effect of increasing the threonine:lysine ratio on weight gain and feed conversion ratio in piglets (9-27 kg; Schutte *et al.*, 1990).

Formulation flexibility

Formulation flexibility depends on the range of feed ingredients available for animal formulation within the framework of nutritional constraints such as determined energy content, minimum total amino acids and maximum crude protein level. Traditionally, cereal-based feeds have been supplemented with some protein-rich sources, such as soya bean meal or fish meal. Advanced nutrition research has shown that a cereal-based diet supplemented with four amino acids, L-lysine, L-threonine, L-tryptophan and DL-methionine support optimal pig growth. Industrial amino acids can replace protein-rich sources to match amino acid requirements, avoiding dietary protein excesses.

Several agricultural products have been adopted more recently by the feed industry, for example legumes (peas, beans), cereal substitution products (grain by-products, corn gluten feed, bran or manioc) and oil cakes such as rapeseed and sunflower. On the other hand, improved animal production has increased amino acid requirements of farm animals and introduced new constraints in feed formulation. For example, limitation of the inclusion of certain raw materials containing anti-nutritional factors, or an upper limit of crude protein concentration.

Development of the usage of alternative feedstuffs, together with the increasing commercial availability of industrial amino acids, offer to the feed industry a large choice of formulation solutions, combining optimal nutritional specifications and lowest feed cost.

Reduction of crude protein levels

Practical animal feeds contain large excesses of most amino acids. Protein overload is partly responsible for several problems encountered in animal productions, e.g. diarrhoea, ammonia emissions and N-pollution. Reduction of the crude protein level of animal feeds is therefore motivated by nutritional, economic and environmental factors (Table 8).

Table 8.   Advantages of dietary protein reduction.

Technical or nutritional	Improve animal production performance Better feed efficiency

	Reduce protein oversupply to the animal
	    Reduce digestive problems
	    Reduce stress from ammonia emission
	    Adaptation of feeds to hot climates
	    Antibiotic-free feeds
	    Phase feeding

Economical	Reduction of feed cost Reduction of water consumption Adaptation to ecological tax
Environmental	Reduction of nitrogen pollution

Guarantee of amino acid supply

Raw materials are analysed routinely for individual amino acids and crude protein content. Total amino acid composition is determined by chemical analysis while digestible amino acid composition is estimated by direct measurements on experimental animals. Feedstuffs are not fully digestible. The non-digestible protein fraction of a raw material can represent from 10% up to 40-50% of the total protein content (Fig. 3).

The total amino acid composition of a raw material is variable according to its origin, crop quality and harvest year. Moreover, amino acid digestibility depends on feedstuff processing such as heat treatment.

Imprecision on the amino acid composition and digestibility for each raw material is compensated by the introduction of safety margins at the formulation level to ensure optimal amino acid supply. Industrial amino acid composition is defined   accurately with 100%

availability to the animal. Amino acid incorporation guarantees dietary amino acid supply, reducing the risk associated to the raw material variability.

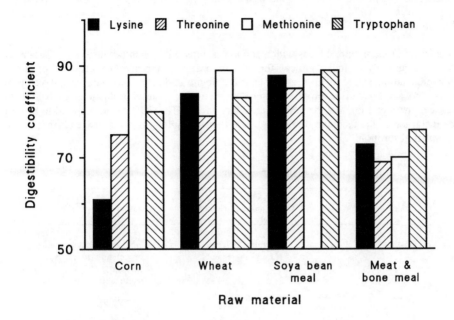

Figure 3. Amino acid digestibility in poultry (CVB Table, Netherlands)

NEW APPLICATIONS OF INDUSTRIAL AMINO ACIDS

As described earlier, industrial amino acids are used mainly in nonruminant feeds as nutritional supplements. Nevertheless, researchers have developed new applications in the animal nutrition area which are now being converted into new products. New applications rely either on applications for different animal species, namely ruminants, or developing alternative uses for amino acids in nonruminant nutrition. In the latter case, industrial amino acids are not only utilised as nutritional supplements for protein synthesis, but for specific chemical properties such as chelation, or as metabolic precursors. L-Tryptophan is a serotonin precursor with implications for the central nervous system and appetite, sleeping cycle, etc.

Rumen-protected amino acids

Supplementation with pure amino acids is not adequate for ruminant animals because they are rapidly degraded by microbes during ruminal transit. In order to overcome this obstacle, amino acid supplementation in the ruminant involves the development of a rumen protection system. Several ways to protect amino acids from rumen degradation have been studied during the last 20 years (Table 9).

Commercial rumen-protected methionine and lysine products are being developed for ruminant nutrition, mainly dairy cows and beef cattle. Industrially available products are essentially based on coating techniques, based on either the chemical polymer or natural ingredients. This topic is dealt with in more detail in Chapter 7.

Amino acid chelates

Supplementation of animal feeds with metal ions is often inefficient because of the instability of the commonly found chemical forms. In order to improve the efficacy of metal supplementation, including iron, copper and zinc, amino acid complexes have been developed. As amino acids have the property to chelate metal ions, the coordination bonds formed between the metal ion and the amino acid functions ($-NH_2$, $-COOH$) are reported to protect the metal ion in the feed and during digestive transit, resulting in an increased efficiency of intestinal absorption.

Table 9.   Main strategies to protect amino acids from ruminal degradation.

Strategy	Agent/modification	Example
Coating	Chemical polymer	Vinylpyridine/styrene
	Natural ingredients	Long chain-fatty acids
		Chitosan
		Stearic acid
Complexation	Metal chelation	Zinc-chelate
Chemical modification	N-modification	N-acetyl-DL-methionine
	Isopeptide	N-ε-MetLys isopeptide

From Patents FR 2 606 597-A1, EP 0 371 878 A1, Intl Cl: A23K1/18, USP: 5227166; also Amos *et al.* (1974), Bercovici *et al.* (1989), Wallace *et al.* (1993).

Alternative usage of amino acids

L-Tryptophan is an essential amino acid, limiting in certain animal feeds. It is a precursor of serotonin (5-hydroxytryptamine) one of the neurotransmitters of the central nervous system. Serotonin is involved in animal behaviour, especially appetite and the sleep/waking cycle. For that reason, an L-tryptophan dietary imbalance can have a negative effect on animal production.

Dietary supplementation with pure amino acids, together with various forms of carbohydrates, has been reported to induce the production of an antisecretory factor, ASF, which is reported to prevent diarrhoea in humans and pigs (Dunn, 1993).

Summary

The benefits of using industrial amino acids in animal feeds can be summarised under the following headings.

They guarantee the supply of limiting amino acids to the animal. There can be substantial variation in the total and, even more, in the digestible amino acid concentrations in feedstuffs. It is expensive and time-consuming to analyse the amino acid composition of every batch of raw material and feed manufacturers often use average values. This means that a particular batch of a raw material may supply significantly less of an amino acid than the average. Knowing this, the addition of industrial amino acid helps to guarantee that the finished feed meets the designed specification. This allows the feed manufacturer to produce a diet with an optimal supply of limiting amino acids whilst still taking advantage of the diversity of raw materials available to him.

They allow the dietary protein to be adjusted to the optimal level. Animals require diets with a particular pattern of amino acids, as described above. In formulating diets from normal ingredients alone it is practically impossible to meet the requirements for all amino acids without some being in considerable excess. The use of industrial amino acids allows this excess to be minimised. This has several consequences. First, because of the imbalances and antagonisms between amino acids described above, the utilisation of the limiting amino acid may be impaired by excesses of other amino acids. Second, free amino acids are completely digestible whereas protein concentrates and other feedstuffs are not; indeed, in some raw materials the ileal digestibility of amino acids may be as low as 50%. Thus, the inclusion of industrial amino acids coupled with the reduced inclusion of such poorly digested feedstuffs leads to a lower elimination of nitrogen in faeces. Third, because the excess amino acids are necessarily degraded by oxidation in the animal tissues, there is reduced elimination of nitrogen in urine. The amount of nitrogen excreted in faeces and urine is important not only because of the wastage of resources but also, and increasingly in areas of intensive animal production, because of the pollution they cause.

Acknowledgements

This work was supported in part by the Scottish Office Agriculture and Fisheries Department.

REFERENCES

Aida, K., Chibata, I., Nakayama, K., Takinami, K. and Yamada, H. 1986. *Biotechnology of Amino Acid Production.* Elsevier, Amsterdam, Netherlands.

Amos, H.E., Little, C.O., Digenis, G.A., Schelling, G.T., Tucker, R.E. and Mitchell, G.E. 1974. Methionine, DL-homocysteine thionolactone and N-acetyl-DL-methionine for ruminants. *J. Anim. Sci.* **39**, 612-617.

Baker, D.H. 1994. Utilization of precursors for L-amino acids. In *Amino Acids in Farm Animal Nutrition* (J.P.F. D'Mello, ed.) pp. 37-61. CAB International, Wallingford, UK.

Baker, D.H., Hahn, J.D., Chung, T.K. and Han, Y. 1993. Nutrition and growth: the concept and application of an ideal protein for swine growth. In *Growth of the Pig* (G.R. Hollis, ed.) pp. 133-139. CAB International, Wallingford, UK.

Bercovici, D., Gaertner, H.F. and Puigserver, A.P.   1989.   Poly-L-lysine and multioligo (L-methionyl)poly-L-lysine as nutritional sources of essential amino acids. *J. Agric. Food Chem.* **37**, 873-877.

Block, R.J. and Mitchell, H.H.   1946.   The correlation of the amino-acid composition of proteins with their nutritive value. *Nutr. Abstr. Rev.* **16**, 249-278.

Chung, T.K. and Baker, D.H.   1992.   Ideal amino acid pattern for 10 kilogram pigs. *J. Anim. Sci.* **70**, 3102-3111.

Cole, D.J.A. and Bong, L.   1989.   Ideal protein in pig nutrition with special reference to threonine. *Feed Compounder* **9 (Oct.)**, 24-27.

D'Mello, J.P.F   1994a.   Amino acids imbalances, antagonisms and toxicities.   In *Amino Acids in Farm Animal Nutrition* (J.P.F. D'Mello, ed.) pp. 63-97.   CAB International, Wallingford, UK.

D'Mello, J.P.F.   1994b.   *Amino Acids in Farm Animal Nutrition.* CAB International, Wallingford, UK.

Dunn, N.   1993.   Alternative solutions. *Int. Milling* **187 (Apr.)**, 26-28.

Esteve, E.   1990.   Threonine requirement of the weaning pig. *XIth ANAPORC Symposium*, Elcaniz, Spain, pp. 119-128.

Gatel, F. and Fekete, J.   1989.   Lysine and threonine balance and requirements for weaned piglets 10-25 kg. *Livest. Prod. Sci.* **23**, 195-206.

Gatel, F. and Grosjean, F.   1992.   Performance of pigs from 2 genotypes in relation to the amino acid content of the diet. *Livest. Prod. Sci.* **30**, 129-140.

Langer, S. and Fuller, M.F.   1994.   The effect of excessive amounts of branched-chain amino acids on amino acid utilization in growing pigs. *Proc. Nutr. Soc.* **53**, 108A.

Latimier, P., Dourmad, J-Y. and Corlouer, A.   1993.   Effect of three protein feeding strategies, for growing-finishing pigs, on growth performance and nitrogen output in the slurry. *J. Rech. Porcine en France* **25**, 295-300.

Lenis, N.P. and van Diepen, J.Th.M.   1990.   Amino acid requirements of pigs. 3. Requirement for apparent digestible threonine of pigs in different stages of growth. *Netherlands J. Agric. Sci.* **38**, 609-622.

Longland, A.C.   1991.   Digestive enzyme activities in pigs and poultry. In *In Vitro Digestion for Pigs and Poultry* (M.F. Fuller, ed.) pp. 3-18. CAB International, Wallingford, UK.

Low, A.G. and Zebrowska, T.   1989a. Digestion in pigs. In *Protein Metabolism in Farm Animals. Evaluation, Digestion, Absorption, and Metabolism* (H-D. Bock, B.O. Eggum, A.G. Low, O. Simon and T. Zebrowska, eds) pp. 53-121. Oxford University Press, Oxford, UK.

Low, A.G. and Zebrowska, T.   1989b. Digestion in poultry. In *Protein Metabolism in Farm Animals. Evaluation, Digestion, Absorption, and Metabolism* (H-D. Bock, B.O. Eggum, A.G. Low, O. Simon, and T. Zebrowska, eds) pp. 122-142. Oxford University Press, Oxford, UK.

Meyer, C.E. and Rose, W.C.   1936.   The spatial configuration of α-amino-β-hydroxy-n-butyric acid. *J. Biol. Chem.* **115**, 721-729.

Moran, E.T.   1982.   *Comparative Nutrition of Fowl and Swine. The Gastrointestinal Systems.* University of Guelph, Canada.

National Research Council.   1988.   *Nutrient Requirements of Swine*, 9th Edition.   National Academy Press, Washington, DC, US.

National Research Council.   1994.   *Nutrient Requirements of Poultry*, 9th Edition.   National Academy Press, Washington, DC, US.

Noblet, J., Shi, X.S. and Dubois, S.   1994.   Effect of body weight on net energy value of feeds for growing pigs. *J. Anim. Sci.* **72**, 648-657.

Schutte, J.B., Bosch, M.W., Lenis, N.P., de Jong, J. and van Diepen, J.Th.M.   1990.   Amino acid requirements of pigs.   2. Requirement for apparent digestible threonine of young pigs. *Netherlands J. Agric. Sci.* **38**, 597-607.

Sève, B., Garnier, P. and Henry, Y.   1993.   Response curve of growth performance to true digestible threonine measured at the ileal level. *J. Rech. Porcine en France* **25**, 255-262.

Valaja, J., Alaviuhkola, T. and Suomi, K.   1993.   Reducing crude protein content with supplementation of synthetic lysine and threonine in barley-rapeseed meal-pea diets for growing pigs. *Agr. Sci. Finland* **2**, 117-123.

Wallace, R.J., Frumholtz, P.P. and Walker, N.D.   1993.   Breakdown of N-terminally modified peptides and an isopeptide by rumen microorganisms. *Appl. Environ. Microbiol.* **59**, 3147-3149.

Wang, T.C. and Fuller, M.F.   1989.   The optimum dietary amino acid pattern for growing pigs. 1. Experiments by amino acid deletion. *Br. J. Nutr.* **62**, 77-89.

7 Protected proteins and amino acids for ruminants

Charles G. Schwab

University of New Hampshire, Durham, NH 03824, US

INTRODUCTION

The fundamental goal of ruminant protein nutrition is to optimize the efficiency of utilization of dietary N to maximize growth and milk production per unit of N consumed. This requires fine-tuning of protein nutrition in two ways. Firstly, it requires feeding the correct types and amounts of ruminally degradable protein (RDP) that will meet but not exceed the requirements of ruminal microorganisms for N substrates as dictated by the types and amounts of ruminally fermentable carbohydrates in the diet. Secondly, it requires feeding ruminally undegraded dietary protein (UDP), with an amino acid (AA) balance that complements that of ruminally synthesized microbial protein in amounts which, when combined with microbial protein, provides the desired protein to energy ratio in absorbed nutrients.

Improvement of ruminant protein nutrition is a matter of practical concern. The increasing attention that must be given to ration formulation to support increasing levels of meat and milk production, the increasing concerns of waste N disposal, and the growing emphasis on lean tissue growth and milk protein production all provide incentives to seek ways to maximize efficiency of N utilization.

The purpose of this chapter is to review the technologies that have been evaluated for protecting feed proteins and AA from ruminal degradation. A brief review of ruminant AA nutrition is presented first to highlight the nutritive value of ruminally synthesized microbial protein and UDP.

AMINO ACID NUTRITION OF RUMINANTS

Essentiality of amino acids

Like all mammals, ruminants have specific metabolic requirements for AA for maintenance and productive functions. Amino acids are uniquely essential as precursors for protein synthesis. They also serve for the synthesis of other N-containing metabolites as precursors for gluconeogenesis, and as sources of metabolic energy when oxidized to CO_2. Research is too limited to categorize precisely the AA commonly found in absorbable protein as being "essential" or "nonessential" for ruminants. However, the early isotopic tracer studies of Black *et al.* (1957) and Downes (1961), using dairy cattle and sheep, indicated that the classification is similar to that of non-ruminants. Limited research also indicates that the nutritive value of absorbed protein for ruminant production, like that of non-ruminants, is influenced by both the balance of essential AA (EAA) and the contribution of total EAA to total AA (Merchen and Titgemeyer, 1992; Rulquin and Vérité, 1993). Ruminants have not responded to postruminal supplements of nonessential AA when fed conventional feedstuffs (Oldham *et al.*, 1983; Schwab *et al.*, 1976).

Sources of absorbable amino acids

Absorbable AA are provided by microbial protein synthesized in the rumen, UDP, and endogenous secretions. Ruminally synthesized microbial protein typically supplies 50% or more of the AA when production-type diets are fed. Microbial protein is supplied by predominantly fermentative populations of bacteria, protozoa, and fungi. Over 200 species of bacteria, more than 20 species of protozoa, and at least 12 species of fungi have been found in ruminal digesta. Bacteria generally constitute most of the microbial biomass in the rumen. Protozoa typically represent less than half and sometimes less than 10% and fungi less than 2-3% of the microbial biomass.

The second major source of absorbable AA is UDP. The quantity of UDP flowing from the rumen for a feedstuff depends on the proportion of the total protein that is degradable, the rate at which the degradable fraction is degraded, and the residence time of the protein source in the rumen. Primary factors influencing one or more of these processes include microbial proteolytic activity in the rumen, microbial access to the protein, level of feed intake, the ingredient composition of the rest of the diet, physical form of the feedstuff, protein solubility, and ruminal pH. Proteolytic activity in the rumen surprisingly is quite variable and is influenced largely by dietary factors that affect the type and number of microorganisms in the rumen (Broderick *et al.*, 1991).

Endogenous secretions and abraded epithelial cells provide some absorbable AA but quantitative information describing this supply in ruminants is extremely limited, except that it is influenced largely by intake and diet composition, for example the intake of digestible organic matter. However, it is likely that this source of protein has little influence on the pattern of absorbable AA.

Nutritive value of microbial protein

The distribution of N in ruminal bacteria is variable and influenced by species and conditions of growth. Data from 62 literature reports indicated that of total N, AA-N averaged 82.5% (SE = 28.3), RNA-N averaged 10.0% (SE = 8.3), and DNA-N averaged 5.2% (SE = 9.4) (Storm and Ørskov, 1983). The same authors found values of 80.9% for AA-N in bacterial biomass of high purity isolated from ruminal contents of slaughtered cattle and sheep. A literature review by Clark *et al.* (1992) involving 34 observations indicated that AA-N constituted only 66.5% of total N (range = 54.9 to 86.7%). Ruminal protozoa contain more AA-N, relative to total N, than ruminal bacteria because of lower concentrations of nucleic acid N (about 11% of total N rather than 15%) and cell wall-associated nonprotein N compounds (Ørskov, 1992).

There are few direct determinations of the intestinal digestibility of ruminally synthesized microbial true protein. Storm *et al.* (1983) infused incremental levels of freeze-dried preparations of rumen bacteria into the abomasum of sheep sustained entirely by intragastric infusion. By regressing input on passage to the ileum, true digestibilities of AA were calculated to be 85%. By employing the same approach, but with sheep fed conventional diets, Tas *et al.* (1981) calculated AA digestibility to be 87%. However, Tas *et al.* (1981) did not include Cys, Trp, Pro, and diaminopimelic acid (DAPA) in their estimate; true digestibilities of these AA in the study by Storm *et al.* (1983) all were below the average of 85% for all AA. Also in the study by Storm *et al.* (1983), the digestibility of individual AA varied little (80 to 88%); the only exceptions were that of Pro (76%), Cys (73%), His (68%), and DAPA (37%).

Microbial protein is considered to be of high quality because of apparent high digestibility and an EAA composition that is similar to that of lean body tissue and milk (Table 1). Although there are apparent differences in EAA composition between ruminal bacteria (higher Met content) and protozoa (higher Lys content), it is assumed that variation in the EAA profile of mixed microbial protein leaving the rumen is fairly small and not influenced markedly by changes in population structure. This assumption is based on three observations: (1) a multitude of different microorganisms inhabit the rumen; (2) the variation in AA profiles between the major groups of microorganisms, as well as among the predominant strains within each group, are small to moderate (Purser and Buechler, 1966); and (3) protozoa are retained selectively in the rumen and do not contribute to postruminal AA supply in proportion to their contribution to the total microbial biomass in the rumen (Veira *et al.*, 1983; John and Ulyatt, 1984). Weller and Pilgrim (1974) estimated that the contribution of protozoa to DM leaving the rumen was less than 20% of their contribution to DM in the rumen. Harrison *et al.* (1979) estimated that 41% of protozoal AA-N left the rumen. Therefore, it is not surprising that a comparison of the average EAA profiles of duodenal digesta from defaunated and faunated sheep in three studies showed no effect of defaunation (Merchen and Titgemeyer, 1992).

Although it appears that the AA composition of microbial protein can be dealt with as the content in mixed rumen bacteria without introducing any major error, it is difficult at present to measure accurately the AA profile of microbial protein leaving the rumen. Moreover, the variations in AA profiles of rumen bacterial cells as noted in extensive literature summaries (Clark *et al.*, 1992; Ørskov, 1992) cannot be ignored, particularly because sizeable variations also are found within laboratories where isolation and analytical procedures have remained the same (Clark *et al.*, 1992).

Nutritive value of UDP

There are few direct estimates of the intestinal digestibility of UDP. The most direct approach is to increase the amount of UDP entering the duodenum in graded fashion while measuring the increment of UDP passing to the terminal ileum. Using this regression approach, Titgemeyer *et al.* (1989) estimated the intestinal digestibilities of N and total AA associated with UDP of soybean meal (SBM), corn gluten meal, blood meal, and fish meal in beef steers to be 63 and 55, 80 and 80, 74 and 72, and 74 and 72%, respectively.

Several workers have used the mobile bag technique for measuring digestibility of UDP. This method generally consists of incubating feedstuffs in nylon bags in the rumen for 12 to 16 h to obtain undegraded residues, incubating the residues in a pepsin + HCl solution to mimic the conditions in the abomasum, and then allowing the bags to pass from the proximal duodenum to either the terminal ileum or feces. A summary of several of these studies (Hvelplund, 1985; Rae and Smithard, 1985; de Boer *et al.*, 1987; Frydrych, 1992) indicates that the UDP-digestibilities of most feed proteins are similar (80 to 90%). However, there are exceptions, such as SBM and fish meal, where estimates of digestibility are generally higher than 90%, and rapeseed meal and meat and bone meal, where the estimates vary between 60 and 80%.

Table 1. A comparison of the essential AA (EAA) profiles of lean body tissue and milk with that of ruminal bacteria and protozoa and common feeds.

	(% of total EAA)										EAA[2] (%CP)
Source	Arg	His	Ile	Leu	**Lys**	**Met**	Phe	Thr	Trp	Val	
Animal products											
Lean tissue[1]	16.8	6.3	7.1	17.0	**16.3**	**5.1**	8.9	9.9	2.5	10.1	-
Milk[2]	7.2	5.5	11.4	19.5	**16.0**	**5.5**	10.0	8.9	3.0	13.0	-
Rumen microbes											
Bacteria[3]	10.2	4.0	11.5	16.3	**15.8**	**5.2**	10.2	11.7	2.7	12.5	-
Bacteria[4]	10.6	4.3	11.6	15.5	**17.3**	**4.9**	10.0	11.0	2.6	12.2	40.0
Protozoa[5]	9.3	3.6	12.7	15.8	**20.6**	**4.2**	10.7	10.5	2.8	9.7	-
Forages[6]											
Alfalfa	10.9	5.2	10.9	18.4	**11.1**	**3.8**	12.2	10.6	3.4	13.5	40.7
Corn silage	6.4	5.5	10.3	27.8	**7.5**	**4.8**	12.0	10.1	1.4	14.1	
Haycrop silage	8.9	5.3	11.0	18.9	**10.3**	**3.8**	13.5	10.3	3.3	14.7	
Grains[6]											
Barley	12.8	5.9	9.6	18.4	**9.6**	**4.5**	13.3	9.1	3.1	13.6	38.5
Corn, yellow	10.8	7.0	8.2	29.1	**7.0**	**5.0**	11.3	8.4	1.7	11.5	42.3
Corn gluten feed	12.0	7.9	8.5	24.6	**8.2**	**4.6**	10.1	9.6	1.6	12.8	38.8
Oats	15.6	5.4	9.5	18.1	**10.0**	**4.3**	11.5	9.2	3.2	13.3	42.8
Sorghum	9.4	5.8	9.4	30.9	**5.6**	**4.3**	12.6	8.0	2.2	11.8	39.8
Wheat	15.2	6.6	9.7	18.9	**8.0**	**4.6**	12.6	8.3	3.4	12.6	31.9
Plant proteins[6]											
Brewer's grain	8.9	6.4	10.6	17.6	**11.4**	**4.8**	10.3	11.4	3.0	15.6	46.3
Corn gluten meal	6.9	4.7	9.3	36.4	**3.8**	**5.5**	13.8	7.5	1.5	10.7	44.2
Corn DDG w/ solubles	7.7	7.2	9.8	26.3	**6.2**	**5.2**	11.1	10.3	2.7	13.4	37.7
Cottonseed meal	25.4	6.0	7.7	13.9	**9.6**	**3.8**	12.2	7.7	2.9	10.8	43.1
DDG w/ solubles	19.9	6.5	15.4	18.7	**6.5**	**3.7**	15.4	8.9	1.6	14.6	43.3
Linseed meal	25.7	5.2	13.3	14.8	**8.1**	**3.5**	11.1	8.9	3.5	11.8	41.1
Peanut meal	13.5	5.4	9.9	15.2	**10.0**	**2.4**	11.5	6.5	2.8	10.6	36.9
Rapeseed meal	14.0	6.7	9.3	16.9	**13.1**	**4.8**	9.5	10.5	3.0	12.4	41.9
Safflower meal	22.3	6.5	8.8	15.1	**7.9**	**3.7**	11.4	7.4	4.6	12.3	40.5
Soybean meal	16.3	5.7	10.8	17.0	**13.7**	**3.1**	11.0	8.6	3.0	10.6	47.6
Sunflower meal	19.4	5.9	10.1	15.5	**8.6**	**5.4**	11.0	9.1	2.8	12.3	45.0
Animal proteins[6]											
Blood meal	7.6	11.2	2.1	22.8	**15.7**	**2.1**	12.3	8.1	2.7	15.4	49.4
Feather meal	14.7	1.1	10.0	29.3	**3.9**	**2.1**	10.0	10.5	1.5	17.1	31.4
Fish meal (menhaden)	13.1	5.7	9.3	16.5	**17.0**	**6.3**	8.8	9.5	2.4	11.3	44.8
Meat meal	18.8	5.2	8.0	17.1	**14.1**	**3.7**	9.7	9.1	2.0	12.4	37.5
Meat and bone meal	20.5	5.5	7.8	16.2	**14.2**	**3.6**	9.2	9.0	1.8	12.1	38.0
Tankage	18.8	5.2	8.0	17.1	**14.1**	**3.7**	9.7	9.1	2.0	12.4	45.1
Whey, dry	5.6	3.7	12.4	20.1	**17.5**	**4.3**	7.4	13.2	3.8	11.9	50.8

[1] From Ainslie *et al.* (1993); average values of empty, whole body carcasses as reported in three studies.
[2] Each value is an average of observations from Jacobson *et al.* (1970), McCance and Widdowson (1978), and Waghorn and Baldwin (1984).
[3] From Clark *et al.* (1992); average values from 61 dietary treatments.
[4] From Storm and Ørskov (1983); average values from 62 literature reports.
[5] From Storm and Ørskov (1983); average values from 15 literature reports.
[6] Calculated from values presented in "European Amino Acid Table: first edition 1992" except for DDG w/ solubles (distillers dried grain with solubles), linseed meal, peanut meal, and feather meal that were calculated from values presented in "Feedstuff Ingredient Analysis Table: 1991 edition".

Using a recently developed *in vitro* approach for both abomasal and intestinal digestion, Calsamiglia and Stern (1993) obtained digestibilities of the UDP in SBM, corn gluten meal, fish meal, blood meal, hydrolyzed feather meal, and meat and bone meal to be 89.8 ± 2.6, 87.6 ± 2.7, 85.4 ± 2.6, 80.1 ± 16.7, 69.5 ± 3.9, and 54.0 ± 6.2%, respectively. Clearly, differences in postruminal protein digestion between various sources must be considered when determining protein value for ruminants.

Because of methodological limitations and the small quantity of available data, the AA composition of the digestible UDP fraction of feed proteins is uncertain. Using the nylon bag technique, several researchers have shown that the AA profile of feed residues following exposure to ruminal fermentation is different from the same feeds before exposure to fermentation (see Rulquin and Vérité, 1993). By using the nylon bag technique and correcting the AA composition of recovered digesta residues for bacterial contamination, University of New Hampshire researchers (Bozak *et al.*, 1986; Schwab *et al.*, 1986; C.G. Schwab, C.K. Bozak and J.E. Nocek, unpublished) found that, for most protein supplements, the contribution of basic AA (Arg, Lys, and His) to total EAA in UDP was slightly lower than in the same feeds before exposure to ruminal fermentation; in contrast, the branched-chain AA were slightly higher. The same workers found that most of the differences occur within the first 1 to 2 h of exposure to ruminal fermentation.

Because the total protein in a feedstuff is composed of different proteins with different degrees of access to proteolytic enzymes and because certain peptide bonds (e.g. with branched-chain AA) or other bonds (e.g. the Maillard reaction sequence between the ε-amino groups of Lys residues and carbonyl compounds) are more resistant than others to hydrolysis, it seems reasonable that the AA composition of digestible UDP may be different from the intact feed protein. However, the author agrees with Rulquin and Vérité (1993) in that differences in AA profiles between a feed protein and the corresponding digestible UDP are small in comparison with the large differences that exist among feeds.

Factors affecting intestinal balance of amino acids

Multivariate analysis of measurements of AA passage to the small intestine in ruminants (Rulquin and Vérité, 1993) confirmed that the AA composition of UDP and the proportional contribution that UDP makes to total protein flow accounts for most of the variation in AA balance of duodenal digesta. This would be expected because feed proteins vary greatly in AA composition and generally differ from microbial protein in AA composition (Table 1). As a consequence, the greatest influence of diet on AA profiles of duodenal digesta is seen when large amounts of high-UDP feeds with AA profiles most different from microbial protein (e.g., corn gluten meal, blood meal, and feather meal) are fed (Stern *et al.*, 1983; Titgemeyer *et al.*, 1989; Waltz *et al.*, 1989).

RUMEN PROTECTED PROTEINS

The need for rumen protected proteins

There are several reasons and advantages for decreasing the rate and extent of ruminal degradation of selected feed proteins and for having a variety of high-UDP feeds available to the producer. First, there are feeding situations in which the diet does not contain adequate quantities of absorbable AA relative to the supply of absorbable energy. This can occur because of: (1) too many ingredients in the diet which contain insufficient UDP relative to RDP, (2) some limitation on ruminal synthesis of microbial protein (e.g. insufficient supplies of fermentable carbohydrates or of RDP), (3) feeding supplemental fats which are dense sources of metabolizable energy but which are not used for microbial cell growth, or (4) some dependence on mobilized body fat for metabolizable energy, such as in the early lactation dairy cow. Second, high quality pastures, hays, and particularly silages often contain so much RDP that any required protein supplementation must be limited to high UDP feeds if the diet is to be balanced for both RDP and UDP. And third, the use of higher UDP feeds permits greater use of NPN supplements and less reliance on more degradable sources of true protein for ruminal synthesis of microbial protein. It also must be remembered that requirements for absorbable AA, relative to absorbable energy, are highest when ruminants are fed for maximum milk protein production and lean tissue growth and that metabolism enhancers such as bovine somatotropin may further increase AA requirements.

One approach to increasing the contribution of UDP to total CP in the diet, as alluded to already, is to feed high-protein by-product feeds (e.g. corn gluten, meat, hydrolyzed feather, fish, and blood meals) that are already of lower ruminal degradability. However, cost, commercial availability, uniformity, AA balance and intestinal digestibility and palatability of product dictate their use. The alternate approach is to reduce artificially the rate of ruminal degradation of high protein forages, oilseeds, and oilseed meals that possess good AA balance and good intestinal availability but which are rapidly degraded. This approach: (1) increases the number of higher UDP feeds with which to optimize diets for UDP/RDP ratios, intestinal AA balance, and price, (2) has the advantage of being applied to feeds of choice and of providing controlled ruminal protection so as to maximize protection with minimal reduction in intestinal digestion, and (3) reduces the reliance on by-product feeds as the only high UDP feed sources.

Methods for protecting feed proteins

Many methods have been investigated to reduce the rate and extent of ruminal degradation of feed proteins. Many excellent reviews (e.g. Chalupa, 1975; Ferguson, 1975; Waldo, 1977; Beever and Thomson, 1981; Kaufmann and Lüpping, 1982; Broderick *et al.*, 1991) have been published on this subject. This section will highlight those treatments that have been most successful and either have been used or hold promise for commercial acceptance.

Heat treatment. First used by Chalmers *et al.* (1954), heat processing has become one of the most commonly used treatments for reducing ruminal degradation of feed proteins. This has included expeller processing of oilseeds (in contrast to solvent extraction), roasting (flame drying), extrusion, and micronization (infrared cooking). Feeds to which heat has been applied include casein, fish meal and other animal proteins, oilseeds and oilseed meals, and high quality forages. Roasting has gained popularity as a treatment of oilseeds and oilseed meals. It is more energy efficient than most other forms of applying dry heat, the palatability of the resulting product often is enhanced, fat of whole beans generally is more inert in the rumen, and roasters are available for on-farm use. However, infrared cooking (micronization) holds considerable promise, particularly of whole beans, because of excellent control of the heating process, more effective heat transfer than dry roasting, and uniformity of product.

The mechanism of protection with heat processing is the formation of cross-links which are more resistant to enzymatic hydrolysis. The principal reaction is the non-enzymatic Maillard reaction sequence between primary amines (especially the ε-amino groups of Lys residues) and carbonyl groups of reducing sugars such as glucose, fructose, and pentoses (Hurrell and Finot, 1985) and of gossypol in cottonseed meal (Craig and Broderick, 1981). Other AA residues, primarily Cys, also may react with reducing sugars, but they do so to a smaller extent than Lys. The initial reactions include the formation of a Schiff's base followed by the formation of "Amadori products" with little or no browning. Resulting Lys intermediates at this point have the same bioavailability as free Lys in rats (Finot *et al.*, 1977). Later reactions cause formation of reactive polycarbonyl compounds which polymerize and bind simultaneously to the amino groups of different polypeptide chains, bringing about the formation of highly cross-linked protein-carbohydrate polymers (premelanoidins and melanoidins) with low digestibility. Lysine residues also can react with oxidized fats (Carpenter and Booth, 1973). In addition to reactions involving Lys, Cys can undergo condensation to form compounds such as lanthionine, protease-resistant cross-links may form within and between polypeptide chains (e.g., between Lys and Asn and Gln residues) (Feeney, 1977), and partial loss may occur of AA such as Arg, Trp, Met, and Cys (Hurrell and Finot, 1985).

Heating can have two adverse effects: actual loss of certain AA and depressed intestinal digestibility of those that remain. This was demonstrated by Parsons *et al.* (1992) who evaluated the effects of autoclaving (121°C and 1.1 kg cm^{-2}) SBM for 0, 20, 40, and 60 min on AA concentrations and bioavailability for chicks. As autoclaving time increased, concentrations of Lys and Cys, and to a lesser extent Arg, decreased. The effect was greatest for Lys where the concentration was reduced by 22% as a result of heating for 60 min. In addition, autoclaving time reduced the true digestibility of most AA with the effect being greatest for Cys, Lys, Asp, and His.

The challenge of heat treatment, like other methods for protection of feed proteins from ruminal degradation, is to identify the processing conditions that increase UDP to an extent that justifies the cost of the treatment but with minimal adverse effects on loss of AA and on intestinal digestibility of the resulting UDP. Under-heating is of little benefit and over-heating causes significant heat damage and irreversible loss of nutritive value. Therefore, a window of optimal heat treatment appears to exist. This concept was demonstrated by the experiments of Broderick and Craig (1980) and Craig and Broderick (1981) as summarized in Table 2.

Autoclaving cottonseed meal for 60 min caused a marked increase in UDP with little decrease in intestinal digestibility of protein. In contrast, heating for an additional 60 min caused a marked decrease in intestinal digestibility of protein with little increase in UDP. As a consequence, the maximum quantity of digestible UDP (UDP × true digestibility) was obtained by heating for 60 min. However, increasing the autoclaving time had a much greater depressing effect on estimates of intestinal available Lys, as assessed by fluorodinitro-benzene (FDNB) reactivity, than on estimates of intestinal digestible protein (Table 2). As a consequence, the effects of increasing autoclaving time on estimates of postruminally available Lys (UDP × intestinally available Lys) was an obvious quadratic response and therefore the optimum response window to heat treatment was even more obvious.

Table 2. Effect of autoclaving (121°C, 1.1 kg cm^{-2}) cold-extracted cottonseed meal for different periods of time on factors related to protein utilization in ruminants.

	Autoclaving time (min)					
Item	0	15	30	60	90	120
UDP[1], % of CP (1)	21.2	26.1	41.6	69.0	73.2	74.9
True digestibility[2], % (2)	90.6	89.2	87.8	84.1	77.2	70.8
Intestinal digestible UDP, % of CP (1×2)	19.2	23.3	36.5	58.0	56.2	53.0
Lysine, g per 100 g cottonseed meal						
Total	2.79	2.55	2.74	2.42	2.04	1.92
Unavailable[3]	.33	.31	.44	.53	1.02	1.08
Available[3] (3)	2.46	2.24	2.30	1.89	1.02	.84
Postruminal available lysine (1×3),						
** g per 100 g cottonseed meal**	**.52**	**.58**	**.96**	**1.31**	**.75**	**.63**

From Broderick and Craig (1980) and Craig and Broderick (1981).

[1] Ruminally undegraded dietary protein; estimated from *in vitro* degradation fractions and rates and an assumed ruminal turnover rate of .04 h^{-1}.

[2] Determined with rats.

[3] Determined using an indirect fluorodinitrobenzene chemical method. Unavailable lysine was considered to be the lysine that was inaccessible to react with 1-fluoro-2,4-dinitrobenzene (FDNB); available lysine = total lysine - FDNB lysine.

Wisconsin workers extended the approach of combining measurements of UDP (using an *in vitro* ruminal system) and FDNB-determined available Lys to determine the optimal holding time after roasting of soybeans and SBM (Faldet *et al.*, 1991), to evaluate soybeans heat-treated by various methods (Faldet *et al.*, 1992b), and to determine optimal heat treatment of soybeans (Faldet *et al.*, 1992a) (Table 3). Similar to the results in Table 2, and those of Parsons *et al.* (1992), increasing the amount of heat applied to whole soybeans not only decreased Lys concentrations but it also decreased the availability of the remaining Lys (Table 3). As temperature increased, the time required to maximize postruminal available Lys decreased. Of particular interest was that the FDNB chemical method and the rat assay both gave similar estimates of nutritionally available Lys, and therefore of estimated postruminal available Lys.

Collectively, these studies appear to validate the combined use of estimates of ruminal undegradability and of FDNB-available Lys to determine optimal heat treatment of feed proteins for ruminants. The Wisconsin workers consistently have demonstrated that a loss of 15 to 22% of chemically determined available Lys is necessary to achieve the heat treatment of soybean protein that results in maximal postruminal available Lys.

Several additional points are noteworthy regarding heat treatment of feed proteins. First, non-enzymatic browning cannot be described simply as the product of time × temperature (see Table 3 as an example). Second, several factors such as the type and level of reducing sugars per mole of Lys, pH of the reaction mixture, and water activity or moisture level (Cleale *et al.*, 1987b) are important in optimizing non-enzymatic browning. The epsilon amino group of Lys is affected primarily between pH 8 and 9 where proton removal makes it a stronger nucleophile. Adequate moisture (about 20 to 25%) is needed for heat transfer. And last, available evidence suggests that an improved approach for determining the window of optimal heat treatment would be to replace estimates of UDP digestibility with estimates of intestinal digestibility of an AA most likely to be limiting such as Lys or Met. Lysine is the AA of choice because it is the most vulnerable to heat damage and because a method is available (the indirect FDNB method) that provides estimates of intestinally available Lys that correlate well with those obtained *in vivo*.

Chemical treatment. Many chemical agents have been shown to decrease ruminal degradation of feed proteins. These include aldehydes, tannins, alcohols, acids and alkalis, sodium bentonite, cations such as zinc, and reducing sugars. In most cases, these agents have been selected because they create pH-dependent chemical modifications which decrease ruminal degradability but which are, with appropriate processing, largely, if not totally, reversed by the acidic conditions in the abomasum and proximal duodenum.

The most studied and probably still the most widely used of these chemical treatments is formaldehyde (Ferguson, 1975; Waldo, 1977; Tamminga, 1979; Kaufmann and Lüpping, 1982; Broderick *et al.*, 1991). Use of formaldehyde varies among countries. For example, it is used widely in France and the Netherlands but to a much lesser extent in other European countries (H. Rulquin, I.N.R.A., Saint Gilles, France, personal communication). On the other hand, the practice is not permissible in the United States because of concerns of potential risk to those who treat feed with formaldehyde (Broderick *et al.*, 1991). The primary use of formaldehyde is for treatment of oilseed meals such as those of soybean and rapeseed. However, its use has been most effective with ensiled forages, particularly grasses and legumes, that are ensiled with little or no wilting. Without the use of formaldehyde, large amounts of the forage protein undergo autolysis during silage fermentation. As an additive in silage making, formaldehyde has two benefits; it inhibits proteolysis during silage fermentation, and when the silage is fed, it protects some of the silage proteins from ruminal degradation (Siddons *et al.*, 1979; Tamminga, 1979). Strong acids such as formic acid often are used in combination with formaldehyde to preserve silage. The effect of acids is complementary to those of aldehydes (e.g. Siddons *et al.*, 1984); by decreasing the pH of the forage, they restrict silage fermentation and further inhibit autolysis of protein.

Table 3. Effect of temperature and duration of forced-air oven heating of full-fat soybeans on estimated ruminally undegraded dietary protein (UDP) and estimated postruminal available lysine (PRAL).

Temp. (°C)	Duration (min)	UDP[1] (% of CP)	Lysine content of soybean (g per 100 g DM)				
			Lysine			PRAL	
			Total	Unavailable [2]	Available [2]	Calculated[3]	Rat[4]
0	0	29.7	2.57	.14	2.43	.72	.59
140	10	33.9	2.55	.11	2.44	.83	.70
	30	43.9	2.36	.16	2.20	.97	.92
	60	49.4	2.36	.19	2.17	1.07	.97
	90	**55.0**	**2.22**	**.21**	**2.01**	**1.11**	**1.04**
	120	59.2	2.12	.23	1.89	1.12	1.07
150	10	36.6	2.48	.09	2.39	.88	.76
	30	42.4	2.33	.14	2.19	.93	.88
	60	**58.4**	**2.22**	**.23**	**1.99**	**1.16**	**1.08**
	90	64.2	1.88	.32	1.56	1.10	.96
	120	69.9	1.88	.32	1.56	1.09	1.02
160	10	37.4	2.46	.13	2.33	.87	.79
	30	**53.2**	**2.26**	**.19**	**2.07**	**1.10**	**1.11**
	60	72.0	1.81	.40	1.41	1.02	.97
	90	71.1	1.57	.43	1.14	.81	.77
	120	75.1	1.50	.44	1.06	.80	.74

From Faldet *et al.* (1992a).

[1] UDP (% of CP) = $\{B[k_p/(k_p + k_d)] + C\} \times 100$, where fraction B is degraded true protein, C is considered indigestible protein, k_d is the *in vitro* fractional protein degradation rate and k_p is the ruminal passage rate (.06 h^{-1}).
[2] Unavailable lysine was considered to be the lysine that was inaccessible to react with 1-fluoro-2,4-dinitrobenzene (FDNB); available lysine = total lysine - FDNB lysine.
[3] Product of estimated UDP × estimated available lysine.
[4] Predicted from rat growth trials.

Initial studies indicated that other aldehydes such as acetaldehyde, glutaraldehyde and glyoxal were as effective as formaldehyde for protecting dietary protein from ruminal degradation (Ferguson *et al.*, 1967).   Mangan *et al.* (1980) concluded that field spraying with glutaraldehyde is a preferred treatment over spraying with formaldehyde for harvest of fresh alfalfa because it reacts quicker and has no toxic effects to rumen microorganisms. However, Ashes *et al.* (1984) reported that glutaraldehyde and glyoxal may offer less protection of protein in the rumen as well as reduce the availability of those AA (i.e. Lys, Tyr and Cys) that, typically, become increasingly unavailable for absorption with increasing levels of aldehyde treatment. Aldehydes decrease protein solubility and proteolysis by introducing cross-links into proteins. Under typical conditions, it is assumed that they cause the formation of methylol groups on the free α- and ε- amino groups of protein. These groups then condense with other groups such as the amide groups of Asn and Gln and the guanidyl group of Arg to form inter- and intra-molecular methylene bridges. Reactions also may occur with indole (Trp), imidazole (His), phenol (Tyr), and sulfhydryl (Met) groups (Ferguson, 1975).

The window of optimal treatment with aldehydes is rather narrow. For example, Kaufmann and Lüpping (1982) reported that increasing application rates of formaldehyde to SBM up to 2 g kg^{-1} of DM decreased N solubility in phosphate buffer (from 24 to 5%) and ammonia release *in vitro* (from 55 to 15 g N per 100 g N incubated) in a curvilinear manner. Over this range of application rates, intestinal digestibility (as measured by disappearance between the abomasum and feces in sheep) decreased only 3 to 4%. However, with formaldehyde applications of 1.5 to 5.0 g kg^{-1} of DM, intestinal digestibility decreased sharply in a linear fashion from 85 to 30%. The decrese in digestibility associated with over-treatment appears to affect all AA rather than only those that are involved directly in the resulting cross-links (Hvelplund and Hesselholt, 1987).

The greatest challenge associated with formaldehyde treatment in commercial practice is determining the optimal rates of application. Required application rates depend not only on the content of ruminally degradable true protein, but also on factors such as carbohydrate content, moisture level, and particle size (Beever and Thomson, 1981; Kaufmann and Lüpping, 1982). In addition to the lack of a clear understanding of the exact interrelationships among these factors, variable losses of formaldehyde are associated with method of application, seepage, and bacterial metabolism. For example, an ensiled forage may contain only 10 to 20% of the amount of formaldehyde originally used (Kaufmann and Lüpping, 1982).

The future role of tannins as chemical additives for decreasing ruminal degradation of feed proteins remains unclear. Tannins are chemically diverse polyphenolics of plant origin that have a variety of biological activities and vary in their association with other plant components. The pH-dependent hydrogen and hydrophobic bonding that occurs between proteins and tannins is such that the resulting complexes are less soluble and less accessible to proteolytic enzymes at the pH of ruminal contents, thereby slowing the rate of ruminal degradation (Broderick *et al.*, 1991). Condensed tannins (polymers of flavonoid phenols) are more effective in this regard than hydrolyzable tannins (polyesters of gallic acid and sugars) (Reid *et al.*, 1974). Further, it is known that bacteria involved in fiber digestion are more sensitive to condensed tannins than proteolytic bacteria (Bae *et al.*, 1993; Jones *et al.*, 1994). However, it is not known which of the condensed tannins are the most effective for increasing digestible UDP and of these, which are least inhibitory toward microbial cell function or ruminal fiber digestibility (Waghorn and Shelton, 1992). The challenges associated with cost-effective isolation of large quantities of selected tannins from agricultural and forest by-products such that their biological activity is retained (e.g. Makkar and Becker, 1994) will also have to be overcome if tannins are to be used successfully to protect feed proteins.

More intriguing than adding exogenous sources of tannins to feedstuffs is the possibility of genetically engineering major legumes such as alfalfa and white clover to express desired levels of selected condensed tannins in their foliage. Indeed, this represents the overall objective of the present collective efforts of research groups in Canada, Australia, and England (M.Y. Gruber, Agriculture Canada, Saskatoon, personal communication). Both forage legumes contain genes for tannin synthesis, but expression is limited to the seed coat of alfalfa (Koupai-Abyazani et al., 1993) and to the flower of white clover (Jones et al., 1976). As reviewed by Broderick et al. (1991), several other legumes (e.g. birdfoot trefoil, sanfoin, and *Lotus pedunculatus*) also contain variable levels and structures of condensed tannins in their foliage and most important, their presence has been shown to increase rumen escape and delivery of AA to the small intestine (McNabb et al., 1993).

Acids, alkalis, and alcohols, well known for their ability to alter protein structure, also have been shown to reduce solubility and ruminal degradation of feed proteins. Some of the more effective treatments for solvent-extracted SBM have included spraying with 5% acetic or propionic acids, soaking in 0.5 N HCl or NaOH (Waltz and Loerch, 1986), or soaking in 40 to 60% (v/v) solutions of ethanol, propanol, or isopropanol (van der Aar et al., 1982). Although not as effective as heat or formaldehyde for increasing ruminal escape of SBM (Waltz and Stern, 1989), the benefit of these and similar treatments is the lack of apparent adverse effects on intestinal availability of AA (Lynch et al., 1987; Mir et al., 1984a, b; van der Aar et al., 1983; Waltz and Loerch, 1986). Therefore, it seems reasonable to expect that opportunities may exist for using these agents in conjunction with milder forms of heat treatment that would be more successful than any one of the treatments alone.

Heat treatment in combination with other treatments. This is an attractive approach if similar or enhanced levels of protection can be obtained with less heat and therefore without the adverse effects of AA loss and decreased intestinal digestibilities of the resulting UDP. Although published research in this area is limited, this approach has been pursued more vigorously by companies wishing to market "high rumen-bypass" plant proteins.

An excellent example of this approach is the addition of reducing sugars (extracted from sulfite pulping liquors) to SBM prior to heating to induce non-enzymatic browning. Currently marketed throughout North America and Europe (Lignotech Inc., Kansas), the UDP content of the resulting product is 65 to 80% of CP as compared to 20-35% for solvent extracted SBM or 50 to 60% for expeller (heat-treated) SBM. Using *in vitro* ammonia release as the response criterion for induction of non-enzymatic browning of SBM, initial research indicated that: (1) sugar addition, pH, and moisture level augment each other, (2) xylose was more effective than glucose, fructose or lactose as a reducing sugar, and (3) 3 moles of added xylose/mole of SBM-Lys was as effective as 5 moles of xylose (Cleale et al., 1987b). Continuation of these studies indicated that feeding a product heated under conditions that promoted enzymatic browning (SBM adjusted to pH 8.5 with NaOH, addition of water to achieve 83% DM, and xylose added at 3 mol per mol of SBM-Lys and heating for 30 min at 150°C in a forced-air oven) increased ruminal escape of digestible UDP in steers (Cleale et al., 1987a) and doubled the efficiency of gain of lambs (Cleale et al., 1987c) as compared to feeding commercial SBM. Windschitl and Stern (1988) fed diets containing untreated SBM, water-SBM, xylose-SBM, and pulp liquor derived sugars-SBM to lactating dairy cows and found that ruminal protein degradation was 71, 70, 56 and 54%, respectively; approximately 50% of dietary protein was supplied by the SBM sources.

A second example is the addition of $ZnSO_4$ to oilseed meals prior to applying moist heat and either pelleting or extruding under controlled conditions of time, temperature and pressure. The resulting Zn-treated SBM is expected to be on the market within a year and has a UDP content of about 70% CP (D. Longmire, Central Soya, Decatur, IN, personal communication). Heavy metals are known to precipitate soluble proteins, and previous research has indicated that: (1) treating SBM with Zn salts at 1 to 2% of feed DM reduced *in vitro* degradation of SBM-protein, (2) $ZnSO_4$ was more effective than other Zn salts, and (3) feeding Zn-treated SBM or high concentrations of Zn (1142 ppm) increased passage of UDP-AA to the small intestine (D. Longmire, personal communication; see Cecava *et al.* 1993 for references). Evidence suggests that Zn functions as an equalizer in the multi-treatment process, thereby reducing the preciseness required for the remaining treatments and as a result, the window of optimal treatment is increased.

Other examples are the additive effects of heat and alcohol, or of heat, pH, and moisture. For example, van der Aar *et al.* (1984) and Lynch *et al.* (1987) demonstrated that the effects of ethanol and heat were additive in reducing ruminal degradation of SBM without apparent adverse effects on AA availability as determined by chick performance (Lynch *et al.*, 1987). Stockman (Supersweet Feeds, Omaho, Nebraska, personal communication) has observed that optimizing pH, moisture, and heat treatment of SBM results in a product with a rumen-escape of 70 to 75% without affecting intestinal digestibility as measured in swine.

RUMEN PROTECTED AMINO ACIDS

The most limiting amino acids for ruminants

Direct evidence as provided by abomasal or duodenal infusion studies indicates that Lys and Met are generally the two most limiting AA for protein synthesis in growing ruminants (Merchen and Titgemeyer, 1992) and lactating dairy cows (Rulquin and Vérité, 1993; Schwab *et al.*, 1993). This should not be too surprising given the combined observations that: (1) Met and Lys are first and second limiting in microbial protein for N retention in growing sheep (Nimrick *et al.*, 1970; Storm and Ørskov, 1984) and cattle (Richardson and Hatfield, 1978), (2) most feed proteins have lower amounts of Lys and Met, particularly of Lys, than ruminally synthesized bacterial protein (Table 1), (3) the contribution of Lys to total EAA in UDP often is slightly lower than in the same feeds before exposure to ruminal fermentation, and (4) Lys and Cys are more susceptible to processing effects and may have lower intestinal digestibilities than other EAA in UDP. Regarding the last point, it is noteworthy that intestinal digestibilities of Lys and Cys usually are lower than of other AA for swine and poultry.

The sequence of Lys and Met limitation is determined by their relative concentrations in UDP. For example, Lys is first-limiting when corn and corn-byproducts provide most of the UDP for growing cattle and lactating dairy cows whereas Met is first-limiting when little UDP is fed or when most of the UDP is provided by legume or animal-derived proteins (Merchen and Titgemeyer, 1992; Rulquin and Vérité, 1993; Schwab *et al.*, 1992a). Feeds of corn origin are low in Lys and higher in Met while legume and animal-derived proteins are low in Met and higher in Lys (Table 1).

The need for ruminally protected lysine and methionine

There is a need for ruminally protected forms of Lys (RPLys) and Met (RPMet) because most feeds contain low amounts of Lys, Met, or both. In turn, the need is greatest when rations are balanced for high levels of production and UDP provides a larger portion of total absorbable AA. This is most evident by comparing the required contributions of Lys and Met to total EAA in duodenal digesta of lactating dairy cows (Table 4) with measurements of the same when cows were fed a variety of corn-based diets (Table 5). Collectively, the data presented in Tables 1, 4, and 5 indicate the difficulty of meeting the desired levels of both Lys and Met in duodenal digesta when corn-based diets are fed. Moreover, the data indicate

Table 4. Determination of the required contributions (%) of Lys and Met to total EAA[1] in duodenal digesta of lactating dairy cows for maximum yield of milk protein when cows consumed conventional corn-based diets.[2]

Lys	Reference	Met	Reference
14.9	Rulquin *et al.* (1990)[3]	≥ 5.1	Rulquin *et al.* (unpublished)[5]
14.8			
		≥ 5.3	Socha and Schwab[6]
15.2	Schwab *et al.* (1992b)[4]	5.3	(unpublished)
14.0			
14.5			
14.7	Average	≥ 5.3	Average

[1] Essential AA; includes Arg, His, Ile, Leu, Lys, Met, Phe, Thr, and Val.
[2] The experiments involved graded infusions of Lys (in the presence of constant supplemental Met) and Met (in the presence of constant supplemental Lys) into the duodenum with simultaneous measurement of milk and milk protein production and AA flows to the small intestine.
[3] Midlactation cows were injected with 30 mg d^{-1} bST and fed protein at 90 or 110% of CP requirements. Each experiment was a replicated 4 x 4 Latin square.
[4] Four cows were assigned to 4 x 4 Latin squares at 4 wk, 14-16 wk, and 21-23 wk postcalving. Rations were balanced to meet 90-100% of CP requirements.
[5] Five cows were assigned to a 5 x 5 Latin square at 4-6 wk postcalving. The ration was formulated to meet 115% of CP requirements.
[6] Five cows were assigned to 5 x 5 Latin squares at 2 wk and 11-13 wk postcalving. Rations were formulated to meet or slightly exceed protein requirements.

Table 5. Comparison of seven studies of the effect of ration composition (excluding fat, mineral and vitamin supplements) on measured passage of Lys and Met to the duodenum of Holstein cows during the first 150 d of lactation.[1]

Item	References[2]						
	1[2]	2	3	4	5	6	7
Diet ingredients (% DM)							
Alfalfa hay			10.0		13.3	26.0	45.4
Alfalfa silage	25.0			30.0			
Corn silage	25.0	26.2	28.7	20.0	28.5	5.0	
Grass-legume silage		14.2					
Corn	40.9	24.7	25.5	40.0	27.1	30.2	34.6
Wheat byproducts		9.4					
Beet pulp						12.3	
Soyhulls			12.5		4.0		8.3
Soybean meal		9.0	16.1	4.0	8.5	4.0	
Roasted soybeans					4.8		6.0
Whole cottonseed					9.0	9.0	
Distiller's grains		9.8	4.7		1.8		1.8
Brewer's grains						8.0	
Corn gluten meal	.9						
Blood meal	2.1						
Feather meal	.3						
Fish meal	1.5			4.0			
Meat meal	.6						
Animal/fish blend						1.5	
Urea	.2						
Diet CP (% DM)	16.2	17.3	17.3	18.1	19.6	19.7	19.0
Flow to duodenum (g d⁻¹)							
Total EAA	1619	1353	1384	1395	1840	1836	1924
Lys	217	179	194	164	249	235	246
Met	61	55	61	52	64	64	63
Flow to duodenum (% EAA)							
Lys	13.4	13.2	14.0	11.8	14.1	13.7	13.9
Met	3.8	4.1	4.4	3.7	4.5	4.6	4.6

[1] Intakes of DM averaged 21.3 kg d⁻¹ (range = 18.2 to 23.5).
[2] References: (1) Christensen *et al.*, 1993; (2) Schwab *et al.*, 1992b; (3) Cunningham *et al.*, 1993; (4) Klusmeyer *et al.*, 1991; and (5, 6 and 7) Cunningham *et al.*, 1991.

that complementary sources of supplemental UDP can be selected to achieve the desired Lys to Met ratio in duodenal digesta of lactating cows but levels of neither will be high enough in total ration UDP to optimize intestinal AA balance. It is expected from studies designed to determine the sequence of AA limitation in ruminants (Schwab *et al.*, 1976, 1992a;

Rulquin, 1987; Fraser *et al.*, 1991) along with the compositional data presented in Table 1 that balancing UDP for other EAA can be accomplished by complementary feed proteins without the use of large amounts of high-UDP, unbalanced feed proteins (e.g., corn gluten meal, blood meal, and feather meal).

Methods for protecting free amino acids

Numerous approaches have been evaluated during the last 25-30 years for protecting selected AA from ruminal degradation. Technologically, most of the approaches fall into one of three categories; synthesis of analogs and derivatives, encapsulation with lipids, and encapsulation with ruminally inert, pH-sensitive materials.

Amino acid derivatives and analogs. Free AA are unstable and degraded rapidly in the rumen. However, it was hypothesized by some researchers in the early 1970's that AA derivatives (a free AA to which a chemical blocking group is added to the α-amino group or in which the acyl group is modified) or analogs (e.g. substitution of the α-amino group with a non-nitrogenous group) might be identified that would be resistant to ruminal degradation, be absorbable from the small intestine, and be capable of conversion to the desired AA either before or after absorption. As a result, many derivatives and analogs, particularly those of Met, have been screened for their resistance to destruction by ruminal microorganisms. Most of these are listed in Table 6, categorized by Loerch and Oke (1989) for expected potential to escape ruminal degradation.

Although data are limited and different methods of evaluation were used, Loerch and Oke (1989) concluded from their literature review that of the derivatives, those with long side-chains such as N-stearoyl-DL-Met, N-oleoyl-DL-Met, and capryl-caproylic-Met are the most resistant to ruminal degradation. All three derivatives produced less methyl mercaptan than free Met in the rumen of sheep (Buttery *et al.*, 1977; Ayoade *et al.*, 1982). Depending on the level of the dose, ruminal administration of stearoyl-Met increased the amount of total Met reaching the duodenum of sheep by 20 to 50% (Langar *et al.*, 1978). Passage of Met to the duodenum of steers was greater for oleoyl-Met than for either free Met or N-hydroxymethyl-Met (Heath *et al.*, 1977). In contrast, feeding or intraruminal dosing of the other derivatives and analogs such as N-acetyl-DL-Met and DL-homocysteine thiolactone HCl (Amos *et al.*, 1974) and Met hydroxy analog (DL-α-hydroxy-γ-mercaptobutyrate) (MHA) (Langar *et al.*, 1978; Jones *et al.*, 1988) resulted in little or no recovery from abomasal or duodenal digesta.

The most studied AA analogs are MHA, N-hydroxymethyl-DL-Met-Ca, and di-hydroxymethyl-L-Lys-Ca. Because of apparent low abomasal recoveries, these analogs cannot be considered protected forms of Met and Lys (Kenna and Schwab, 1981; Loerch and Oke, 1989). Nevertheless, the calcium salt of MHA has been studied extensively as a supplement for increasing milk and milk fat production. Metabolically, MHA is equivalent to Met in both chicks and rats. Although little or no MHA escapes ruminal degradation, there is evidence of preintestinal absorption of MHA and as well as of several esters of Met (Ferguson, 1975; Ayoade *et al.*, 1982). Feeding MHA often influences ruminal fermentation (e.g. increased counts of protozoa or bacteria and altered concentrations of volatile fatty

Table 6. Methionine derivatives and analogs which have been investigated for level of rumen protection.

Some protection	Little or no protection	Conflicting evidence
N-stearoyl-DL-methionine	N-acetyl-DL-methionine	DL-homocysteine thiolactone HCL
N-oleoyl-DL-methionine	N-formyl-DL-methionine	N-hydroxymethyl-DL-
Capryl-caproylic-methionine	Poly-L-methionine	methionine Ca salt
Methionine ethyl ester HCl	Methionine hydroxy analog	
Methionyl DL-methionine	Methionine hydroxy analog	
Benzoyl-L-methionine	methyl ester	
N-phthalyl-DL-methionine	3-hydroxydihydro-2(3H)-thiophenone	
	Phenyl-γ-methyl mercapto-α-	
N-t-butyloxycarbonyl-L-methionine-	hydroxybutyrate	
dicylohexyl ammonium salt	Methyl-γ-methyl mercapto-α-	
N-t-butyloxycarbonyl-L-methionine-	hydroxybutyrate	
ρ-nitrophenyl ester	Methionine sulfoxide	
N-propionyl-DL-methionine	DL-methionine amide HCL	
N-carbobenzoxy-DL-methionine	DL-methionine sulfone	
3-benzoyloxydihydro-2-(3-H)-	DL-methionine methyl ester HCl	
thiophenone	DL-2-ureido-4-methylthiobutyric	
Glycyl-DL-methionine	acid	
	N-acetyl-DL-homocysteine	
	thiolactone	
	N-formyl-DL-methionine	
	DL-methionine	
	N-benzoyl-DL-methionine amide	
	N-benzoyl-DL-methionine methyl	
	ester	
	DL-methionine methyl sulfonium	
	chloride	
	DL-homocysteine	
	N-octanoyl-DL-methionine	
	N-lauryl-DL-methionine	
	N-lauryl-DL-homocysteine	
	thiolactone	
	N-benzoyl-DL-homocysteine	
	thiolactone	
	N-lauryl-DL-methionine methyl	
	ester	
	N-lauryl-DL-methionine ethyl ester	
	N-acetyl-DL-methionine ethyl ester	

From Loerch and Oke (1989).

acids), diet digestibility, and lipid metabolism (e.g. changes in serum lipoproteins). For more details on MHA, the reader is referred to the excellent review by Loerch and Oke (1989).

Encapsulation with lipids. Many laboratories have pursued the use of fats and oils, often in combination with inorganic materials and carbohydrates as stabilizers, softening agents and fillers, for protecting free AA from ruminal degradation. This approach is attractive because coating materials are readily available and because the ingredients are generally recognized as safe, allowing for rapid government approval. With few exceptions, this technology has been limited to the protection of Met.

Early studies provided encouragement. Delmar Chemicals of Canada developed a product composed of 20% DL-Met, 20% colloidal kaolin, and 60% tristearin (Sibbald *et al.*, 1968). Physically, the product consisted of a core of Met, kaolin, and tristearin enveloped in a continuous film of tristearin. The final material was small beads ranging from 0.3 to 1.0 mm in diameter with a specific gravity of 1.18 - 1.20. Neudoerffer *et al.* (1971) reported that 70% of the Met remained with the beads following suspension for 18 h in nylon bags in the rumen and that about 12% remained encapsulated after successive incubations in abomasal and intestinal juices. The authors concluded that 60 - 65% of the Met would be available for intestinal absorption. Grass and Unangst (1972) reported that the intestinal release of Met from the product was poor and that it could be improved, without compromising ruminal protection, by substituting kaolin and some of the tristearin with $CaCO_3$ and oleic acid. Rumen Kjemi a/s, Oslo, Norway introduced a product (Ketionin®) of two particle sizes (2.1 and 3.5 mm) that contained 30% DL-Met, 2% glucose, 4% flavoring, antioxidant and stabilizing agents, 6% $CaCO_3$, and 58% fatty acids (U.S. Patent No. 3,959,493). Daugaard (1978) concluded that 80% of the product escaped ruminal degradation and that 20% was lost in the feces of lactating dairy cows. Arambel *et al.* (1987) reported similar findings when the protected Met product was fed to growing heifers; 72% escaped ruminal degradation and 19% was excreted in the feces. As expected, all of these as well as similar other products are effective in increasing plasma Met in ruminants (Loerch and Oke, 1989).

Since the introduction of these early lipid-protected Met products, many others have been developed. Several patents have been issued and numerous growth and lactation experiments have been conducted to demonstrate production responses and product efficacy. In some cases, marketing has been attempted. However, for most products, strict *in vivo* determinations of ruminal escape and intestinal availability are not available. Incubation in the rumen for short periods of time, quick *in vitro* tests, and measurements of plasma levels of the test AA are all useful techniques for demonstrating that ruminal escape and intestinal release occurs and for comparing the relative efficacy of RPAA products. However, these techniques do not replace the use of duodenally and ileally cannulated animals for quantification and claims of ruminal escape and intestinal release. Certainly, milk production and milk fat responses are not appropriate response criteria for evaluating sources of RPMet as free Met or analogs of Met such as MHA may provide similar responses (Kaufmann and Lüpping, 1982; Loerch and Oke, 1989).

The challenge of protecting free AA with lipids has been to identify a combination of process and coating materials that will provide a consistent product with both high ruminal escape and intestinal release, a high payload of AA, and resistance to the mechanical and thermal stresses of storage and handling. Recently, Degussa Corp. introduced a protected Met product (Mepron®85) which contains 85% DL-Met and small amounts of ash, starch, fat and cellulose. Physically, the product consists of a nucleus of Met and starch enveloped with several thin coats of stearic acid and ethylcellulose. The small pellets measure 1.8 mm in diameter and 3-4 mm in length and have a specific gravity (density) of 1.2 g cm^{-3}. The technology is a novel combination of coating ingredients and application that increases the payload of AA but which, like other lipid-coated products, relies on the sensitivity of the coating to digestive enzymes for ruminal protection and intestinal release. The result is a slow-release product; nylon bag studies indicate protection rates that approximate 90% at 2 h, 80% at 6 h, and 70% at 15 h (Degussa bulletin Ch 691-1-205-294V).

Encapsulation with ruminally-inert, pH-sensitive polymers. To date, this approach has been the most efficient means of delivering supplemental AA and other rumen-labile compounds to the small intestine. By coating (or overcoating) ruminally degradable materials with enzymatically-inert materials that are insoluble in the more neutral pH environment of ruminal digesta (pH = 5 to 7) but which are soluble in the acidic abomasum (pH = 2 to 3), a postruminal delivery system is achieved that is independent of digestive enzyme function and, therefore, of residence time in the rumen. The result is a rumen-stable product rather than a slow-release product. While this approach has the advantage of biological effectiveness, it has the disadvantages of being more costly and requiring governmental approval.

Early studies by Australian and German scientists indicted that imidamine polymers, cellulose propionate-3-morpholino butyrate, and the copolymers poly(*t*-butylaminoethyl methacrylate: styrene) and poly(dimethylaminoethyl methacrylate:styrene) all provided good ruminal protection (Chalupa, 1975; Ferguson, 1975). The use of these and other pH-sensitive polymers was pursued by Eastman Kodak Co., USA. The evaluation of a Met product composed of DL-Met coated with cellulose propionate morpholinobutyrate indicated excellent ruminal protection and intestinal release. *In vitro* incubation (17 h in pH 5.5 rumen fluid) and nylon bag studies (24 h in the rumen of sheep) both resulted in recoveries of greater than 96%, while exposure to abomasal fluid for 30 min completely removed the coating (Komarek and Jandzinski, 1978). Coating DL-Met or L-Lys with a copolymer of styrene and 2-methyl-5-vinyl pyridine also provided impressive results (Dannelly *et al.*, 1980). Both products were 94-95% stable in acetate buffer (pH 5.4 for 24 h) and 94-95% of each AA was released in citrate buffer (pH 2.9 for 1 h) (Papas *et al.*, 1984; Polan *et al.*, 1991); 96% of the RPMet-N remained in dacron bags after 48 h of ruminal incubation (Wright and Loerch, 1988). Follow-up studies indicated that both of the polymer coating systems developed by Eastman Kodak Co. were highly effective in increasing the supply of absorbable Met and Lys to the small intestine of sheep, cattle, and lactating dairy cows (Wright and Loerch, 1988; Loerch and Oke, 1989).

A concern of the Kodak products was their stability in silage-containing diets. Published data in this regard appears to be limited to the copolymer of styrene and 2-methyl-5-vinyl pyridine.

Papas *et al.* (1984) reported Met recoveries of greater than 80% and 70% after incubating RPMet in a silage-diet of pH 4.5 - 4.7 for 2 h and 18 h, respectively; the recovery was 60 - 70% after 18 h in a silage-diet of pH 4.1 - 4.3. In contrast, Polan *et al.* (1991) reported that incubating RPMet and RPLys in silage-containing total mixed rations or in corn silage alone for 8-12 h consistently resulted in AA recoveries exceeding 90%.

The patent rights for the use of pH-sensitive polymers in postruminal delivery systems are currently held by Rhone-Poulenc Animal Nutrition. This has led to the introduction of Smartamine™ M and Smartamine™ ML, rumen-stable forms of Met and Met plus Lys. The products contain 70% DL-Met or 15% DL-Met plus 50% L-Lys-HCl and consist of a core of AA plus ethylcellulose which is covered with a coat of stearic acid containing small droplets of poly(2-vinylpyridine-co-styrene). The small beads measure 2 mm in diameter and contain 3% by weight of the copolymer. Nylon bag studies indicate ruminal stability exceeding 90% at 24 h and intestinal availability values approximating 90% (determined either by the amount released after 1 h in a pH 2.0 HCl-pepsin solution or by the mobile bag technique following exposure to the HCl-pepsin solution) (Rhone-Poulenc bulletin). The technology is currently approved and marketed within the EC, it was recently approved for beef and dairy in Canada and for beef in the U.S., and approval is pending for dairy in the U.S.

Responses to improved Lys and Met nutrition

Production responses to improved Lys and Met nutrition include variable increases in growth rates of lightweight cattle (e.g. Oke *et al.*, 1986; Lubsy, 1993; Van Amburgh *et al.*, 1993), wool and mohair growth of sheep and angora goats (Loerch and Oke, 1989), and content and yield of milk protein, milk production, and feed intake of dairy cows. As summarized by Rulquin and Vérité (1993) and Schwab *et al.* (1993), experiments with dairy cows confirm the expected; namely, that responses to postruminal Lys and Met supplementation are greater when basal levels of Lys and Met in UDP are low rather than high, when intake of UDP is high rather than low, when cows are in early lactation rather than mid or late lactation, and in high producing cows rather than low producing cows. Further, it is noteworthy that: (1) content of milk protein is more sensitive than milk yield to duodenal concentrations of Lys and Met, (2) increasing duodenal concentrations of Lys and Met increase only the casein fraction of milk protein and not the whey and NPN fractions, (3) increasing duodenal concentrations of Lys and Met often increase content of milk protein more than would be expected by increasing ration CP, (4) the relationship between duodenal concentrations of Lys and Met and content and yield of milk protein is described by typical curves of diminishing increments (Rulquin *et al.*, 1993), and (5) increases in milk yield to supplemental Lys and Met generally are limited to cows in early lactation when the need for absorbable AA, relative to absorbable energy, is greatest.

The obvious advantage of improving the balance of absorbable AA is the increased efficiency of use of absorbed AA for protein production. It has been demonstrated that improved Lys and Met nutrition reduces the amount of dietary CP needed to achieve similar yields of milk and milk protein. A reduction of ration CP not only improves efficiency of protein synthesis but it also provides more "room" in the diet to meet other critical needs of ruminal fermentation or of the host animal.

There may be other more subtle or indirect benefits of optimizing Lys and Met nutrition. As examples, Durand *et al.* (1992) observed an enhanced ability of the liver to secrete triglyceride-rich VLDL when 20 g per day of Lys and 10 g per day of Met were infused into the mesenteric veins of early lactation dairy cows, C. Chapoutot, P. Schmidely, D. Sauvant, P. Bousquin, J.C. Robert and B.K. Sloan (unpublished) observed a significant reduction in blood nonesterfied fatty acids when Smartamine™ ML was fed to lactating dairy cows, and Rulquin (personal communication) observed a reduction in post-calving metabolic disorders when dairy cows were fed Smartamine™ ML from about two weeks before calving through the first four weeks of lactation. These observations may be related and result, at least in part, from a normalization of lipid metabolism.

CONCLUSIONS

Many of the challenges associated with protecting feed proteins and selected AA from ruminal degradation have been overcome. Nevertheless, technologies must continue to be refined. Researchers must continue to seek methods of protecting feed proteins that will decrease postruminal losses and of encapsulating free AA that will increase delivery of absorbable AA per unit cost of product. After nearly three decades of research, suitable sources of RPAA are becoming available for commercial use. With the use of sound models for predicting their need, RPAA give producers their first opportunity to optimize the balance of AA in UDP. This has the advantages of reducing the amount of UDP required to achieve a given level of protein production and of improving the prediction of animal responses from UDP.

ACKNOWLEDGMENTS

The author gratefully acknowledges Nancy Whitehouse for her dedicated assistance with manuscript preparation.

REFERENCES

Ainslie, S.J., Fox, D.G., Perry, T.C., Ketchen, D.J. and Barry, M.C. 1993. Predicting amino acid adequacy of diets fed to Holstein steers. *J. Anim. Sci.* **71**, 1312-1319.

Amos, H.E., Little, C.O., Digenis, G.A., Schelling, G.T., Tucker, R.E. and Mitchell, Jr., G.E. 1974. Methionine, DL-homocysteine thiolactone and N-acetyl-DL-methionine for ruminants. *J. Anim. Sci.* **39**, 612-617.

Arambel, M.J., Bartley, E.E., Camac, J.L., Dennis, S.M., Nagaraja, T.G. and Dayton, A.D. 1987. Rumen degradability and intestinal availability of a protected methionine product and its effects on rumen fermentation, and passage rate of nutrients. *Nutr. Rep. Int.* **35**, 661-672.

Ashes, J.R., Mangan, J.L. and Sidhu, G.S. 1984. Nutritional availability of amino acids from protein cross-linked to protect against degradation in the rumen. *Br. J. Nutr.* **52**, 239-247.

Ayoade, J.A., Buttery, P.J. and Lewis, D. 1982. Studies on methionine derivatives as possible sources of protected methionine in ruminant rations. *J. Sci. Food Agric.* **33**, 949-956.

Bae, H.D., McAllister, T.A., Yanke, J., Cheng, K.J. and Muir, A.D. 1993. Effects of condensed tannins on endoglucanase activity and filter paper digestion by *Fibrobacter succinogenes* S85. *Appl. Environ. Microbiol.* **59**, 2132-2138.

Beever, D.E. and Thomson, D.J. 1981. The potential of protected proteins in ruminant nutrition. In *Recent Developments in Ruminant Nutrition* (W. Haresign and D.J.A. Cole, D.J.A. eds) pp. 82-98. Butterworths, London, UK.

Black, A.L., Kleiber, M., Smith, A.H. and Stewart, D.N. 1957. Acetate as a precursor of amino acids of casein in the intact dairy cow. *Biochim. Biophys. Acta.* **23**, 54-59.

Bozak, C.K., Schwab, C.G. and Nocek, J.E. 1986. Changes in amino acid pattern of feed proteins upon exposure to rumen fermentation using the *in situ* bag technique. *J. Dairy Sci.* **69** (Suppl. 1), 108. (Abstract).

Broderick, G.A. and Craig, W.M. 1980. Effect of heat treatment on ruminal degradation and escape, and intestinal digestibility of cottonseed meal protein. *J. Nutr.* **110**, 2381-2389.

Broderick, G.A., Wallace, R.J. and Ørskov, E.R. 1991. Control of rate and extent of protein degradation. In *Physiological Aspects of Digestion and Metabolism in Ruminants* (T. Tsuda, Y. Sasaki, and R. Kawashima, eds) pp. 541-592. Academic Press, Tokyo, Japan.

Buttery, P.J., Manomai-Udom, S. and Lewis, D. 1977. Preliminary investigations on some potential sources of protected methionine derivatives for ruminant rations. *J. Sci. Food Agric.* **28**, 481-485.

Calsamiglia, S. and Stern, M.D. 1993. A three step procedure to estimate postruminal protein digestion in ruminants. *J. Dairy Sci.* **76** (Suppl. 1), 176. (Abstract).

Carpenter, K.J. and Booth, V.H. 1973. Damage to lysine in food processing: its measurement and significance. *Nutr. Abstr. Rev.* **43**, 423-451.

Cecava, M.J., Hancock, D.L. and Parker, J.E. 1993. Effects of zinc-treated soybean meal on ruminal fermentation and intestinal amino acid flows in steers fed corn silage-based diets. *J. Anim. Sci.* **71**, 3423-3431.

Chalmers. M.I., Cuthberston, D.P. and Synge, R.L.M. 1954. Ruminal ammonia formation in relation to the protein requirement of sheep. I. Duodenal administration and heat processing as factors influencing fate of casein supplements. *J. Agric. Sci., Camb.* **44**, 254-262.

Chalupa, W. 1975. Rumen bypass and protection of proteins and amino acids. *J. Dairy Sci.* **58**, 1198-1218.

Christensen, R.A., Cameron, M.R., Klusmeyer, T.H., Elliott, J.P., Clark, J.H., Nelson, D.R. and Yu, Y. 1993. Influence of amount and degradability of dietary protein on nitrogen utilization by dairy cows. *J. Dairy Sci.* **76**, 3496-3513.

Clark, J.H., Klusmeyer, T.H. and Cameron, M.R. 1992. Microbial protein synthesis and flows of nitrogen fractions to the duodenum of dairy cows. *J. Dairy Sci.* **75**, 2304-2323.

Cleale, R.M., Britton, R.A., Klopfenstein, T.J., Bauer, M.L., Harmon, D.L. and Satterlee, L.D. 1987a. Induced non-enzymatic browning of soybean meal. II. Ruminal escape and net portal absorption of soybean protein treated with xylose. *J. Anim. Sci.* **65**, 1319-1326.

Cleale, R.M., Klopfenstein, T.J., Britton, R.A., Satterlee, L.D., and Lowry, S.R. 1987b. Induced non-enzymatic browning of soybean meal. I. Effects of factors controlling non-enzymatic browning on *in vitro* ammonia release. *J. Anim. Sci.* **65**, 1312-1318.

Cleale, R.M., Klopfenstein, T.J., Britton, R.A., Satterlee, L.D., and Lowry, S.R. 1987c. Induced non-enzymatic browning of soybean meal. III. Digestibility and efficiency of protein utilization by ruminants of soybean meal treated with xylose or glucose. *J. Anim. Sci.* **65**, 1327-1335.

Craig, W.M. and Broderick, G.A. 1981. Effect of treatment on true digestibility in the rat, *in vitro* proteolysis and available lysine content of cottonseed meal protein. *J. Anim Sci.* **52**, 292-301.

Cunningham, K.D., Lykos, T.L., Whitehouse, N.L. and Schwab, C.G. 1991. Effect of ration on amino acid flow to the small intestine in early lactation Holstein cows. *J. Dairy Sci.* **74** (Suppl. 1), 179. (Abstract).

Cunningham, K.D., Cecava, M.J. and Johnson, T.T. 1993. Nutrient digestion, nitrogen, and amino acid flows in lactating cows fed soybean hulls in place of forage or concentrate. *J. Dairy Sci.* **76**, 3523-3535.

Dannelly, C.C., Ardell, R.E. and Parr, G. E. 1980. Rumen-stable pellets. U.S. Patent 4,181,710.

Daugaard, J. 1978. Investigation on methionine supplement to lactating cows. Ph.D. Thesis, The Royal Veterinary and Agricultural University, Copenhagen, Denmark.

de Boer, G., Murphy, J.J and Kennelly, J.J. 1987. Mobile nylon bag for estimating intestinal availability of rumen undegradable protein. *J. Dairy Sci.* **70**, 977-982.

Downes, A.M. 1961. On the amino acids essential for the tissues of the sheep. *Aust. J. Biol. Sci.* **14**, 254-259.

Durand, D., Chilliard, Y. and Bauchart, D. 1992. Effects of lysine and methionine on *in vivo* hepatic secretion of VLDL in the high yielding dairy cow. *J. Dairy Sci.* **75** (Suppl. 1), 279. (Abstract).

Faldet, M.A., Voss. V.L., Broderick, G.A. and Satter, L.D. 1991. Chemical, *in vitro*, and *in situ* evaluation of heat-treated soybean proteins. *J. Dairy Sci.* **74**, 2548-2554.

Faldet, M.A., Satter, L.D. and Broderick, G.A. 1992a. Determining optimal heat treatment of soybeans by measuring available lysine chemically and biologically with rats to maximize protein utilization by ruminants. *J. Nutr.* **122**, 151-160.

Faldet, M.A., Son, Y.S. and Satter, L.D. 1992b. Chemical, *in vitro*, and *in vivo* evaluation of soybeans heat-treated by various processing methods. *J. Dairy Sci.* **75**, 789-795.

Feeney, R.E. 1977. Chemical changes in food proteins. In *Evaluation of Proteins for Humans* (C.E. Bodwell, ed.) pp. 233-254. AVI, US.

Ferguson, K.A. 1975. The protection of dietary proteins and amino acids against microbial fermentation in the rumen. In *Digestion and Metabolism in the Ruminant* (I.W. McDonald and A.C.I. Warner, eds) pp. 448-464. University of New England Unit, Armidale, NSW, Australia.

Ferguson, K.A., Hemsley, J.A. and Reis, P.J. 1967. Nutrition and wool growth. The effect of protecting dietary protein from microbial degradation in the rumen. *Aust. J. Sci.* **30**, 215-217.

Finot, P.A., Bujard, E., Mottu, F. and Mauron, J. 1977. Availability of the true Schiff's bases of lysine. Chemical evaluation of the Schiff's base between lysine and lactose in milk. *Adv. Exp. Med. Biol.* **86B**, 343-365.

Fraser, D.L., Ørskov, E.R., Whitelaw, F.G. and Franklin, M.F. 1991. Limiting amino acids in dairy cows given casein as the sole source of protein. *Livest. Prod. Sci.* **28**, 235-252.

Frydrych, Z. 1992. Intestinal digestibility of rumen undegraded protein of various feeds as estimated by the mobile bag technique. *Anim. Feed Sci. Tech.* **37**, 161-172.

Grass, G.M. and Unangst, R.R. 1972. Glycerol tristearate and higher fatty acid mixtures for improving digestive absorption. US patent 3,655,864.

Harrison, D.G., Beever, D.E. and Osbourn, D.F. 1979. The contribution of protozoa to the protein entering the duodenum of sheep. *Br. J. Nutr.* **41**, 521-527.

Heath, D.G., Owens, F.N. and Weakley, D.C. 1977. Methionine complexes for steers. *J. Anim. Sci.* **45** (Suppl. 1), 239. (Abstract).

Hurrell, R.F. and Finot, R.A. 1985. Effect of food processing on protein digestibility and amino acid availability. In *Digestibility and Amino Acid Availability in Cereals and Oilseeds* (J.W. Finley and D.T. Hopkins, eds) pp. 233-258. American Association of Cereal Chemists, St. Paul, MN, US.

Hvelplund, T. 1985. Digestibility of rumen microbial protein and undegraded protein estimated in the small intestine of sheep and by *in sacco* procedure. *Acta Agric. Scand. Suppl.* **25**, 132-144.

Hvelplund, T. and Hesselholt, M. 1987. Digestibility of individual amino acids in rumen microbial protein and undegraded dietary protein in the small intestine of sheep. *Acta Agric. Scand.* **37**, 469-477.

Jacobson, D.R., Van Horn, H.H. and Sniffen, C.J. 1970. Lactating ruminants. *Fed. Proc.* **29**, 35-40.

John, A. and Ulyatt, M.J. 1984. Measurement of protozoa, using phosphatidyl choline, and of bacteria, using nucleic acids, in the duodenal digesta of sheep fed chaffed lucerne hay (*Medicago sativa* L.) diets. *J. Agric. Sci., Camb.* **102**, 33-44.

Jones, B.A., Mohamed, O.E., Prange, R.W. and Satter, L.D. 1988. Degradation of methionine hydroxy analog in the rumen of lactating cows. *J. Dairy Sci.* **71**, 525-529.

Jones, G.A., McAllister, T.A., Muir, A.D. and Cheng, K.J. 1994. Effects of sainfoin (*Onobrychis viciifolia* Scop.) condensed tannins on growth and proteolysis by four strains of ruminal bacteria. *Appl. Environ. Microbiol.* **60**, 1374-1378.

Jones, W.T., Broadhurst, R.B. and Lyttleton, J.W. 1976. The condensed tannins of pasture legume species. *Phytochemistry*, **15**, 1407-1409.

Kaufmann, W. and Lüpping, W. 1982. Protected proteins and protected amino acids for ruminants. In *Protein Contribution of Feedstuffs for Ruminants: Application to Feed Formulation* (E.L. Miller, I.H. Pike and Van Es A.J.H., eds) pp. 36-75. Butterworth Scientific, London, UK.

Kenna, T.M. and Schwab, C.G. 1981. Evaluation of N-hydroxymethyl-DL-methionine-Ca and di-hydroxymethyl-L-lysine-Ca in a blended corn based ration for lactating cows. *J. Dairy Sci.* **64**, 775-781.

Klusmeyer, T.H., Lynch, G.L., Clark, J.H. and Nelson, D.R. 1991. Effects of calcium salts of fatty acids and protein source on ruminal fermentation and nutrient flow to duodenum of cows. *J. Dairy Sci.* **74**, 2206-2219.

Komarek, R.J. and Jandzinski, R.A. 1978. Rumen stability and postruminal delivery of methionine in rumen-protected form. *J. Anim. Sci.* **47** (Suppl. 1), 426. (Abstract).

Koupai-Abyazani, M.R., McCallum, J., Muir, A.D., Lees, G.L., Bohm, B.A., Towers, G.H.N. and Gruber, M.Y. 1993. Purification and characterization of a proanthocyanidin polymer from seed of alfalfa (*Medicago sativa* Cv. Beaver). *J. Agric. Food Chem.* **41**, 565-569.

Langar, P.N., Buttery, P.J. and Lewis, D. 1978. N-Stearoyl-D,L-methionine, a protected methionine source for ruminants. *J. Sci. Food Agric.* **29**, 808-814.

Loerch, S.C. and Oke, B.O. 1989. Rumen protected amino acids in ruminant nutrition. In *Absorption and Utilization of Amino Acids Vol III* (M. Friedman, ed.) pp. 187-200. CRC Press, Boca Raton, FL, US.

Lubsy, K.S. 1993. Rumen-stable methionine improves gain of lightweight cattle. *Feedstuffs* **65**, 14-16.

Lynch, G.L., Berger, L.L. and Fahey, Jr., G.C. 1987. Effects of ethanol, heat, and lipid treatment of soybean meal on nitrogen utilization by ruminants. *J. Dairy Sci.* **70**, 91-97.

Makkar, H.P.S. and Becker, K. 1994. Isolation of tannins from leaves of some trees and shrubs and their properties. *J. Agric. Food Chem.* **42**, 731-734.

Mangan, J.L., Jordan, D.J., West, J. and Webb, P.J. 1980. Protection of leaf protein of lucerne (*Medicago sativa* L.) against degradation in the rumen by treatment with formaldehyde and glutaraldehyde. *J. Agric. Sci., Camb.* **95**, 603-617.

McCance, R.A. and Widdowson, E. 1978. *The Composition of Foods, 4th ed.* (D.A.T. Southgate, and A.A. Paul, eds) HMSO, London, UK.

McNabb, W.C., Waghorn, G.C., Barry, T.N. and Shelton, I.D. 1993. The effect of condensed tannins in *Lotus pedunculatus* on the digestion and metabolism of methionine, cystine and inorganic sulfur in sheep. *Br. J. Nutr.* **70**, 647-661.

Merchen, N.R. and Titgemeyer, E.C. 1992. Manipulation of amino acid supply to the growing ruminant. *J. Anim. Sci.* **70**, 3238-3247.

Mir, Z., MacLeod, G.K., Buchanan-Smith, J.G., Grieve, D.G. and Grovum, W.L. 1984a. Effect of feeding soybean meal protected with sodium hydroxide, fresh blood, or fish hydrolyzate to growing calves and lactating dairy cows. *Can. J. Anim. Sci.* **64**, 845-852.

Mir, Z., MacLeod, G.K., Buchanan-Smith, J.G., Grieve, D.G. and Grovum, W.L. 1984b. Methods for protecting soybean and canola protein from degradation in the rumen. *Can. J. Anim. Sci.* **64**, 853-865.

Neudoerffer, T.S., Duncan, D.B. and Horney, F.D. 1971. The extent of release of encapsulated methionine in the intestine of cattle. *Br. J. Nutr.* **25**, 333-341.

Nimrick, K., Hatfield, E.E., Kaminski, J. and Owens. F.N. 1970. Qualitative assessment of supplemental amino acid needs for growing lambs fed urea as the sole nitrogen source. *J. Nutr.* **100**, 1293-1300.

Oldham, J.D., Bines, J.A. and MacRae, J.C. 1983. Milk production in cows infused abomasally with casein, glucose or aspartic and glutamic acids early in lactation. *Proc. Nutr. Soc.* **43**, 65A.

Oke, B.O., Loerch, S.C. and Deetz, L.E. 1986. Effects of rumen-protected methionine and lysine on ruminant performance and nutrient metabolism. *J. Anim. Sci.* **62**, 1101-1112.

Ørskov, E.R. 1992. *Protein Nutrition in Ruminants, 2nd ed.,* Academic Press, London, UK.

Papas, A.M., Sniffen, C.J. and Muscato, T.V. 1984. Effectiveness of rumen-protected methionine for delivering methionine postruminally in dairy cows. *J. Dairy Sci.* **67**, 545-552.

Parsons, C.M., Hashimoto, K., Wedekind, K.-J., Han, Y. and Baker, D.H. 1992. Effect of ovenprocessing on availability of amino acids and energy in soybean meal. *Poultry Sci.* **71**, 133-140.

Polan, C.E., Cummins, K.A., Sniffen, C.J., Muscato, T.V., Vicini, J.L., Crooker, B.A., Clark, J.H., Johnson, D.G., Otterby, D.E., Guillaume, B., Muller, L.D., Varga, G.A., Murray, R.A. and Peirce-Sandner, S.B. 1991. Responses of dairy cows to supplemental rumen-protected forms of methionine and lysine. *J. Dairy Sci.* **74**, 2997-3013.

Purser, D.B. and Buechler, S.M. 1966. Amino acid composition of rumen organisms. *J. Dairy Sci.* **49**, 81-84.

Rae, R.C. and Smithard, R.R. 1985. Estimation of true nitrogen digestibility in cattle by a modified nylon bag technique. *Proc. Nutr. Soc.* **44**, 116A.

Reid, C.S.W., Ulyatt, M.J. and Wilson, J.M. 1974. Plant tannins, bloat, and nutritive value. *Proc. NZ Soc. Anim. Prod.* **34**, 82-93.

Richardson, C.R. and Hatfield, E.E. 1978. The limiting amino acid in growing cattle. *J. Anim. Sci.* **46**, 740-745.

Rulquin, H. 1987. The determination of certain limiting amino acids in the dairy cow by post-ruminal administration. *Reprod. Nutr. Dev.* **27**, 299.

Rulquin, H. and Vérité, R. 1993. Amino acid nutrition of dairy cows: production effects and animal requirements. In *Recent Advances in Animal Nutrition* (P.C. Garnsworthy and D.J.A. Cole, eds) pp. 55-77. Nottingham University Press, UK.

Rulquin, H., Le Henaff, L. and Vérité, R. 1990. Effects on milk protein yield of graded levels of lysine infused into the duodenum of dairy cows fed diets with two levels of protein. *Reprod. Nutr. Dev.* (Suppl 2), 238S.

Rulquin, H., Pisulewski, P.M., Vérité, R. and Guinard, J. 1993. Milk production and composition as a function of postruminal lysine and methionine supply: a nutrient-response approach. *Livest. Prod. Sci.* **37**, 69-90.

Schwab, C.G., Satter, L.D. and Clay, A.B. 1976. Response of lactating dairy cows to abomasal infusion of amino acids. *J. Dairy Sci.* **59**, 1254.

Schwab, C. G., Bozak, C.K. and Nocek, J.E. 1986. Change in amino acid pattern of soybean meal and corn gluten meal upon exposure to rumen fermentation. *J. Anim. Sci.* **63** (Suppl. 1), 158. (Abstract).

Schwab, C.G., Bozak, C.K., Whitehouse, N.L. and Mesbah, M.M.A. 1992a. Amino acid limitation and flow to the duodenum at four stages of lactation. I. Sequence of lysine and methionine limitation. *J. Dairy Sci.* **75**, 3486-3502.

Schwab, C.G., Bozak, C.K., Whitehouse, N.L. and Olson, V.M. 1992b. Amino acid limitation and flow to the duodenum at four stages of lactation. II. Extent of lysine limitation. *J. Dairy Sci.* **75**, 3503-3518.

Schwab, C.G., Socha, M.T. and Whitehouse, N.L. 1993. Opportunities for rumen protected lysine and methionine in lactating dairy cow nutrition. Rhône-Poulenc Animal Nutrition Symposium, April 20, Guelph, Ontario, Mississauga, Ontario, pp. 3-28.

Sibbald, I.R., Loughheed, T.C. and Linton, J.H. 1968. A methionine supplement for ruminants. Proc. 2nd World Conf. Anim. Prod. pp. 453-457. Univ. of Maryland, College Park, MD, US.

Siddons, R.C., Arricastres, C., Gale, D.L. and Beever, D.E. 1984. The effect of formaldehyde or glutaraldehyde application to lucerne before ensiling on silage fermentation and silage N digestion in sheep. *Br. J. Nutr.* **52**, 391-401.

Siddons, R.C., Evans, R.T. and Beever, D.E. 1979. The effect of formaldehyde treatment before ensiling on the digestion of wilted grass silage by sheep. *Br. J. Nutr.* **42**, 535-545.

Stern, M.D., Rode, L.M., Prange, R.W., Stauffacher, R.H. and Satter, L.D. 1983. Ruminal protein degradation of corn gluten meal in lactating dairy cattle fitted with duodenal T-type cannulae. *J. Anim. Sci.* **56**, 194-204.

Storm, E. and Ørskov, E.R. 1983. The nutritive value of rumen micro-organisms in ruminants. 1. Large scale isolation and chemical composition of rumen micro-organisms. *Br. J. Nutr.* **50**, 463-470.

Storm, E. and Ørskov, E.R. 1984. The nutritive value of rumen micro-organisms in ruminants. 4. The limiting amino acids of microbial protein in growing sheep determined by a new approach. *Br. J. Nutr.* **52**, 613-620.

Storm, E., Brown, D.S. and Ørskov, E.R. 1983. The nutritive value of rumen micro-organisms in ruminants. 3. The digestion of microbial amino and nucleic acids in, and losses of endogenous from, the small intestine of sheep. *Br. J. Nutr.* **50**, 479-485.

Tamminga, S. 1979. Protein degradation in the forestomachs of ruminants. *J. Anim. Sci.* **49**, 1615-1630.

Tas, M.V., Evans, R.A. and Axford, R.F.E. 1981. The digestibility of amino acids in the small intestine of the sheep. *Br. J. Nutr.* **45**, 167-174.

Titgemeyer, E.C., Merchen, N.R. and Berger, L.L. 1989. Evaluation of soybean meal, corn gluten meal, blood meal and fish meal as sources of nitrogen and amino acids disappearing from the small intestine of steers. *J. Anim. Sci.* **67**, 262-275.

van Amburgh, M., Perry, T. , Fox, D. and Ducharme, G. 1993. Growth response of Holstein steers supplemented with rumen protected lysine and methionine. *J. Anim. Sci.* **71**, (Suppl. 1), 260. (Abstract).

van der Aar, P.J., Berger, L.L. and Fahey, Jr., G.C. 1982. The effect of alcohol treatments on solubility and *in vitro* and *in situ* digestibilities of soybean meal protein. *J. Anim. Sci.* **55**, 1179-1189.

van der Aar, P.J., Berger, L.L., Fahey, Jr., G.C. and Loerch, S.C. 1983. Effects of alcohol treatments on utilization of soybean meal by lambs and chicks. *J. Anim. Sci.* **57**, 511-518.

van der Aar, P.J., Berger, L.L., Fahey, Jr., G.C. and Merchen, N.R. 1984. Effect of alcohol treatments of soybean meal on ruminal escape of soybean meal protein. *J. Anim. Sci.* **59**, 483-489.

Veira, D.M., Ivan, M. and Jui, P.Y. 1983. Rumen ciliate protozoa: effects on digestion in the stomach of sheep. *J. Dairy Sci.* **66**, 1015-1022.

Waghorn, G.C. and Baldwin, R.L. 1984. Model of metabolite flux within mammary gland of the lactating cow. *J. Dairy Sci.* **67**, 531-544.

Waghorn, G.C. and Shelton, I.D. 1992. The nutritive value of *Lotus* for sheep. *Proc. N.Z. Soc. Anim. Prod.* **52**, 89-92.

Waldo, D.R. 1977. Potential of chemical preservation and improvement of forages. *J. Dairy Sci.* **60**, 306-326.

Waltz, D.M. and Loerch, S.C. 1986. Effect of acid and alkali treatment of soybean meal on nitrogen utilization by ruminants. *J. Anim Sci.* **63**, 879-887.

Waltz, D.M. and Stern, M.D. 1989. Evaluation of various methods for protecting soya-bean protein from degradation by rumen bacteria. *Anim. Feed Sci. Tech.* **25**, 111-122.

Waltz, D.M., Stern, M.D and Illg, D.J. 1989. Effect of ruminal protein degradation of blood meal and feather meal on the intestinal amino acid supply to lactating cows. *J. Dairy Sci.* **72**, 1509-1518.

Weller, R.A. and Pilgrim, A.F. 1974. Passage of protozoa and volatile fatty acids from the rumen of the sheep and from a continuous in vitro fermentation system. *Br. J. Nutr.* **32**, 341-351.

Windschitl, P.M. and Stern, M.D. 1988. Evaluation of calcium lignosulfonate-treated soybean meal as a source of rumen protected protein for dairy cattle. *J. Dairy Sci.* **71**, 3310-3322.

Wright, M.D. and Loerch, S.C. 1988. Effects of rumen-protected amino acids on ruminant nitrogen balance, plasma amino acid concentrations and performance. *J. Anim. Sci.* **66**, 2014-2027.

8 Antibacterials in poultry and pig nutrition

Gordon D. Rosen

66 Bathgate Road; Wimbledon, London SW19 5PH, UK

INTRODUCTION

The boundaries between nutritional and veterinary sciences and between health and disease are difficult, if not impossible, to define (Blaxter, 1979). Disease-free is an ideal most nearly approached in germ-free animals. In this review 'apparently-healthy' animals are those used in nutrition tests, reported without veterinary diagnoses or professional opinions of the presence of overt or sub-clinical disease. Nutrition improvers are defined as trace quantities of non-nutrient, antibacterial, medicinal substances used in the feed of apparently healthy poultry and pigs to provide specified nutritional and econometrical effects at defined rates of production or reproduction.

The nutritional effects of antibacterials in chicken feed were first reported by Moore *et al.* (1946). An early review by Braude *et al.* (1953) of antibiotics in swine nutrition contained tabulated data showing that responses varied greatly. In 91% of over 200 trials weight gain was improved but only 78% had improved feed efficiency. The magnitude of response was negatively (not inversely) proportional to control pig performance and the responses were increased by sub-optimum feeding, the presence of disease and in animals of low initial weight. Mixtures of antibiotics conferred no advantage; and the reduction of feed concentration in follow-on feeds reduced response. However the raw data were not statistically analysed and the reliance on overall mean relative response indices vitiates the comparison of effectiveness. Hence broad-spectrum antibiotics were erroneously judged superior to others, without any allowance for the influence of relative pig performance levels or applied feed concentrations.

Subsequently Vanschoubroek and de Wilde (1969) surveyed antibiotics in pig nutrition via 66 reports (27 of European origin). Overall results were described as very variable. Coefficients of variation in daily liveweight gain response for penicillin, tetracyclines, tylosin and zinc bacitracin ranged from 66-110%. They regarded observed differences between antibiotics as not greatly significant.

A report prepared for the US Congress Office of Technology Assessment reviewed the effectiveness of antibacterial feed additives in pig and poultry production over 27 years, with major emphases on modes of action and continued effectiveness (Hays, 1981). It listed 598 references, mostly US, with 25 of European origin. Tabulated summaries of 2,405 phases of tests up to 1977 on pigs, chicks, layers and turkeys versus negative controls substantially amplified earlier findings that antibacterials largely improved performance by control or prevention of disease. Responses were greater in starter than in finisher feeds. There was some evidence of a decreased response over the years. Hays stressed that concentrations recommended or selected for practical use did not necessarily elicit maximum response and that the decline in price of active ingredients allowed the use of higher feed concentrations than at the outset. Precise drug comparisons were not attempted, but Hays' data from 279 tests on 5,666 growing-finishing pigs illustrated topics in need of elucidation. Groupings of arsenicals, bacitracins, nitrofurans and tetracyclines prevent molecular distinctions; and differences in initial (15-27 kg) and final (61-94 kg) liveweights, as well as the absence of mean feed concentrations, preclude valid comparisons of relative effectiveness. Cromwell (1991) has recently extended Hays' studies for pigs by inclusion of more recent data for 1978-1986.

Only a very small fraction of known biosynthetic (antibiotic) and chemosynthetic antibacterials is used as nutrition improvers. They include arsenilic acid, avilamycin, avoparcin, bacitracin methylene disalicylate, carbadox, chlortetracycline, colistin, copper (sulfate, etc.), dimetridazole, efrotomycin, enramycin, erythromycin, flavophospholipol, furazolidone, ipronidazole, kitasamycin, lincomycin, neomycin, nitrovin, nosiheptide, olaquindox, oleandomycin, oxytetracycline, penicillin, polynactin, ronidazole, roxarsone, salinomycin, sedecemycin, spiramycin, streptomycin, thiopeptin, tylosin, virginiamycin and zinc bacitracin.

The estimation of nutritional dose-response relationships for antibacterials and the quantitative influence of other independent variable factors (Rosen, 1983, 1984) are basic objectives of continuing research towards more efficient use in practice of antibacterials in nutrition, avoiding pitfalls from the use of superficial or selected data. The latter influence is well illustrated in egg production response:control performance ratios for bacitracin in layers (Rosen, 1982). The average response over 79 tests (1.8/66, +2.7%) could be substantially improved by omission of the 20 worst results (3.1/65, +4.8%), while the 18 best responses (6.4/58) showed +11% improvement. The relevant nutritional literature on poultry and pigs has thousands of publications with a wealth of performance data from diverse conditions of use (Table 1).

Modes of action

More than four decades' research on modes of action has been reviewed from time to time, for example, by the National Academy of Sciences - National Research Council (1956), Menke & Krampitz (1973), O'Connor (1980), Hays (1981) and Muir (1985). While the main focus of this review is action, rather than modes of action, Table 2 contains an illustrative, non-exhaustive list of 43 such modes in four categories.

The demonstration of so many diverse modes accounts for the large variations observed in animal responses to dietary antibacterials. Presence or absence of any given mode or modes is normally unknown in the circumstances of a feeding test. As intestinal and environmental flora are incompletely characterised, differ widely and can fluctuate rapidly in numbers, this may predestine little or no difference between the mean nutritional values of antibacterials, as assessed from large collections of individual tests.

It may also explain why research on modes of action has not yet yielded improved antibacterial molecules for nutritional use. Bunyan et al. (1977) and Jeffries et al. (1977) were unable to correlate antibacterial spectra and mammalian absorption characteristics of 52 antimicrobial substances with their effects on chick feed consumption or bodyweight. The notion that a broad antibacterial spectrum means greater nutritional effectiveness has often been followed without substantive proof. In this context also no comprehensive quantitative relationships have yet been elaborated, relating mode(s) of action, or absorption dynamics, to nutritional dose-response functions.

Table 1. Numbers of controlled tests and published reports (1949-91)[1].

Substance	No. of tests			
	Chicken	Pig	Turkey	Layer
Avoparcin	379	154	24	-
Bacitracin	115	19	12	18
Bacitracin methylene disalicylate	554	47	171	54
Carbadox	-	527	-	-
Chlortetracycline	898	758	-	-
Chlortetracycline/sulphamethazine/ penicillin	-	322	-	-
Cyadox	-	70	-	-
Flavophospholipol	697	-	-	106
Lincomycin	121	-	-	-
Nitrovin	643	-	-	-
Olaquindox	-	268	-	-
Oxytetracycline	605	250	-	-
Tylosin	-	743	-	-
Virginiamycin	560	421	103	35
Zinc bacitracin	2,429	551	390	109
Total (12,153)	7,001	4,130	700	322
Number of published reports (4,301)	1,717	2,116	208	260

[1]From the author's data bank from 55 countries

Economics

Antibacterials as nutrition improvers are used to reduce animal production costs. The economic benefits gained spread across the food chain, split, according to local circumstances, between antibacterial manufacturers and distributors, animal feed premixers and compounders, animal producers, food processors, wholesalers and retailers and consumers.

Hays (1981) noted that improved methods of production and competition had reduced 1975 prices of commonly-used, feed-grade antibacterials to only 13-18% of those obtaining in 1950, thereby allowing consideration of the use of higher feed concentrations, as distinct from need due to any decline in effectiveness. Inflation in feedstuffs cost has also had important consequences for the use of antibacterials as exemplified for zinc bacitracin in broilers (Table 3).

Respective antibacterial and feed cost movements (1955-81) of -92% and +500% meant that 0.4% improvement in feed conversion in 1981 could defray the cost of 50 g tonne^{-1}, compared with 24% in 1955. Increases in antibacterial and feed price since 1981 have barely changed this scenario. Such changes demand a better understanding of dose-response relationships, in order to maximise the productivity benefits of antibacterials in nutrition.

Total feed additive use (nutritional and medicinal, non-prescription) in the US was 1,000 tonnes activity by 1963 and rose to 3,900 tonnes in 1987 (Cromwell, 1991). A world-wide order of magnitude of the quantities used in pig and poultry production can be assessed

Table 2. Modes of action of in-feed antibacterial nutritional additives.

Microbiological		Physiological	
Beneficial bacteria	+[1]	Gut food transit time	-
Adverse bacteria	-	Gut wall diameter	-
Transferable resistance	+ - 0	Gut wall length	-
Competition for nutrients by gut flora	-	Gut wall weight	-
Gut floral nutrient synthesis	+	Gut absorptive capacity	+
		Feed intake	+ - 0
Clostridium perfringens	-	Faecal moisture	-
Pathogenic *E. coli*	-	Mucosal cell turnover	-
Pathogenic streptococci	-	Stress	-
Beneficial lactobacilli	+		
Beneficial *E. coli*	+		
Debilitation of pathogens	+		

Nutritional		Metabolic	
Energy retention	+	Ammonia production	-
Gut energy loss	-	Toxic amine production	-
Nitrogen retention	+	Alpha-toxin production	-
Limiting amino acid supply	+	Mitochondrial fatty acid oxidation	-
Vitamin absorption	+	Bacterial cell wall synthesis	-
Trace element absorption	+	Bacterial DNA synthesis	-
Fatty acid absorption	+	Bacterial protein synthesis	-
Glucose absorption	+	Faecal fat excretion	-
Calcium absorption	+	Liver protein synthesis	+
Plasma nutrients	+	Gut alkaline phosphatase	+
		Gut urease	-

[1]+ denotes an increase; - a reduction; 0 no change.

as shown in Table 4. The total usage so indicated is of the order of 10,000 tonnes antibacterial activity per annum.

When the United States Food & Drug Administration (1972) Task Force reported on various aspects of the use of antibiotics in animal feeds it estimated economic values to animal producers for 1970 and the pharmaceutical industry for 1968-69 respectively as $33M and $2M for broilers, $14M and $0.6M for turkeys and $202M and $46M for pigs. The Council for Agricultural Science and Technology report (CAST, 1981) identified major problems in six published economic studies of the value to consumers of the sub-therapeutic use of antibiotics in US livestock and poultry feeds. From manifest over- and under-estimates, mean annual values for pork, broiler and turkey were $963M, $699M and $156M respectively. More recently, Craene and Viaene (1992) calculated that losses of economic benefit in the European Union, attributable to a withdrawal of antibacterial feed additive performance enhancers from broiler, pig and layer feeds, would total 763 and 701 million ECU per annum respectively for animal producers and consumers.

Table 3. Change in the cost and value of inclusion of zinc bacitracin in broiler diets between 1955 and 1993.

	1955	1968	1981	1993
Cost of antibacterial (£ g^{-1})	.12	.03	.01	.015
Feed cost (£ tonne^{-1})	25	35	125	175
Cost of 50 g activity tonne^{-}	6.0	1.5	0.5	0.75
Improvement needed (%)[1]	24	4.3	0.40	0.43

[1] Improvement in feed conversion needed to defray cost of antibacterial.

METHODOLOGY

Measurement of effectiveness and elaboration of nutritional models

The nutritional value of antibacterial feed additives are determined by means of properly designed feeding tests, as the differences between the performances of treated animals and otherwise-identical, untreated controls. Performance may be measured in terms of feed consumption, liveweight gain, feed conversion ratio, mortality, carcass characteristics, egg or piglet mass or progeny performance.

Table 4. An assessment of the world-wide use of antibacterials in diets for pigs and poultry.

Species	Feed production (10^6 tonnes)	Feed supplemented (%)	Mean concentration in feed (mg kg^{-1})	Quantity of antibacterial per annum (tonnes activity)
Broiler	100	90	30	2,700
Turkey	15	80	20	240
Pig	225	60	40	5,400
Layer	100	35	40	1,400

Efficacy tests need to encompass a wide range of breeds, feeds and management and environmental conditions in order to take into account the large variations in response with time and place. Typical variations are shown in Table 5. The coefficients of variation for the effects on gain and conversion are 110-199%, while those for effects on feed consumption are larger, up to 705%.

Following the setting of maximum safe levels of use of antibacterials, determination of the dose-response function is paramount, in conjunction with the quantification of the influence of other key independent variable factors. The latter are listed in Table 6, identified by the symbols used in this text. Level of control performance normally contributes most to variation in response in apparently healthy stock. Changes in response over the years (EXDAT +ve or -ve) may also be important, as well as form of feed, housing systems, presence of a coccidiostat and/or a second antibacterial and also the presence of disease.

Table 5. Variations in feed intake, liveweight gain and feed conversion ratio responses to in-feed antibacterials in broilers and pigs as number of tests (n), mean values, ranges and coefficients of variation (CV).

Response		Mean	Range	CV(%)
Broiler virginiamycin (n = 560)				
Feed intake	(g)	10	-234 - 345	604
Liveweight gain	(g)	40	-120 - 379	136
Feed conversion ratio		-.061	-.93 - .12	163
Broiler zinc bacitracin (n = 1,001)				
Feed intake	(g)	18	-725 - 850	705
Liveweight gain	(g)	33	-113 - 297	140
Feed conversion ratio		-.058	-.73 - .36	176
Pig chlortetracycline (n = 648)				
Feed intake	(kg day^{-1})	.094	-.97 - .86	176
Liveweight gain	(kg day^{-1})	.052	-.113 - .427	110
Feed conversion ratio		-.134	-2.70 - .78	199
Pig tylosin (n = 619)				
Feed intake	(kg day^{-1})	.052	-.58 - .65	232
Liveweight gain	(kg day^{-1})	.042	-.111 - .319	111
Feed conversion ratio		-.125	-2.00 - .74	155

Antibacterial effectiveness in nutrition can then best be evaluated by computation of mathematical models from all available data (Rosen, 1983), using conventional multiple regression methods (Draper and Smith, 1981), in the following stages:

1. Comprehensive collection of author-attributed, published reports on controlled feeding tests and abstraction of response data, as dependent variables (effects on control performances), and all other relevant independent numeric and descriptive (dummy) variables.
2. Systematic entry of variables on recording forms for subsequent computer filing and statistical analysis, using a suitable programme suite (e.g. Nie *et al.*, 1975). Checking for elimination of errors and data repeats in separate publications.
3. Multiple regression analysis relating dependent to independent variables for the development of best-fit algebraic equations (nutritional models) for the total data bank. Statistical validity requires the use of tests from start (O) to finish (F) only. Hence for lesser starter (S) or starter-grower (G) phase models, use of intermediate response values are based on O → S and O → G, because S → G and G → F have no valid untreated controls.
4. Thereafter, models for sub-classes can be investigated for categories which might differ significantly from the total (e.g. a growth phase, a geographic region).
5. Choice of significant regressions with minimum standard deviations (SD) and maximum multiple correlation coefficient squares (R^2), containing significant partial regression coefficients, after removal of aberrant responses (having residuals > 3 x SD about the regression).
6. Use of these models to estimate nutritional responses and associated confidence limits for specific required values of the component independent variables.

Table 6. Variables in the multi-factorial analysis of nutritional responses

Symbol	Unit	Variable	Broiler	Pig	Layer
n		number of tests	+	+	+
X	(mg kg^{-1})	feed concentration of substance X	+	+	+
FDIC[1]	(g)	feed consumption of control	+	kg day^{-1}	kg cycle^{-1}
LWGC[1]	(g)	liveweight gain of control	+	kg day^{-1}	+
FCRC[1]		feed conversion ratio of control	+	+	+
EGMASC[1]	(kg)	egg mass of control/cycle	-	-	+
EGGC[1]	(%)	egg numbers of control, hen-housed	-	-	+
MORTC[1]	(%)	mortality of control	+	+	+
DURC	(day)	duration of feeding X	+	+	+
LWIC	(kg)	initial control liveweight	-	+	+
LWFC	(kg)	final control liveweight	+	+	+
EXDAT	(year)	date of completion of test	+	+	+
REST	0 or 1	restricted feeding	+	+	+
DISC	0 or 1	discontinuous X	+	+	+
EXT	0 or 1	extruded feed	+	+	+
VET	0 or 1	disease diagnosed	+	+	+
CTY	0 or 1	test in country CTY	+	+	+
IND	0 or 1	independent test	+	+	+
COX	0 or 1	male	+	-	-
PUL	0 or 1	females	+	-	-
BRD	0 or 1	breeder	+	+	+
INST	0 or 1	research facility	+	+	+
FL	0 or 1	solid floor	+	+	+
CA	0 or 1	cage, wire or slatted floor	+	+	+
BRA	0 or 1	specified brand of X	+	+	+
SPD	0 or 1	semi-purified diet	+	+	+
COC	0 or 1	coccidiostat in feed	+	-	-
F2	0 or 1	second additive present (Y)	+	+	+
F2Y	(mg kg^{-1})	feed concentration of Y	+	+	+
N	(mg kg^{-1} or %)	nutrient N feed concentration	+	+	+
STD	(n m^2)	stocking density	+	+	+

Interactions are products e.g. FCRCxDUR, COCxX

[1] Corresponding dependent variable, replace C with EFF, e.g. FDIEFF, for effect on feed consumption or with X, e.g. FDIX, for treated feed consumption.

Comparison of antibacterials

Comparison of percentage or absolute overall mean values of nutritional effects of two or more antibacterials is inadequate, because of large differences in circumstances of the tests. Direct within-test comparisons are the ideal, but generally quite impractical because much larger tests are needed to prove statistically significant differences of effects which are smaller than those for individual antibacterials versus negative controls. That, and the substantial variations observed in such tests imply the need for very considerable replication (Roberts, 1983). In addition, it is virtually impossible to test a minimum of zero (suitably replicated) and at least three concentrations of each candidate in dose-response comparisons.

The published literature on within-test comparisons contains many examples of highly discordant efficacy ratings of pairs and groups of antibacterial substances. Hence comprehensive nutritional models for substances to be compared are used to estimate responses and confidence limits for each substance, relative to any required conditions of use, which estimates are then subjected to a statistical test of the significance of observed differences (Rosen, 1984). Comparisons thus made are normally based on equal feed concentration and/or equal investment cost considerations. The latter gives the "animal verdict" on the outcome of equal investment, without the need to consider reasons for, and the influence of, wide disparities in the unit cost of antibacterials.

Econometrics

Nutritional gain or conversion responses cannot alone provide an adequate evaluation of antibacterials as nutrition improvers. The partial contributions of nutritional improvements in rate of gain and feed conversion to net productivity vary in magnitude and correlation and are not additive. The relationship differs for production to target liveweight and target duration. Net cost reduction calculations (net profit) are therefore needed to provide a unique productivity index. The use of so-called "Production Numbers" (Voeten and Brus, 1986), and related "European Performance Efficiency Factors", in broilers, is inappropriate, due to bias introduced by the use of liveweight squared in the calculation. Its lack of value has been confirmed by Akkerman (1993).

Net cost reduction to target weight (NCRw) is cost of feed saved by better conversion plus other costs (non-feed, non-animal) saved by accelerated output, minus the cost of antibacterial, per crop or cycle or per annum. Net cost reduction to target duration (NCRd) is the sales value of extra weight plus or minus the cost of feed saved or added, less the cost of antibacterial, per crop or cycle or per annum. Commonly, errors in econometric indices come from arithmetic addition of unconnected liveweight and conversion financial benefits and from a failure to distinguish between NCRw and NCRd.

The value of NCRd/NCRw usually exceeds one, because the unit financial value of produce is greater than that of feed. For example, the NCRd/NCRw value for broilers of control slaughter weight 2.1 kg for 20-100 mg zinc bacitracin kg^{-1} feed is 1.26 (Rosen, 1992a), as compared with 2.02 for turkeys of 4-13 kg control slaughter weight and 2.09 for pigs of 100 kg slaughter weight (Rosen, 1994a). NCRd is, however, normally used for layers and breeding pigs.

POSOLOGY

Nutritional considerations

Posology is the science of dosage. Selection of an optimal dose requires data relating the amount of response to the level of dose administered. For antibacterials (feed concentration up to 110 mg kg^{-1}) logarithmic dose-response functions are the most common, as illustrated in Fig. 1. The latter also contains an objective criterion for selection of a minimum level, as the dosage at which the lower gain or upper conversion 95% confidence limit is zero, i.e. 11 mg kg^{-1} for FCREFF and 14 mg kg^{-1} for LWGEFF. Fig. 1 also shows why use of higher feed concentrations reduces the chances of zero or adverse responses, (see confidence intervals at 4 or 5 and at 75 mg kg^{-1}). This aspect of the practical application of antibacterials in nutrition is often overlooked. The percentage of zero or adverse gain and conversion responses of the subjects of Table 5 are shown in Table 7. For the 14 antibacterials (Table 1) the overall percentage of zero and adverse responses in gain and/or conversion in growing pigs and poultry is 28%, about two in seven. This proportion can be improved by the use of higher feed concentrations.

Table 7. Percentage of adverse and zero response by pigs and broilers to the in-feed antibacterials shown in Table 5.

Species and substance	LWGEFF (%)	FCREFF (%)	n
Broiler - virginiamycin	14.4	18.9	560
Broiler - zinc bacitracin	17.6	23.7	1,001
Pig - chlortetracycline	13.2	23.3	648
Pig - tylosin	12.3	21.1	619

Economic aspects

Net cost reduction by dietary antibacterials is mainly influenced by the unit cost of feed for production to target liveweight, and by the unit value of the produce for production to target duration. For cost-effective dosage the key economic factor is unit cost per gram of activity of the antibacterial. Fig. 2 projections (Rosen, 1989) are from tylosin models (Rosen and Jansegers, 1988) for 10-100 mg kg^{-1} in control growing-fattening pigs (27-105 kg liveweight) gaining 0.654 kg day^{-1} at a feed conversion of 3.17. At notional prices of 1.3, 0.65, 0.325 and 0.13 French francs g^{-1} activity, the maximum economic benefits of FF 7.4, 11.0, 14.4 and 17.9 per pig respectively are obtained at 15, 33, 60 and 95 mg tylosin kg^{-1} feed.

In broilers, slaughter liveweight markedly affects net profit posology. Mean econometric data (Rosen, 1988b), based on nutritional models for Flavomycin® flavophospholipol (473 tests), Stafac® virginiamycin (326 tests) and Albac® zinc bacitracin (777 tests), showed that increasing slaughter liveweight from 1.5 kg (35 days) to 2.6 kg (56 days) elevated annual net profit per 1,000 birds from £104 to £164 and that a mean £137 net profit per 1,000 birds per annum requires 39 mg antibacterial kg^{-1} feed for birds of 1.5 kg and 14 mg kg^{-1} for 2.6 kg.

There are large differences in recommended dosages and costs per g activity of antibacterials. In practice the quotients use concentration x cost g^{-1}, tend to converge to similar feed

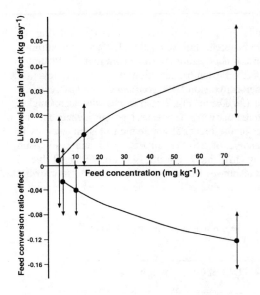

Figure 1. Dose-response relationships and 95% confidence limits

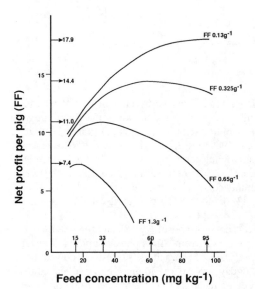

Figure 2. The relationship between antibacterial unit cost (French francs g⁻¹), concentration in feed and net profit. Figures above the X axis are feed concentrations for maximum net profits indicated by arrows on the Y axis.

costs per tonne. Hence the latter is used as a base line to elucidate posological aspects of net productivity in comparing antibacterial nutrition improvers (see Broilers).

Mortality

Prophylaxis for mortality reduction against specified bacteria normally uses higher feed concentrations than for nutrition improvement but the concentrations used for the latter do reduce mortality. Mortality effects (MORTEFF) in broilers are inherently highly variable with coefficients of variation of 225-2, 150% (mean 675%) for the substances in Table 8, which compares the effects of lower and higher concentrations of the antibacterial in the feed. In each case the higher level improved mortality reduction. Overall mean MORTEFF values are -0.9% for lower use levels (mean 11 mg kg^{-1}) and -2.5% for higher feed concentrations (mean 36 mg kg^{-1}).

Table 8. Comparison of the effects of antibacterials at lower and higher feed concentrations on non-specific mortality in broilers.

Substance	Concentration in feed		Number of controlled trials	Control mortality (%)	Effect on mortality (% absolute)
	Range (mg kg^{-1})	Mean (mg kg^{-1})			
Avoparcin	5 - 10	10	91	5.8	+1.1
	15 - 50	20	22	6.1	-2.0
Chlortetracycline	6 - 22	13	64	5.0	-1.7
	25 - 55	37	19	6.3	-2.4
Nitrovin	2 - 15	11	136	4.7	-1.4
	18 - 80	28	11	5.8	-4.4
Oxytetracycline	5 - 22	14	63	7.7	-2.0
	25 - 50	37	6	5.2	-2.8
Virginiamycin	1 - 10	6	80	3.7	-0.5
	12 - 110	21	24	5.1	-1.2
Zinc bacitracin	4 - 11	12	264	4.3	-0.9
	50 - 110	71	89	5.7	-2.4

EFFECTIVENESS OF ANTIBACTERIALS IN NUTRITION

Feed intake

Dietary antibacterials stimulate feed intake in pigs and turkeys, but not in broilers and layers. Overall the 14 antibacterials in Table 1 gave mean improvements in liveweight gain/feed conversion of +8.1/-4.8% in pigs and +3.6/-2.2% in turkeys, as against +3.6/-3.4% in broilers and +2.8/-2.7% in laying hens. A larger feed intake differential occurs in piglets than in slaughter pigs for which the respective average values from the reviews of Hays (1981), Jost (1983) and Gropp *et al.* (1991) are +15.7/-8.6% and +3.2/-2.0% respectively.

In pigs, a general model for FDIEFF, based on 1,500 controlled tests on carbadox, chlortetracycline, oxytetracycline, tylosin and zinc bacitracin (Rosen, 1994a) has three highly significant independent variables.

$$FDIEFF = .134 - .0678FDIC - .0721REST + .000969LWFC$$

Feed concentration functions did not approach statistical significance. The partial regression coefficient for feed restriction systems as against *ad libitum* indicates lower FDIEFF by an average of -.072 kg per day, while the counter-active FDIC and LWFC terms are negative up to slaughter weight for normal daily intakes.

For apparently healthy broilers, an analogous model for feed intake effect, based on 1,429 tests on chlortetracycline, oxytetracycline, virginiamycin and zinc bacitracin includes a significant feed concentration function:

$$FDIEFF = - 40.8 + 20.8\log(X+1) - .0400FDIC + 3.18DUR + 29.3EXT - 25.3COC$$

Level of control feed intake and duration of feeding are counter-active and positive above 32 and 57 days of age for birds consuming 2,500 and 4,500 g respectively. The feed intake response is greater in extruded feeds and is reduced in the presence of a coccidiostat.

Influence of independent variables

Quantification of the influence of key independent variables is important for the comprehensive assessment of nutrition improvement over a wide range of practical conditions.

Feed concentration (X mg kg^{-1}). For nutritional levels (Ferrando, 1979) up to 110 mg kg^{-1} in the diet, $\log(X+1)$ is the most common dose-response function. Interactions of terms in X in broilers with other variables are rare and contribute little to total R^2.

Control performance (LWGC, FCRC, EGMASC). Terms for control performance are major contributors to R^2. Negative partial regression coefficients accord with diminished responses for better control performances. In broilers, LWGC partial regression coefficients range from -0.01 to -0.05 (mean -0.026 g g^{-1} liveweight gain) and FCRC from -0.10 to -0.20 (mean -0.15 per unit feed conversion). Corresponding means for layers are -0.13 g day^{-1} for EGMASC and -0.16 for FCRC. In pigs, control performance terms are more complex insofar as LWGEFF and FCREFF models usually contain pairs from LWGC, FCRC and DFIC.

Duration of inclusion in diet (DUR). Positive DUR terms in LWGEFF and FCREFF broiler models are counter-active to LWGC and FCRC. Typical partial correlation coefficients for DUR are 0.9 to 2.7 (mean 1.5 g day^{-1}) for LWGEFF and -0.0018 to -0.0033 (mean -0.0026) for FCREFF.

Sex. LWGEFF is greater in males than in females or as-hatched birds by 13-43 g (mean 26 g).

Presence of coccidiostat (COC). LWGEFF is less in the presence of certain coccidiostats by 11 to 26 g (mean -17 g), due perhaps to contributory antibacterial activity.

Year of test (EXDAT). Some reduced responses over the years in pigs are revealed for LWGEFF and FCREFF respectively by EXDAT coefficients of -0.0012 to -0.0018 (mean - 0.0014 kg day^{-1} per annum) and +0.0013 to +0.0038 (mean 0.0023 per annum).

Broilers

Table 9 and Figs. 3 and 4 summarise a comprehensive comparison of the nutritional and econometrical effectiveness of four antibacterials in broiler nutrition (Rosen, 1990), based on nutritional models for Albac® zinc bacitracin (777 tests), Avotan® avoparcin (254), Flavomycin® flavophospholipol (473) and Stafac® virginiamycin (326). At each level of investment, price per gram defines the quantity of antibacterial afforded. For nine investment levels, columns give the dose-response patterns and rows compare equal investment, including those for normally recommended use levels. For inputs of 2.5-12.5 French francs per tonne, ascending dose-response curves do not reach a maximum. Lowest unit price per gram of activity gives the best net cost reduction.

Feed conversion response in broilers is affected by the presence of disease (VET), as illustrated for virginiamycin (V) and zinc bacitracin (Z).

$$FCRV = .271 - .05891og(V+1) - .774FCRC + .00407DUR - .197VET$$
$$FCRZ = .196 - .04891og(Z+1) - .132FCRC + .00159DUR - .0819VET$$

These models indicate, for apparently healthy birds (VET = 0), respective responses of -0.077 and -0.074 at 50 mg kg^{-1} in 49 day-old birds for FCRC = 2 and substantially larger FCREFF responses in the presence of disease (VET = 1). The magnitude of the partial regression coefficients for VET depends upon the severity of the condition. The values of -0.197 and -0.0819 are for necrotic enterites having respective mean control mortalities of 24 and 12% in the data banks.

Consideration of the posology of prophylaxis in broilers is limited by the scarcity of controlled tests in disease. Although mortality can be reduced by as little as 3-6 mg bacitracin kg^{-1} diet, the notional, "mean dose-response curve" from five individual tests indicates that, while 20 mg kg^{-1} is largely effective, better coverage is more likely at 70-100 mg kg^{-1} (Fig. 5).

Turkeys

The US Food and Drug Administration (1972) summarised 21 responses in turkeys at market weight to dietary bacitracin (16) and penicillin (5), with mean values of +222 for control liveweight of 7,763 g (+3.3%) and -0.168 for control feed conversion of 3.51 (-4.8%). In contrast, the means of 85 tests surveyed by Hays (1981) for bacitracin (80) and penicillin (5) were +644 for control liveweight of 8,981 g (+7.2%) and -0.060 for control feed conversion of 3.18 (-1.9%). A recent summary (Rosen, 1994a) of 373 term studies in turkeys (1952-92) for the five antibacterials in Table 1 has mean responses of +184, for control liveweight of 6,848 g (+3.6%) and -0.052 for control feed conversion of 2.35 (-2.2%). These differences in response data underline the need for diagnostic models in turkeys such as for zinc bacitracin (ZB) (n = 236, Rosen, 1994b).

$$LWGZ^{.35} = .0983 + .1691og(ZB+1) + .980LWGC^{.35} + .00307DUR$$
$$FCRZ = .151 - .04061og(ZB+1) + .879FCRC + .00170DUR$$

Save for the necessary LWG$^{.35}$ transformations (to eliminate heterogeneity of residuals), these models closely resemble the format of broiler analogues. Productivity calculations using these

Table 9. Dosage, FCREFF, days saved to production liveweight and reduction in net cost per 1000 birds for Albac® zinc bacitracin (ZB), Avotan® avoparcin (A), Flavomycin® flavophospholipol (F) and Stafac® virginiamycin (V) in broilers[1]. Investment costs and net cost reductions are in French francs (FF)

Investment cost per tonne	ZB	A	F	V	ZB	A	F	V
	Dosage (mg kg^{-1})				FCREFF			
2.50	20	-	-	-	-.060	-	-	-
3.13	-	-	2.5	5	-	-	-.052	-.018
4.10	50/20	-	5/2	-	-.073	-	-.055	-
4.69	-	7.5	-	-	-	-.023	-	-
6.25	50	10	5	10	-.087	-.035	-.060	-.044
7.56	-	15/10	-	-	-	-.038	-	-
8.94	-	-	-	20/10	-	-	-	-.057
9.38	75	15	-	-	-.103	-.042	-	-
12.50	100	-	10	20	-.113	-	-.070	-.070
	Days saved				Net cost reduction per 1000 birds			
2.50	0.75	-	-	-	202	-	-	-
3.13	-	-	0.3	0.4	-	-	162	57
4.10	0.8	-	0.4	-	239	-	170	-
4.69	-	0.7	-	-	-	75	-	-
6.25	0.9	0.7	0.5	0.5	280	108	182	131
7.56	-	0.8	-	-	-	115	-	-
8.94	-	-	-	0.6	-	-	-	166
9.38	1.0	0.8	-	-	322	121	-	-
12.50	1.1	-	0.6	0.65	343	-	194	195

[1] LWGC = 1,875 g; DURC = 45 days; FCRC = 1.97; ZB cost = 0.125FF g^{-1}; A cost = 0.625FF g^{-1}; F cost = 1.25FF g^{-1}; V cost = 0.625FF g^{-1}
Feed = 1.73FF kg^{-1}; other costs = .0284FF per bird per day; terminal rate of gain = 58 g per day

models suggest the need for 50-55 mg kg^{-1} for routine use from start to finish. Larger data banks than currently available are required for models of other antibacterials in turkeys.

Snetsinger (1970) surveyed the use of chlortetracycline, oxytetracycline and zinc bacitracin in turkey breeders, indicating improved egg production and more poults per hen via better output and/or hatchability. Hays (1981) summarised 15 tests on 8 antibacterials, reporting a reduction in feed per egg, with proportionate increase in egg production and no effect on hatchability. However, more modern studies are required.

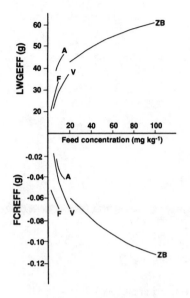

Figure 3. LWGEFF and FCREFF dose-response relationships in broilers for Albac® zinc bacitracin (ZB), Avotan® avoparcin (A), Flavomycin® flavophospholipol (F) and Stafac® virginiamycin (V).

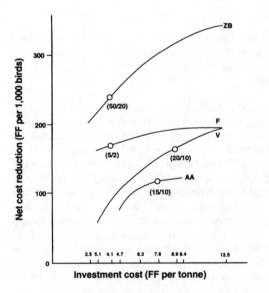

Figure 4. Econometrical dose-response relationships in broilers for Albac® zinc bacitracin (ZB), Avotan® avoparcin (AA), Flavomycin® flavophospholipol (F) and Stafac® virginiamycin (V) Values are in French francs (FF). The open circles represent the normally recommended dose.

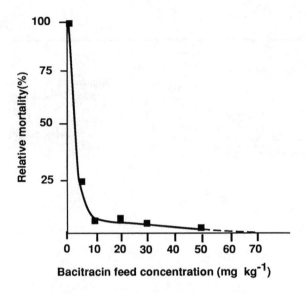

Figure 5. The effect on mortality of bacitracin in necrotic enteritis in broilers.

Pullets

Assessment of the use of antibacterials in pullet nutrition requires expensive, whole-life studies. It is complicated by the need to establish the potential influence of multi-phase growth functions (Kwakkel, 1993) in rearing and their sequelae during lay. Factorial 2 x 2 tests on rearing and laying phases are rare.

Early US reports on chlortetracycline in pullets were conducted on admixtures with vitamin B12 to 4-8 weeks of age and lacked data on feed consumption. Hoie and Lund (1963) found that LWGEFF = +50 g, at 16 weeks of age for oxytetracycline (10-15 mg kg^{-1}), was lost by point-of-lay. Tueller (1973) observed improved feed conversion by Flavomycin® (2.5 mg kg^{-1}), Payzone® nitrovin (24 mg kg^{-1}) and A.L.® zinc bacitracin (15 mg kg^{-1}) in pullets from day-old to 20 weeks of age, without influence on weight gain or mortality. From 8 to 20 weeks of age Miles *et al.* (1984) reported that virginiamycin at 20 mg kg^{-1} provided significantly heavier pullets, in sub-optimal protein regimes and also improved feed conversion overall. Studies by Groote (1983) on avoparcin (10 mg kg^{-1}), flavophospholipol (3 mg kg^{-1}), lincomycin (4.4 mg kg^{-1}), virginiamycin (7.5 mg kg^{-1}) and zinc bacitracin (20 mg kg^{-1}) in pullets from day-old to 20 weeks of age yielded mean values of +10 g on a mean control liveweight gain of 620 g, a reduction of 0.07 on control feed conversion of 4.97 and +0.2% on a control mortality of 0.6%. Subsequent responses during lay were +0.21 kg for control egg mass of 17.31 kg, a reduction of 0.05 for control feed conversion ratio of 2.40 and a reduction of 0.6% on control mortality of 6.7%. Regression analysis of 109 tests in layers on the use of zinc bacitracin (5-100 mg kg^{-1} feed with a of mean 28 mg kg^{-1}, including nine whole-life studies, showed a significant (p<0.025) increase of 1.1% hen-housed egg production due to pullet feed supplementation (Rosen, 1994a).

Layers

Branion *et al.* (1956) reviewed the effects of bacitracin, chlortetracycline, oxytetracycline, penicillin and streptomycin in layers feeds. They found positive egg production responses in 14 of 30 tests, including 10 of 21 for tetracyclines. Havermann and Wegner (1958) surveyed 52 US and eight European tests. Of the former, they noted no positive results in ten tests and only a small positive response in a further ten tests. Definite responses were seen with nutritionally deficient rations (7); in the presence of disease (7); in unfavourable weather (4); and in normal conditions (14), thus pin-pointing some factors governing response. The European tests gave positive results.

For layers in flocks, Rosen *et al.* (1960) found a significant correlation for oxytetracycline (25 mg kg^{-1}) administration, R = 2,530 - 42.0E, between net return per 1,000 birds (£R) and hen-housed egg production (E%). In a test on individually fed, caged layers the poorest egg producers pre-test (11 weeks) failed to respond, as compared with the average and good performers. Correspondingly, large-scale field trials on 22,000 birds given 25, 50 and 100 mg chlortetracycline kg^{-1} feed continuously, revealed a linear dose-response and significant improvements for hen-housed control production levels less than 50% (Smith *et al.*, 1961). Responses were greater in the presence of pullet and upper respiratory diseases and at low temperatures.

A summary table by Hays (1981) of weighted mean responses in 244 tests in layers showed +2.4% over 59.9% control egg production (n = 244) and a reduction of 0.11 from 2.40 kg per dozen eggs in feed conversion (n = 122). Continuing reports on the use of bacitracins (n = 109 between 1953-91, Rosen *et al.*, 1976; Rosen, 1982), flavophospholipol (n = 106 from 1967-85, Rosen, 1988a) and virginiamycin (n = 35 from 1968-88, Rosen, 1986) contained enough data to provide the following models for responses in laying fowl.

$$EGGEFF = 11.6 + .0236Z - .154EGGC^1$$

[1]Bacitracin has no effect on feed consumption or egg weight, so EGMASEFF and FCREFF are calculable from EGGEFF.

$$EGMASEFF = 5.50 + 1.71log(F+1) - .126EGMASC - 1.61BRD$$
$$FCREFF = .339 + .358log(F+1) - .139FCRC - .132 \ FCRCxlog(F+1) + .119BRD$$
$$EGMASEFF = 4.14 + .159V - .00293V^2 - .143EGMASC$$
$$FCREFF = .437 - .011OV + .000173V^2 - .124FCRC$$

The dose-response function for bacitracin is linear (to the maximum fed of 110 mg kg^{-1}), logarithmic for flavophospholipol and quadratic for virginiamycin (maximum responses at 32-33 mg kg^{-1}). Virginiamycin significantly reduces mean egg weight (Groote, 1983). Flavophospholipol responses are significantly less in breeding stock.

These models have been used, for equal cost per tonne investment, to establish the comparative value for table egg production of the use of three antibacterials as summarised in Fig. 6.

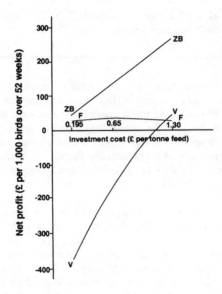

Figure 6. Equal investment dose-response comparison of flavophospholipol (F), virginiamycin (V) and zinc bacitracin (ZB) in layers feed for table egg production in terms of net profit per 1000 birds per year for EGMASC = 45 g per day and FCRC = 2.50. Feed cost £0.15 kg^{-1}, egg value £0.60 kg^{-1}, ZB cost £0.013 g^{-1} activity, V cost £0.065g^{-1} activity, F cost £0.13 g^{-1} activity. The EU approved feed concentrations for ZB (15-100 mg kg^{-1} feed), F (2-5 mg kg^{-1} feed) and V (20 mg kg^{-1} feed) require investments of £0.195-1.30, £0.195-0.65 and £1.30 per tonne feed respectively.

The dose-response curves reflect the European Union approved levels of usage of 20 mg kg^{-1} for virginiamycin, 2-5 mg kg^{-1} for flavophospholipol and 15-100 mg kg^{-1} for zinc bacitracin. Net profits from the maximum approved levels for flavophospholipol and virginiamycin and for the minimum of zinc bacitracin are approximately equal, while the use of elevated levels of zinc bacitracin of 50-100 mg kg^{-1} affords substantially better returns.

Responses in breeding hens in egg production, fertility and hatchability are especially important because of the higher unit value of live progeny than table eggs. Branion *et al.* (1956) reported no response to chlortetracycline and penicillin in three tests on breeders. Smith *et al.* (1961) also reported no significant difference in hatchability from chlortetracycline at 25-100 mg kg^{-1}. The summary of 69 tests by Hays (1981), mainly conducted on the tetracyclines, arsenicals and penicillin, indicated an increase in hatchability of 2.6% over control values of 76.2%. Nine tests on zinc bacitracin at 11-110 mg kg^{-1} (mean 51 mg kg^{-1}) for 30-60 weeks (mean 44 weeks) gave an average improvement of 2.9% for fertility and 2.2% in hatchability of fertile eggs on control values of 90% and 80% respectively (Rosen, 1994a). More recently, Krueger *et al.* (1983) and Damron *et al.* (1991) reported significant improvements in overall hatchability due to the inclusion of 28-110 mg zinc bacitracin kg^{-1} in broiler breeders, with modest egg production responses, whereas Brake (1990) with higher control hatchability found no response therein from 10-50 mg kg^{-1} in the face of greatly improved hen-housed egg production of +4.9%. As yet no guide exists to factors determining differential responses in egg production and hatchability.

Minor poultry species

Relatively few reports have described the use of antibacterials in minor poultry. More are available for ducks than for geese, guinea fowl and quail and none for pheasants or pigeon.

Ducks. Early US studies on ducks to six weeks of age by Branion *et al.* (1953) showed no response to chlortetracycline (10 mg kg^{-1}), penicillin (25 mg kg^{-1}), oxytetracycline (100 mg kg^{-1}) or streptomycin (25 mg kg^{-1}). Subsequent test reports on the continuous administration from day-old of nutritional levels of 5-100 mg kg^{-1} of avoparcin, cyadox, flavophospholipol, nitrovin, kormogrisin, oxytetracycline, virginiamycin and zinc bacitracin have insufficient data as yet for nutritional models, so mean liveweight gain and conversion responses are summarised in Table 10. The proportionate liveweight gain (3.5%) and feed conversion (3.1%) improvements are similar to broilers (3.6 and 3.4% respectively). Table 10 shows that higher mean feed concentrations of cyadox (23 mg kg^{-1}) and zinc bacitracin (38 mg kg^{-1}) produce greater responses than other substances tested at 14-15 mg kg^{-1}. Chen *et al.* (1981) conducted a dose-response study at 20, 50, 100 and 150 mg zinc bacitracin kg^{-1} which showed maximum responses at 80-100 mg kg^{-1}. Copper sulfate at 250-375 mg Cu kg^{-1} is effective in ducks (Helder, 1968; Jeroch *et al.*, 1973), with mean improvements of 53 g LWGEFF on LWGC of 2.64 kg (2.0%) and FCREFF of -0.05 on FCRC of 3.81 (1.3%). Zinc bacitracin has also been shown to improve egg yield (Solntsev, 1988).

Table 10. Mean liveweight gain (LWGEFF) and feed conversion (FCREFF) responses of ducks to antibacterial feed supplements.

Antibacterial	No. of tests	Feed concentration (mg kg^{-1})	Duration (days)	LWGC (g)	LWGEFF (g)	FCRC	FCREFF
Cyadox[1]	8	23	50	2921	196	3.50	-.175
Nitrovin[2]	13	15	53	2608	62	3.55	-.066
Zinc bacitracin[3]	9	38	58	2303	69	3.65	-.140
Others[4]	7	14	63	2227	45	3.52	-.086
All	37	22	55	2529	89	3.56	-.111

[1]Kaplan *et al.*, 1985.
[2]Jeroch *et al.*, 1980/81; Tejnora *et al.*, 1977.
[3]Chen *et al.*, 1981; Jeroch *et al.*, 1981; Satava, 1973; Schubert *et al.*, 1981.
[4]Bergero *et al.*, 1993, flavophospholipol, virginiamycin; Gruhn *et al.*, 1961/62, oxytetracycline; Pan *et al.*, 1985, avoparcin; Schubert et al., 1981, kormogrisin.

Geese. Papers by Branion and Hill (1952), Slinger *et al.* (1953) and Tejnora *et al.* (1978) contain the results of 13 tests on chlortetracycline (50 mg kg^{-1}), nitrovin (10 and 20 mg kg^{-1}), oxytetracycline (50 mg kg^{-1}), penicillin (4 and 50 mg kg^{-1}) and streptomycin (50 mg kg^{-1}). These provide mean responses of 3.6% for LWGEFF and 4.3% for FCREFF from 26 mg kg^{-1} fed for 58 days. Kostadinov *et al.* (1985) have reported increased liver weight and quality in force-fattened geese fed flavophospholipol (4-16 mg kg^{-1}) or zinc bacitracin (30 mg kg^{-1}) for 27 days pre-slaughter.

Guinea fowl. The high mean nutritional improvements in guinea fowl of 160 g over a control value of 0.924 kg (17%) in LWGEFF and -0.52 over a control value of 3.87 (13%) in

FCREFF reported by Bonomi *et al.* (1975) and Oguntona (1988a,b,c), for flavophospholipol (4 mg kg[-1]), oxytetracycline (5-20 mg kg[-1]), roxarsone (50 mg kg[-1]) and zinc bacitracin (11-45 mg kg[-1]) addition from day-old to 87 days may relate to the relatively slow rate of gain and poor conversion characteristics of this species. Flavophospholipol at 3 mg kg[-1] enhanced hatchability of guinea-fowl breeders over a 37-week test period (Bolognesi *et al.*, 1977).

Quail. Guerocak (1970) tested flavophospholipol, oxytetracycline and zinc bacitracin to 42 days of age with mean responses of +1.5% for gain (1.5 g over 100 g) and -1.1% (-0.054 over 4.82) for conversion. This small bird, however, may require higher feed concentrations than other species because flavophospholipol (20 mg kg[-1]), zinc bacitracin (25 mg kg[-1]) and oxytetracycline (50 mg kg[-1]) gave improvements of +3.3% (3.3 g over 100 g) and -2.1% (-0.098 over 4.73) respectively compared with flavophospholipol (1-8 mg kg[-1]) and oxytetracycline (10 mg kg[-1]) which were ineffective.

This pointer for optimum dosage in quail is supported in the screening tests of Schulz and Gropp (1973), in which 14-21 day tests indicated little or no mean overall improvement. But gain and conversion responses to chlortetracycline at 200 mg kg[-1], nitrovin at 20 mg kg[-1], penicillin at 10 mg kg[-1] and zinc bacitracin at 25 mg kg[-1] were reported, as against zero or adverse outcomes in gain and/or conversion from lower inclusions of chlortetracycline (20-50 mg kg[-1]), flavophospholipol (2 mg kg[-1]) and virginiamycin (10 mg kg[-1]). In quail copper sulfate from 7-42 days of age at 200-600 mg Cu kg[-1] feed improved respective gain and conversion responses by 9.2 g over a control value of 139 g (+6.6%) and -0.99 over a control value of 6.83 (14%) (Yannakopoulos *et al.*, 1990).

Pigs

Nutritional responses of pigs to antibacterials in the diet are clearly sensitive to environmental influence. Two summaries of efficacy in research station versus farm tests (Cromwell, 1991) have shown that percentage improvements are virtually doubled on farms. It remains to determine the quantitative contributions to this differential of the variables, level of performance, range of liveweight and duration of feeding, proportion of discontinuous feeding levels, stocking density and disease status. Table 11 illustrates the influence of such variables in a comparison in piglets and slaughter pigs based on nutritional models for olaquindox (LAQ, n = 126) and carbadox (CAR, n = 309) (Rosen, 1994a).

LWGEFF = .118 + .039log(CAR+1) - .233LWGC - .00236DUR - .0032OLWI + .00377LWF
FCREFF = .371 - .059log(CAR+1) - .471FCRC + .433FDIC + .0102DUR + .0181LWI -.0133LWF + .0333USA
LWGEFF = - .0289 + .038log(LAQ+1) - .0622LWGC + .0217FCRC - .000228DUR
FCREFF = .235 - .108(LAQ+1) - .184FCRC + .572LWGC + .0578DISC

Carbadox for LWGEFF and olaquindox for FCREFF are numerically superior, but the differences are significant only for LWGEFF in slaughter pigs with no pre-slaughter withdrawal. Obligatory withdrawal, at four months of age and/or four weeks pre-slaughter in the European Union would mean, however, that FCREFF responses to discontinuous (DISC) use of, for example, 50/O mg LAQ kg[-1] would be reduced from -.073 to -.015. A similar reduction in response with discontinuous use has also been reported by Jordan and Waitt (1962) for tylosin withdrawal from finisher feed, which lowered mean daily gain response by

-0.045 kg per day and increased feed conversion by 0.08 in tests comparing 44/22/11 with 44/22/O mg tylosin kg^{-1}.

Table 11. Comparison of nutritional responses to carbadox (CAR) and olaquindox (LAQ) in starter piglets and slaughter pigs.

Feed concentration (mg kg^{-1})	LWGEFF (kg day^{-1})		FCREFF	
	CAR	LAQ	CAR	LAQ
Starter piglets[2]				
25	.036 ± .0086[1]	.026 ± .013	.0021 ± .033	.0089 ± .040
50	.048 ± .0078	.038 ± .0098	-.019 ± .030	-.023 ± .030
100	.059 ± .010	.049 ± .012	-.037 ± .037	-.055 ± .036
Slaughter pigs[3]				
12.5	.028 ± .011	.0068 ± .016	-.031 ± .040	-.043 ± .042
25.0	.039 ± .012	.018 ± .015	-.048 ± .042	-.073 ± .030
50	.051 ± .015	.029 ± .017	-.065 ± .050	-.105 ± .032

[1]95% confidence limits.
[2]LWGC .467 kg day^{-1}; FCRC 1.85; FDIC .851 kg day^{-1}; LWI 7 kg; DISC O; USA O; LWF 28 kg; DUR 45 days.
[3]LWGC .677 kg day^{-1} FCRC 2.95; FDIC 2.00 kg day^{-1}; LWI 7 kg; DISC O; USA O; LWF 95 kg; DUR 130 days.

Mellière *et al.* (1973) showed in earlier tylosin models for finishing pigs that response was negatively proportional to control level of performance and that lower feed concentrations of 11-22 mg kg^{-1} would not be expected to improve FCRC less than 3.28. This aspect of response in pigs is further quantified in a model based on 461 tests for 6-110 mg tylosin kg^{-1} (Rosen and Jansegers, 1988).

$$FCREFF = .0991 - .0902\log(T+1) - .0644FCRC + .0390DISC + .00134EXDAT$$

This indicates that:

- more efficient pigs, of FCRC 2.5, will average FCREFF .064 less than pigs of FCRC 3.5
- pigs of FCRC 2.80 need 40 mg tylosin kg^{-1} to equal FCREFF of pigs of FCRC 3.20, fed 20 mg tylosin kg^{-1}
- DISC indicates 0.039 less FCREFF from 40/20 mg tylosin kg^{-1} compared with 30 mg kg^{-1} continuously
- mean FCREFF fell, independently of change in FCRC over the years, by .00134 per annum for 1959-82. In a 1976-80 series of West European trials (Elanco Products Ltd., undated), FCREFF fell significantly from -0.18 to -0.12.

There is no general agreement on the efficacy of antibacterial combinations in pigs. Individual tests give conflicting results and evaluation is handicapped by the confounding of substance and feed concentration in test design. Fully additive effects are rare and synergistic more so. However, the survey of Berende and Schutte (1978) found mixtures somewhat better than components.

Admixtures of antibacterials and copper compounds in pigs diets are especially relevant due to the relatively low cost of copper supplementation. Braude (1967) summarised 83 tests on copper showing widely divergent results in LWGEFF (-12.0 to 25.2%) and FCREFF (-12.6 to 5.2%) and quoted eight cases with improvement in copper sulphate-antibiotic admixture and five without. Cromwell's (1991) citation of additivity for copper and antibiotics is based on only 14 tests from six reports. A more comprehensive modelling study of 159 reports (1966-75) by UKASTA (1978) found insignificant differences for LWGEFF and FCREFF over those of copper for the presence of one or more other additives, of which the partial regression coefficients were +0.011 and +0.071 respectively. The liveweight gain and conversion models from this research for copper (CU) in pig feeds are invaluable for assessment of the practical importance of observed responses to antibacterials in 2 x 2 or larger factorial tests on admixtures.

$$LWGEFF = .0944 + .000324CU - .000000751CU^2 - .151LWGC$$
$$FCREFF = .113 - .000430CU + .000000707CU^2 - .0594FCRC$$

In Beames and Lloyd's (1965) tests on 110 mg kg^{-1} of tylosin and 250 mg Cu kg^{-1}, tylosin improved rate of gain over copper by 0.021 kg per day but the response to copper alone (0.042 kg day^{-1}) was low compared with a predicted mean of 0.073 ± 0.0083. Conversely, tylosin did not improve FCREFF over copper (-0.20), but the latter was well above an expected mean of -0.077 ± 0.021 for copper alone. Similarly, Barber *et al.* (1979) found that 50/0 mg olaquindox kg^{-1} markedly improved upon the effects of 200 mg Cu kg^{-1}. But the LWGEFF and FCREFF additional responses of +0.037 kg day^{-1} and -0.12 over copper effects occurred for the latter well below average, i.e. +0.007 kg per day versus 0.027 ± 0.0051 and -0.04 versus -0.14 ± 0.017. Several more factorial studies are needed to assess the roles of tylosin or olaquindox in admixture with copper in nutrition improvement in pigs and also for other antibacterials.

There appears to be no clear-cut evidence of mortality reduction in apparently healthy pigs by antibacterials used at nutritional levels. Admixtures of antibacterials with sulfur drugs at higher feed concentrations can reduce mortality in piglets, as evidenced by MORTEFF/MORTC values of -2.3/4.3% from 67 commercial field trial experiments with 1,597 starter pigs (1960-82) treated with chlortetracycline/penicillin/sulphamethazine (2:1:2) at a total antibacterial feed concentration of 275 mg kg^{-1} (Zimmerman, 1986). In five farm trials with 638 pigs of mean initial liveweight 8 kg fed the same admixture or tylosin/sulphamethazine (1:1) at 220 mg kg^{-1} for 67 days to piglets under high-disease conditions and environmental stress, the responses were -12.5/15.6% (Cromwell, 1991).

Clausen's early review (1955) of effects of antibacterials on carcass quality pinpointed difficulties in evaluation of many experimental reports because of differences in sex, breeds, feeding, management practices and methods of measurement. He concluded that effects on carcass composition, dressing percentage and quality were variable, but slight, with a tendency towards a higher fat content from *ad libitum* feeding in finisher pigs. Braude (1967) also found no clear picture from 83 tests on copper at 250 mg kg^{-1}, while noting some observations of increased back fat thickness and decreased carcass length. Sporadic claims of carcass improvement have been made by antibacterial manufacturers, based on selected data from few tests. These are not in general borne out by independent scientific reports.

Sows

A smaller numbers of tests on dietary antibacterials in breeding pigs contain rather variable results. Early tests on chlortetracycline and vitamin B12 admixtures (Ellis, 1956) indicated slightly earlier puberty and no disturbance to oestrus or numbers of embryos, but birth weights were unaffected. Number of pigs weaned per litter was increased.

A mean improvement in farrowing rate from 68 to 77% in 13 tests on 2,070 sows fed for one week pre-breeding and two weeks post-breeding 0.5-1.25 g day^{-1} of chlortetracycline, chlortetracycline/penicillin/sulphamethazine, tylosin, tylosin/sulphamethazine or furazolidone was reported by Zimmerman (1986). Similarly for these drugs and oxytetracycline, Cromwell (1991) noted enhanced farrowing rate, in nine tests on 1,931 sows, from 75.4 to 82.1% and an increase in the mean number of live pigs born per litter (10.0 to 10.4). His summary of the effects of 110-275 mg kg^{-1} feed of chlortetracycline, chlortetracycline/penicillin/ sulphamethazine, oxytetracycline, tylosin, copper sulphate and zinc bacitracin, administered to 2,105 sows from three to seven days before farrowing and for 14-21 days during lactation in 11 tests, showed mean treated versus control values of 8.6/8.2 (+4.9%) for piglets weaned per litter, 87.1/84.9 (+2.6%) for percentage survival to weaning and 4.70/4.65 (+1.1%) for weaning weight. More recently, the five-centre test on 850 sows reported by Maxwell *et al.* (1987) showed that chlortetracycline increased litter size at birth and reduced feed consumption and sow weight loss during lactation.

The general presumption in the US is that a high level of an absorbed antibacterial or admixture seems to be needed for such responses in sows, presumably because systemic rather than gastrointestinal problems and mechanisms are involved. Interestingly, however, avoparcin (Korniewicz *et al.*, 1991), bacitracin methylene disalicylate (Aherne, 1985), virginiamycin (Kyriakis *et al.*, 1992) and zinc bacitracin (Briones, 1982; Kadamanova, 1984), which are virtually non-absorbed antibacterials, have produced diverse responses in sows in the improvement of breeding performance. Better definition of optimum feeding regimes and dosage for such responses is required for practical application.

FUTURE RESEARCH AND DEVELOPMENT

Nutritional evaluations. Research on mode(s) of action has not shown new antibacterials as potentially more effective than those used for decades. Newer candidates, (e.g. ardacin, avilamycin, efrotomycin, salinomycin) need more feeding tests, including independent studies, to complement the relative few required for initial registration, in order to furnish comprehensive nutritional models. Additional research is also required for all antibacterials to better quantify:

- effects of nutritional levels on mortality and morbidity
- the importance of key environmental parameters, such as stocking densities, temperatures, lighting systems, measurable causes of stress, and welfare housing
- effects of harsher feed extrusions and phased feeding
- energy- and protein-based economies with antibacterials, including interactions with limiting nutrients, such as performance-promoting synthetic amino acids
- geographical differences and biological explanations

- the use of admixtures of antibacterials *inter se* and with coccidiostats, histomoniastats, microbials, enzymes, organic acids, hormones and partitioning agents.

Admixtures. Due to large observed variations, admixtures require well-replicated, full factorial tests to measure relevant interactions of molecules and dosages. This is especially necessary for lower concentrations of copper salts with antibacterials in pigs, encouraged because of environmental concerns about copper excretion, and for the use in poultry, of those coccidiostats and histomoniastats, which are also antibacterial. Dilworth and Day's (1985) survey of 3-Nitro in broiler diets from 1968 to 1983 illustrates the need to re-appraise concentrations of arsenicals in admixtures. Establishing the optimum dosage in admixtures requires that the traditional basic test, in which A mg kg^{-1} of Substance A is compared with B mg kg^{-1} of Substance B and A+B mg kg^{-1} of A plus B and a negative control, should be expanded to test A+B mg kg^{-1} of A and of B. Larger factorial tests may be required to optimise doses in admixtures if dose-response varies with environment.

Bacteria versus antibacterials. Bacteria as feed additives are often suggested as substitutes for the probiotic benefits of dietary antibacterials, creating a need for comparisons. Questions of dosage of bacteria, and their interaction with antibacterials, urgently require much greater research effort than hitherto reported during more than two decades of use and re-development. Negative results with bacterials may well have been due to sub-optimal dosage and in-feed instability. Teller and Vanbelle (1991) have stressed the irregular and not always positive results of microbials and the need to find preparations equal in zootechnical performances to antibacterials. Failure of bacteria to produce nutritional responses in research facilities is sometimes excused under the aegis of a need for 'field' conditions. Very high coefficients of variation of responses to bacterial additives in pig feeds in a preliminary survey (Rosen, 1992b) are 442-9, 253% for LWGEFF and 167-605% for FCREFF. Mean gain and conversion responses to bacterial additives in medicated piglet and growing-fattening, slaughter pig feeds are small or zero.

Rotation and shuttle programmes for antibacterials. Annual or other regular changes of antibacterials (rotation) and changes within a production cycle in starter, grower and finisher feeds (shuttle) are used in practice. There is, however, little published proof of efficacy or rationale. There is a need for controlled tests on practical feeds to slaughter, in order to compare rotation and continuity and to define possible viable changes of molecules and dosages.

Experimental reports on shuttles are very rare and contentious. In broilers, for example, Dudley-Cash (1991) stated that shuttles are based more on intuition than science and invoke assumptions of bacterial resistance phenomena, but then concluded, from a single test, that shuttles are effective in improving weight gain and feed efficiency. The quoted test was ambiguous in that the bacitracin methylene disalicylate control gave no overall response (an infrequent observation for all antibacterials) and that the dosage also was reduced from 55 mg kg^{-1} to 28 mg kg^{-1} in finisher feed. For growing-finishing pigs, Kornegay *et al.* (1975) reported no significant advantage in the shuttling of tylosin, zinc bacitracin and copper in growth phases to 34 kg, 68 kg and market weight. The high cost of extensive scientific tests to evaluate rotations and shuttles may greatly limit progress therein, also because the potential magnitude of benefits therefrom is unpredictable.

Nutritional requirements for antibacterial feed additives. Nutrients are essential dietary constituents of tissues and organs. Antibacterial additives are not essential, in this sense, but they will continue to be required in widespread use unless they can be replaced cost-effectively by limiting nutrients. Four topics on requirements for antibacterials should be considered for further research and development. Firstly, when nutrient densities of feed formulations are increased, is there a need to adjust antibacterial dosages *pro rata* to maintain response? This can easily be tested experimentally.

Secondly, is the use of a single feed concentration from start to finish optimal? In broilers 20 mg kg^{-1} feed provides a dose to five days of age of approximately 4.8 mg kg^{-1} liveweight day^{-1}, which drops to 1.2 mg kg^{-1} liveweight/day in the five days pre-slaughter at 49 days old, and less, if finisher feed concentration is reduced. Reduction and elimination of antibacterial feed concentration from starter to finisher is known to reduce response but the converse of elevation, to maintain physiological dosage, needs to be tested for those antibacterials without tissue residues and environmental problems, having a low enough unit cost of active ingredient for a cost-effective increased dose.

Thirdly, requirements for antibacterials are routinely recommended as feed concentrations, without reference to level of feed intake or animal performance. Hence, physiological intake is ill-defined with no indication of response as a proportion of the optimum possible. Routine provision of nutritional models to predict responses with confidence limits, related at least to projected animal control performance, for use in feed formulation procedures, could well enhance the value of antibacterials in nutrition. Alternative models will be developed to relate responses to the requisite total or daily intake of antibacterial.

Fourthly, models of responses with ration attributes as independent variables are needed, notably for the limiting factors of energy or protein (presumably amino acid) provision. Feed compositions in experimental reports can be used for the calculation of nutrient contents. Preliminary studies for broiler, turkey, layer and pig feeds have indicated no significant effects for crude protein content (Rosen, 1994a). The role of available as against total nutrient contents will need further experimentation to provide an alternative, perhaps more meaningful, data base.

Future progress in the efficient use of antibacterial feed additives would be facilitated if their nutritional effects were subject to appraisal from time to time by independent expert bodies, such as the USDA and UK Research Councils, alongside and in conjunction with their assessments of nutrient requirements. In future, the latter will be based on curvilinear dose-response models for performance levels nearing nutritional sufficiency. In this region overlapping nutritional effects of nutrients and antibacterials will concentrate our attention on possible interactions and on comparisons of cost effectiveness. As we approach the limits of genetic potential in near-ideal environments and feed formulations, the debate on antibacterials will centre on their capacities for cost economies in nutrient provision or, alternatively, on the replacement of non-nutrient additives by nutrients *per se*.

REFERENCES

Aherne, F.X. 1985. *Antibiotics in sow diets.* Department of Animal Science, Faculty of Agriculture and Forestry, University of Alberta, Edmonton, Canada.

Akkerman, G.A. 1993. Production number has limited utility for reliable financial comparisons. PUF **23**, 10-11.

Barber, R.S., Braude, R., Hosking, Z.D. and Mitchell, K.G. 1979. Olaquindox as performance-promoting feed additive for growing pigs. *Anim. Feed Sci. Technol.* **4**, 117-123.

Beames, R.M. and Lloyd, L.E. 1965. Response of pigs and rats to rations supplemented with tylosin and high levels of copper. *J. Anim. Sci.* **24**, 1020-1026.

Berende, P.L.M. and Schutte, J.B. 1978. Literature review of the effect of combinations of antibiotics with other growth-promoting substances in piglets and broilers. ILOB-report 452, September, 1978. Wageningen, Netherlands

Bergero, D., Romboli, I., Sacchi, P., Turi, R.M. and Ladetto, G. 1993. The use of virginiamycin and Flavomycin in diets for Muscovy ducklings. *Arch. Gefluegelk.* **57**, 131-135.

Blaxter, K. 1979. The role of nutrition in animal disease. *Vet. Rec.* **104**, 595-598.

Bolognesi, P.G., Valerani, L., Mussa, P.P., Boccignone, M. and Quaglino, G. 1977. Field tests with Flavomycin (flavophospholipol) in guinea fowl producing hatching eggs. *G. Allevatori* **27**, 19-27.

Bonomi, A., Ghilardi, G., Bianchi, M. and Mazzocco, P. 1975. Flavomycin in meat-producing guinea fowl feeding. Economy of proteins of animal origin. *Riv. Agric.* **44**, 53-63.

Brake, J. 1990. Effect of bacitracin zinc on broiler breeders. *Poultry Sci.* **69** (Suppl. 1), 23. (Abstract).

Branion, H.D., Anderson, G.W. and Hill, D.C. 1953. Antibiotics and the growth of ducks. *Poultry Sci.* **32**, 335-347.

Branion, H.D. and Hill, D.C. 1952. Antibiotics and the growth of goslings. *Poultry Sci.* **31**, 1100-1102.

Branion, H.D., Hill, D.C. and Jukes, H.G. 1956. Effect of an antibiotic on egg production. *Poultry Sci.* **35**, 783-789.

Braude, R. 1967. Copper as a growth stimulant in pigs (cuprum pro pecunia). *World Rev. Anim. Prod.* **3**, 69-81.

Braude, R., Wallace, H.D. and Cunha, T.J. 1953. The value of antibiotics in the nutrition of swine: a review. *Antibiot. Chemother.* **3**, 271-291.

Briones, E.A.B. 1982. Effect of supplementation by feed grade zinc bacitracin on the weight and litter size of pigs. Thesis. Department of Animal Production, National Agrarian University, La Molina, Lima, Peru.

Bunyan, J., Jeffries, L., Sayers, J.R., Gulliver, A.L. and Coleman, K. 1977. Antimicrobial substances and chick growth promotion: the growth promoting activities of antimicrobial substances, including fifty-two used either in therapy or as dietary additives. *Br. Poultry Sci.* **18**, 283-294.

CAST. 1981. Antibiotics in animal feeds. Council for Agricultural Science and Technology, Report No. 88, Ames, Iowa 50011, US.

Chen, B.J., Lin, C.E., Kan, C.L. and Shen, T.F. 1981. The growth promotion effect of zinc bacitracin on mule ducks. Duck Research Center, 28-1, Je-Sui Village, Wuchieh, I-Lan, Taiwan 268.

Clausen, H. 1956. The influence of antibiotics on carcass quality of pigs. In: *Proceedings First International Conference on the Use of Antibiotics in Agriculture*, pp. 19-32. Publication 397, National Academy of Sciences - National Research Council, Washington, D.C., US.

Cromwell, G.L. 1991. Antimicrobial agents. In *Swine Nutrition* (E.R. Miller, D.E. Ullrey, and A.J. Lewis, eds) pp. 297-314. Butterworth-Heinemann, Stoneham, US.

Craene, A. de and Viaene, J. 1992. Economic effects of technology in agriculture. Do performance enhancers for animals benefit consumers? Faculty of Agricultural Sciences, Department of Agro-Marketing, University of Ghent, Ghent, Belgium.

Damron, B.L., Wilson, H.R. and Fell, R.V. 1991. Growth and performance of broiler breeders fed bacitracin methylene disalicylate and zinc bacitracin. *Poultry Sci.* **70**, 1487-1492.

Dilworth, B.C. and Day, E.J. 1985. Survey of the use of 3-Nitro in broiler diets. *Poultry Sci.* **64** (Suppl. 1), 17. (Abstract).

Draper, N.R. and Smith, H. 1981. *Applied Regression Analysis*, Second Edition. John Wiley and Sons, Inc., New York, US.

Dudley-Cash, W.A. 1991. Shuttling of antibiotics improves weight gain, feed efficiency of poultry. *Feedstuffs* **11**, 18.

Elanco Products Ltd. (undated). Tylamix quality succeeds. Elanco Products Ltd., Basingstoke, UK.

Ellis, N.R. 1956. Antibiotics in reproduction. In *Proceedings First International Conference on the Use of Antibiotics in Agriculture*, pp. 69-72. Publication 397, National Academy of Sciences - National Research Council, Washington 25, D.C., US.

Ferrando, R. 1979. Referred to in Braeunlich, K. 1980. A new look at the problem of nutritional requirements with special reference to vitamins in poultry. Roche Information Animal Nutrition, Hofmann-La-Roche and Co. Basle, Switzerland.

Food and Drug Administration. 1972. Report to the Commissioner of the Food and Drug Administration by the FDA Task Force on the use of antibiotics in animal feeds. 72-6008. US Department of Health, Education, and Welfare, Public Health Service, Food and Drug Administration, Rockville, Maryland, US.

Groote, G. de. 1983. Antibiotics as performance-promoting additives in laying hens. National Institute for Small Animal Breeding, Burg. van Gansberghelaan, Merelbeke, Belgium.

Gropp, J.M., Kruse, G.O.W. and Birzer, D.R.T. 1991. Spotlights on feed additives. *Feed Magazine* **2**, 31-32.

Gruhn, K., Hennig, A. and Albold, A. 1961/2. Supplementation of duck feed by oxytetracycline and sodium salicylate. *Jahrb. Arbeitsgemein. Fuetterungsber.* **4**, 370-381.

Guerocak, B. 1970. The nutritional action of antibiotics in quail rearing. *Arch. Gefluegelk.* **34**, 147-153.

Havermann, H. and Wegner, R.M. 1958. Antibiotics in the feeding of laying hens. *Arch. Gefluegelk.* **22**, 217-239.

Hays, V.W. 1981. Effectiveness of feed additive usage of antibacterial agents in swine and poultry production. Rachelle Laboratories, Inc., Long Beach, California 90801, US.

Helder, J.F. 1968. Supplementation of Peking table duck diets with copper sulphate. In *Report Third European Poultry Conference*, pp. 390-396. Jerusalem, Israel.

Hoie, J. and Lund, S. 1963. Experiments with antibiotics for chicks and laying hens. Report No. 17. The Agricultural College of Norway,. Department of Poultry and Fur Animals. Mariendals Boktrykkeri A/S, Gjøvik, Norway.

Jeffries, L., Coleman, K. and Bunyan, J. 1977. Antimicrobial substances and chick growth promotion: comparative studies on selected compounds *in vitro* and *in vivo*. *Br. Poultry Sci.* **18**, 295-308.

Jeroch, H., Clauss, F. and Friedel, E. 1972/3. The use of copper sulphate as an ergotrophic agent in duck fattening. *Jahrb. Tierernaehr. Fuetter* **8**, 402-406.

Jeroch, H., Berger, H., Keller, G. and Gebhardt, G. 1980/1. The influence of nitrovin on the performance of fattening ducks. *Tierernaehr. Fuetter.* **12**, 216-220.

Jeroch, H., Berger, H., Keller, G., Wilke, A., Pfuetzner, B., Jackisch, B., Weber, K. and Gebhardt, G. 1981. Results obtained by the growth promoter nitrovin (of Czechoslovakian provenance) in rearing calves, laying hens and chickens. *Biol. Chem. Vet. (Praha)* **17**, 143-150.

Jordan, C.E. and Waitt, W.P. 1962. Referred to in Mellière, A.L. and Waitt, W.P. 1971. The effect of discontinuing antibiotics from swine finishing rations on subsequent weight gain and feed efficiency. *Feedstuffs* **23**, 45.

Jost, M. 1983. The use of growth promoters in pigs. *Schweiz. Arch Tierheilk.* **125**, 205-212.

Kadamanova, L.D. 1984. Increase of fertility and litter size of sows through the use of bacitracin. *Sb. Nauch. Tr. Beloruss. Akad.* **118**, 28-32.

Kaplan, R., Polasek, L., Podsednicek, M., Tejnora, J. and Sevcik, B. 1985. Examination of effectiveness of cyadox used for the fattening of ducks. *Biol. Chem. Vet. (Praha)* **21**, 499-506.

Kornegay, T., Thomas, H.R. and Kraemer, C.Y. 1975. Effect on subsequent feed lot performance of rotating or withdrawing dietary antibiotics from swine growing and finishing rations. *J. Anim. Sci.* **46**, 1555-1562.

Korniewicz, A., Korniewicz, D. and Paleczek, B. 1991. The influence of avoparcin on the use value of sows. *Rocz. Nauk. Zootech. Monogr. Rozp.* **29**, 169-179.

Kostadinov, K., Drumev, D. and Pashov, D. 1985. On the ergotrophic action of flavophospholipol in the fattening of geese. *Vet. Sci. Sophia* **22**, 74-80.

Krueger, W.F., Bradley, J.W. and Creger, C.R. 1983. Effect of feeding bacitracin zinc on reproduction in broiler breeders. *Poultry Sci.* **62**, 1450-1451. (Abstract).

Kwakkel, R.P. 1993. Rearing the laying pullet. In *Recent Advances in Animal Nutrition 1993* (P.C. Garnsworthy and D.J.A. Cole, eds.) pp. 109-129. Nottingham University Press, Loughborough, UK.

Kyriakis, S.C., Vassilopoulos, V., Demade, I., Kissels, W., Polizopoulou, Z. and Milner, C.K. 1992. The effect of virginiamycin on sow and litter performance. *Anim. Prod.* **55**, 431-436.

Maxwell, C.V., Dietz, D.N., Knabe, D.A., Combs, G.E., Kornegay, E.T., Noland, P.R. and McNew, R.W. 1987. Effect of dietary chlortetracycline during breeding and/or farrowing and lactation on reproductive performance of sows: a cooperative study. *J. Anim. Sci.* **65** (Suppl. 1), 312. (Abstract).

Mellière, A.L., Brown, H. and Rathmacher, R.P. 1973. Finishing swine performance and responses to tylosin. *J. Anim. Sci.* **37**, 286.

Menke, K.H. and Krampitz, G. 1973. Antibiotic modes of action at nutritional dosages. *Uber. Tierernaehr.* **1**, 255-272.

Miles, R.D., Douglas, C.R. and Harms, R.H. 1984. Influence of virginiamycin in pullets and broilers fed diets containing suboptimal protein and sulphur amino acid levels. *Nutr. Rep. Int.* **30**, 983-989.

Moore, P.R., Evenson, A., Luckey, T.D., McCoy, E., Elvehjem, C.A. and Hart, E.B. 1946. Use of sulphasuccidine, streptothricin and streptomycin in nutrition studies with the chick. *J. Biol. Chem.* **165**, 437-441.

Muir, L.A. 1985. Mode of action of exogenous substances on animal growth - an overview. *J. Anim. Sci.* **61** (Suppl. 2), 154-180.

National Academy of Sciences - National Research Council 1956. *Proceedings of First International Conference on the Use of Antibiotics in Agriculture*. Publication 397. Washington, DC, US.

Nie, N.H., Hadlai-Hull, C., Jenkins, J.G., Steinbrenner, K. and Bent, B.H. 1975. *Statistical Package for the Social Sciences*. Second Edition. McGraw-Hill Book Company, New York, US.

O'Connor, J.J. 1980. Mechanisms of growth promoters in single-stomach animals. In *Growth in Animals* (T.L.J. Lawrence, ed.) pp. 207-277. Butterworths, London, UK.

Oguntona, T. 1988a. Response of guinea fowl (*Numida meleagris*) to antibiotics. *Br. Poultry Sci.* **29**, 683-687.

Oguntona, T. 1988b. Effects of dietary levels of oxytetracycline on the growth and organ weights of guinea fowl (*Numida meleagris*). *J. Agri. Sci., Camb.* **111**, 217-220.

Oguntona, T. 1988c. Research note: response of guinea fowl (*Numida meleagris*) to dietary supplementation of zinc bacitracin. *Poultry Sci.* **67**, 145-148.

Pan, C.-M., Lin, C.-Y., Kan, C.-L., Liu, C.-C. and Shen, T.-F. 1985. The effect of avoparcin as a growth promoting agent for mule ducks. *J. Taiwan Livestock Res.* **18**, 217-229.

Roberts, P. 1983. The number of replicates and other considerations in the design of field trials. In *Recent Advances in Animal Nutrition - 1983* (W. Haresign, ed.) pp. 3-11. Butterworths, London, UK.

Rosen, G.D. 1982. Zinc bacitracin as an egg promoter. *Feed Compounder,* December, 22-25.

Rosen, G.D. 1983. Performance promoters in animal nutrition. I. Quantitative factorial analysis of effectiveness. *Vet. Res. Commun.* **7**, 73-81.

Rosen, G.D. 1984. Performance promoters in animal nutrition. II. Methods of comparison of effectiveness. In *Antimicrobials and Agriculture 1984* (M. Woodbine, ed.) pp. 303-313. Butterworths, London, UK.

Rosen, G.D. 1986. Evaluation of the nutritional effects of virginiamycin in layers feed. In *Seventh European Poultry Conference*, Paris, pp. 538-542. World's Poultry Science Association.

Rosen, G.D. 1988a. Evaluation of the nutritional effects of flavophospholipol in layers feeds. In *Proc. XVIII World's Poultry Congress*, pp. 846-848. Japan Poultry Science Association, Masumida Printing Company, Nagoya, Japan.

Rosen, G.D. 1988b. The influence of level of investment, slaughter age and cost/gram on profitability of broiler growth promoters. In *Proc. XVIII World's Poultry Congress*, pp. 849, 968-969. Japan Poultry Science Association, Masumida Printing Company, Nagoya, Japan.

Rosen, G.D. 1989. Nutritional and econometrical comparison of growth promoters for growing-fattening pigs. *Amicale des Vétérinaires Salariés de l'Ouest,* January.

Rosen, G.D. 1990. Nutritional and econometrical comparison of growth promoters for broilers. *Amicale des Vétérinaires Salariés de l'Ouest,* April.

Rosen, G.D. 1992a. Performance promoters in animal nutrition. IV. Updating of statistics and multi-factorial nutritional models. In *Proc. XIX World's Poultry Congress*, Amsterdam, The Netherlands, pp. 495-498. Ponsen and Looijen, Wageningen, Netherlands.

Rosen, G.D. 1992b. Antibacterials in disease control and performance enhancement. *Feed Compounder.* October, November and December 1992, 22-27, 20-23, 40.

Rosen, G.D. 1994a. Unpublished data.

Rosen, G.D. 1994b. Nutrition improvement models for zinc bacitracin in turkeys. In *Proceedings of 9th European Poultry Conference*, Vol. 1. pp. 453-454. Walker and Connell Ltd., Darvel, UK.

Rosen, G.D. and Jansegers, L. 1988. An evaluation of dietary tylosin as a growth promoter in pigs. In *Proceedings of the X Congress, International Pig Veterinary Society*, p. 374. Rio de Janeiro, Brazil.

Rosen, G.D., Roberts, P. and Widdowson, V.M. 1976. An algebraic model for bacitracin in laying hen nutrition. In *Fifth European Poultry Conference Malta*, pp. 201-212. World Poultry Science Association, Interprint (Malta) Ltd., Marsa.

Rosen, G.D., Vernon, J. and Chubb, L.G. 1960. Continuous feeding of Terramycin to flocks and individually-fed laying hens. In *Proceedings Pfizer European Agricultural Research Conference,* (J. Vernon and G.D. Rosen, eds) pp. 282-290. Pfizer Ltd, Sandwich, UK.

Satava, M. 1973. Results of nutritional application of antibiotics to fattened ducklings. *Agrochem.* **13**, 318-322.

Schubert, R., Hennig, A. and Richter, G. 1981. Studies into the ergotrophic effects of kormogrisin and zinc bacitracin of Moscovy duck (*Cairina moschata*). *Monatsh. Vet.* **36**, 505-508.

Schulz, V. and Gropp, J. 1973. Nutritive effects of antibiotics in rearing quail. *Arch. Gefluegelk.* **37**, 176-179.

Slinger, S.J., Snyder, E.S. and Pepper, W.F. 1953. Effect of penicillin on the growth of goslings. *Poultry Sci.* **32**, 396-400.

Smith, H., Taylor, J.H. and Quenouille, M.H. 1961. The continuous feeding of chlortetracycline to laying fowl. *Br. Poultry Sci.* **2**, 107-132.

Snetsinger, D.C. 1970. Antibiotics for turkey and chicken layers and breeders. Presented to FDA Task Force on the Use of Antibiotics in Animal Feeds, Poultry Presentation and Schedule, August 1970. Atlanta, Georgia, US.

Solntsev, M.K. 1989. Egg yield of ducks in relation to the amount of protein and bacitracin in the feed mixture. *Ref. Zhurnal* **3**, 756.

Teller, E. and Vanbelle, M. 1991. Probiotics: facts and fiction. *Méd. Fac. Landbouww. Rijksuniv. Gent* **56**, 1591-1599.

Tejnora, J., Polasek, L., Kaplan, R. and Bauer, B. 1977. The use of nitrovin in the fattening of ducklings. *Biol. a Chem. Vyz. Zvir.* **13**, 349-356.

Tejnora, J., Polasek, L., Kaplan, R. and Bauer, B. 1978. The use of nitrovin of Czechoslovakian production in gosling feeding. *Biol. Chem. Vet. (Praha)* **14**, 319-325.

Tueller, R. 1973. Influence of the feed additives Payzone nitrovin, Flavomycin and zinc bacitracin on laying hens. *Arch. Gefluegelk.* **4**, 154-159.

UKASTA. 1978. Survey on the response of growing pigs to dietary copper supplementations. UK Agricultural Supply Trade Association Ltd., London.

Vanschoubroek, F. and de Wilde, R. 1969. The use of antibiotics in the nutrition of pigs, particularly that of tylosin. *Vlaams Diergeneesk. Tijdschr.* **38**, 213-240.

Voeten, A.C. and Brus, D.H.J. 1966. The production number as a criterion for the breeding results of broiler chickens. *Tijdschr. Diergeneeskd.* **19**, 1233-1240.

Yannakopoulos, A.L., Tserveni-Gousi, A.S. and Zervas, G. 1990. Effect of dietary copper sulphate on the performance of growing Japanese quail. *J. Agric. Sci., Camb.* **115**, 291-293.

Zimmerman, D.R. 1986. Role of sub-therapeutic levels of antimicrobials in pig production. *J. Anim. Sci.* **62** (Suppl. 3), 6-17.

9 Ionophores and antibiotics in ruminants

T. G. Nagaraja

Department of Animal Sciences, Kansas State University, Manhattan, Kansas 66506-1600 US

INTRODUCTION

Antimicrobial agents are used not only for the control and treatment of infectious diseases, but also for the enhancement of body growth and improvement of feed efficiency of animals. Antibiotic feed supplements for growth promotion have been used extensively in every major livestock-producing country for more than 40 years. It is generally appreciated that the use of antibiotics has contributed to lower animal production costs and ultimately to lower costs to the consumer for meat, milk, and wool. The use of antibiotics as feed additives originated with the observation that spent culture mash from the commercial production of chlortetracycline improved weight gain and increased feed efficiency in chickens. Initially, the recognizable growth promotion was ascribed simply to an "unidentified growth factor". Subsequently, the growth factor was identified as the residual antibiotic remaining in the mash because of an inefficient extraction process (Jukes and Williams, 1953). The growth-promoting effect was confirmed quickly in pigs and turkeys and also was produced by the addition of other antibiotics to the feed. The small amounts of antibiotic required to elicit the growth promotion meant that it was economically feasible to add to livestock feed. In ruminant animals, however, it was conjectured that antibiotics would not be beneficial because they might interfere with the nutrition of the host animal by suppressing microbial fermentation in the foregut. Because the newborn calf behaves like a nonruminant animal with regard to feed digestion, initial investigations were directed towards determining whether or not antibiotics included in the diet would stimulate growth of calves. Bartley *et al.* (1950) and Loosli and Wallace (1950) reported that daily chlortetracycline administration produced a marked increase in the growth of dairy calves. Subsequent studies showed that adult ruminants could tolerate the antibiotics with no deleterious effects. Thus began the widespread use of antibiotics for growth promotion in ruminant diets (Lassiter, 1955).

Literally hundreds of antibiotics that promote growth have been reported in the scientific literature and in patents worldwide, but only a few have been approved by various governmental agencies in different countries. These antibiotics represent a diverse group and can be grouped broadly into ionophores and nonionophores.

IONOPHORE ANTIBIOTICS

Discovery and development

In order to maximize the efficiency of feed utilization in ruminants, research in the past two decades has focussed on chemicals that promote adjustments in ruminal fermentation to decrease losses in energy and nitrogen but not impede beneficial processes of microbial activity, such as fiber degradation, synthesis of B vitamins, and microbial protein synthesis from nonprotein nitrogen, and ultimately to improve animal performance. Dr. A.P. Raun and his colleagues at Lilly Research Laboratories (Greenfield, Indiana, US), using an *in vitro* fermentation system, began screening compounds that would enhance propionate production (Raun, 1990). They theorized that a significant increase in ruminal propionate production would increase the energy available from a given amount of feedstuffs and, hence, would translate to an economically significant effect. The research resulted in the discovery that monensin, an ionophore antibiotic, could beneficially modify ruminal fermentative activity (Raun *et al.*, 1976). It was approved as a feed additive in the US in 1976 for increasing feed efficiency in feedlot cattle and in 1978 for increasing rate of gain of pasture cattle.

Ionophore antibiotics, so named because of their ion bearing property, are members of a large and growing group of compounds possessing the ability to form lipid-soluble complexes with cations and mediate their transport across lipid barriers. Because of the multiplicity of cyclic ethers in structures of some ionophores, they are also called "polyether" antibiotics. Although ionophores were isolated first in the early 1950s, it was not until 1967 that the first structure, that of monensin, was described (Agtarap *et al.*, 1967). This class of compound attracted considerable attention because of the report that monensin and other ionophores, when added to the ration, were effective in preventing coccidiosis in poultry (Shumard and Callender, 1968). Subsequently, it was shown that monensin improves utilization of feedstuffs in ruminants by altering ruminal fermentation. However, these compounds continue to be used as valuable biochemical tools to perturb gradients of H^+ or mono- or divalent cations across membranes and thus probe the role of key cations in biology.

All of the ionophores currently in use or being investigated as growth promotants for ruminants (Table 1) are classified as carboxylic ionophores (they possess a carboxyl group). These form electrically neutral complexes with mono- or divalent cations (i.e. they shed a proton to form neutral cation-ionophore complexes) and catalyze electrically silent exchanges of cations for protons or other cations across a variety of biological membranes. All these antibiotics can complex with monovalent cations, but lasalocid, lysocellin, and tetronasin are able to complex with divalent cations that have binding constants of the same order as those of monovalent cations (Westley, 1983). Laidlomycin propionate, a chemically derived (semisynthetic) ionophore, is more potent than the naturally occurring parent compound (Spires and Algeo, 1983) and its cation selectivity has not been determined.

Performance response in adult ruminants

Ionophore antibiotics, particularly monensin, have gained wide acceptance in the cattle feeding industry. The success of monensin has spurred interest in the investigations of several new ionophores (Table 1). Generally, dietary inclusion of ionophores has improved feed efficiency but effects on body weight gain and feed intake have been variable. In grain-fed animals, ionophores generally depress feed intake, but body weight gain is increased or unaffected and feed efficiency (feed/gain) is improved. In pasture-fed cattle, ionophores do not reduce intake but body weight gain is increased, thus resulting in improved feed efficiency (Table 2). Reductions in feed intake may be due to flavors of ionophore compounds or to animals regulating intake to maintain body energy balance. Reduced feed intake has been observed most consistently with cattle fed monensin. Baile *et al.* (1979) suggested that the immediate aversion to feed shown by cattle fed high-concentrate diets was attributable to the flavor of the monensin premix. However, an aversion to monensin by cattle fed high-roughage diet was not immediate and apparently developed as a conditioned stimulus resulting from prior exposure.

Table 1. Ionophore antibiotics used or under investigation for use in ruminant diets.

Ionophore	Producing organism	Molecular weight	Cation selectivity sequence[a]
Monensin	*Streptomyces cinnamonensis*	671	$Na^+>K^+$, $Li^+>Rb^+>Cs^+$
Lasalocid	*Streptomyces lasaliensis*	591	Ba^{++}, $K^+>Rb^+>Na^+>Cs^+>Li^+$
Laidlomycin	*Streptoverticillum eurocidicum*	721	ND
Lysocellin	*Streptomyces longwoodensis*	660	$Na^+>K^+$, Ca^{++}, Mg^{++}
Narasin	*Streptomyces aureofaciens*	765	$Na^+>K^+$, Rb^+, Cs^+, Li^+
Salinomycin	*Streptomyces albus*	751	Rb^+, $Na^+>K^+>>Cs^+$, Sr^+, Ca^{++}, Mg^{++}
Tetronasin	*Streptomyces longisporoflavus*	628	$Ca^{++}>Mg^{++}>Na^+$, $K^+>Rb^+$

[a] Selectivity sequence of cation flux across bilayer membranes.
ND = Not determined.

The nature and magnitude of the response to ionophores are dependent upon the type of ionophores, dose of ionophore (Fig. 1), cattle type, geographical location, management system, and duration of feeding. Goodrich *et al.* (1984) summarized 228 experiments conducted in

Table 2. General responses of beef cattle to ionophore antibiotics.

Ionophore	Grain-fed			Pasture-fed	Dose per head per day	
	Intake	Gain	Efficiency	Gain	Grain-fed (mg/kg of feed)	Pasture-fed (mg)
Monensin	↓	0	↑	↑	5.5 - 33	50 - 200
Lasalocid	0,↑	↑	↑	↑	11 - 33	60 - 200
Laidlomycin propionate	0,↑	↑	↑	NA	6 - 12	25 - 50
Lysocellin	↓	0,↑	↑	↑	11 - 33	80 - 100
Narasin	↓	0	↑	NA	8 - 16	-
Salinomycin	0, ↓	0,↑	↑	↑	5.5 - 16.5	50 - 100
Tetronasin	↓	0,↑	↑	↑	7.5 - 15	30 - 60

↑, Increase; ↓, Decrease; 0, No change; NA, Data not available

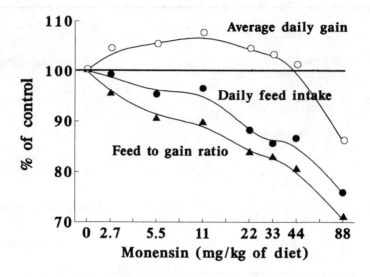

Figure 1. Effect of varying doses of monensin on average daily gain, daily feed intake and feed to gain ratio in feedlot cattle (adapted from Raun *et al.*, 1976).

the US in which the average feed efficiency response was 7.5% in cattle fed an average of 246 mg of monensin per day (Table 3). Results from 35 experiments conducted in nine countries in Europe showed that monensin (25-33 mg per kg of feed) decreased feed intake

Table 3. Performance response of feedlot and pasture cattle fed monensin.

Location	Type of cattle	Response	Control	Monensin	% Change
US[a]	Feedlot	Daily gain, kg	1.09	1.10	1.6
		Daily feed intake, kg DM	8.27	7.73	-6.4
		Feed/gain	8.09	7.43	-7.5
	Pasture	Daily gain, kg	0.609	0.691	13.5
Europe	Feedlot[b]	Daily gain, kg	1.153	1.213	5.2
		Daily feed intake, kg	7.45	7.15	-4.0
		Feed/gain	6.59	6.02	-8.7
	Pasture[c]	Daily gain, kg	0.786	0.893	13.7

[a] Goodrich *et al.* (1984).
[b] Wilkinson *et al.* (1980).

[c] Hawkridge (1980).

by 4%, increased gain by 5%, and improved feed efficiency by 9% (Hawkridge, 1980). In a summary of 24 trials conducted in the USA, monensin at an average dose of 154.5 mg per day increased gain by 13.5% (Goodrich *et al.*, 1984). In 12 pasture studies in Europe, monensin at 200 mg per head daily increased gain by 14% (Wilkinson *et al.*, 1980). The performance response with lasalocid is similar or slightly greater than that of monensin (Stuart, 1982). Reports on ionophores other than monensin or lasalocid are limited, but the overall responses appear to be similar, and new ionophores are generally two to five-fold more potent than either lasalocid or monensin (Table 2).

MODE OF ACTION OF IONOPHORES

The effectiveness of ionophores in achieving increased efficiency of feed conversion and, under some conditions, improving the rate of gain is attributed principally to alterations in ruminal fermentation. Because ionophores have activity against both prokaryotic and eukaryotic cells, part of the performance response may be due to metabolic changes that do not involve alterations in ruminal microbial fermentation.

Ruminal effects

Most studies on changes in ruminal fermentation that are associated with ionophore feeding have been done with monensin or lasalocid (Russell and Strobel, 1989). The studies dealing with other ionophores generally have indicated that the fermentation changes induced are similar to those of monensin or lasalocid except for the difference in potency of the antibiotic (Nagaraja *et al.*, 1987). Bergen and Bates (1984) listed fermentation changes associated with ionophore feeding in three major areas:
- increased production of propionate and decreased production of methane, resulting in increased efficiency of energy metabolism of the rumen and/or animal
- decreased protein degradation and deamination of amino acids, resulting in the improvement of nitrogen metabolism in the rumen and/or animal
- decreased lactic acid production and froth formation in the rumen, leading to reduction of ruminal disorders.

Increased propionate and decreased methane production. The most consistent and well-documented fermentation alterations observed when ionophores are fed are the increased molar proportion of propionic acid and decrease in the molar proportions of acetate and butyrate in the VFA produced in the rumen (Raun *et al.*, 1976). Changes reported in acetate and butyrate molar proportions with ionophore feeding are not consistent. The magnitude of increase in the molar percent of propionate generally is inversely related to energy density of the diet. The relative enhancement is lower in cattle consuming high-energy feeds (high grain) that already have large amounts of propionic acid in the rumen than in cattle consuming low-energy feeds (high roughage). However, changes in propionate molar percentages do not reflect accurately changes in propionate production (Table 4; Prange *et al.*, 1978; Rogers and Davis, 1982; Van Maanen *et al.*, 1978).

Increased propionic acid accumulation in the rumen of ionophore-fed animals may be a consequence of redirected hydrogen utilization caused by lower methane production. However, monensin has been shown to shift the acetate:propionate ratio even in cultures not producing methane, suggesting that part of the increase in propionate is independent of its effect on

Table 4. Concentration, molar proportion and production of ruminal volatile fatty acids in cattle fed diets with or without monensin.

VFA	70% Roughage + 30% Concentrate[a]			50% Roughage + 50% Concentrate[b]		
	Control	Monensin	% change from control	Control	Monensin	% change from control
Concentration, mM						
Acetate	70	61[c]	-13	65.8	55.9	-15
Propionate	19	23[c]	+21	41.1	41.9	+2
Butyrate	10	8	-20	13.5	9.1	-33
Proportion, %						
Acetate	71.0	66.8	-6	53.5	51.3[c]	-4
Propionate	19.1	24.7[c]	+29	33.4	38.4[c]	+15
Butyrate	9.9	8.5[c]	-14	11.0	8.3	-25
Production, moles per day						
Acetate	-	-	-	7.32	8.68	+19
Propionate	7.74	11.2[c]	+46	4.82	7.30	+52
Butyrate	-	-	-	2.12	1.76	-17

[a] Adapted from Prange et al. (1978).
[b] Adapted from Rogers and Davis (1982).
[c] Different from control, $P<0.05$.

methane production (Slyter, 1979). The concept that propionate is utilized more efficiently than acetate by the host tissue is subject to dispute (Ørskov et al., 1991). However, flexibility in the use of propionate (gluconeogenesis or oxidation via the Krebs cycle) by the host tissue offers a distinct advantage over acetate. Also, propionate production in the rumen results in improved fermentation efficiency because of greater recovery of metabolic hydrogen (Chalupa, 1984).

The increase in rumen propionate is accompanied by a reduction, ranging from 4 to 31%, in the amount of methane produced in the rumen (Schelling, 1984; Rumpler et al., 1986). Because ionophore antibiotics are not inhibitory to methanogenic bacteria (Chen and Wolin, 1979), the lower methane production is believed to be due to a decreased rate of production of its precursors (H_2 and formate), an idea that is supported by the observation that when substrates (CO_2 and H_2) are provided, ionophores have no effect on methane production (Van Nevel and Demeyer, 1977; Russell and Martin, 1984). However, monensin inhibits methanogenesis from formate (Van Nevel and Demeyer, 1977; Dellinger and Ferry, 1984). Inhibition of methanogenesis may be partly because nickel uptake is inhibited by monensin in methanogenic bacteria (Jarrell and Sprott, 1983). Nickel is required for synthesis of coenzyme F_{430} and the hydrogenase enzyme (Daniels et al., 1984), and therefore monensin could have direct effects on metabolism in ruminal methanogens. However, nickel supplementation with or without monensin had no effect on ruminal methane production in cattle (Oscar et al., 1987).

Effect on nitrogen metabolism. The earliest evidence that nitrogen metabolism is affected by feeding ionophores came from the report of Dinius *et al.* (1976) who found a decreased ruminal ammonia concentration in cattle fed forage-based diet supplemented with monensin. A number of *in vitro* and *in vivo* studies (Dinius *et al.*, 1976; Van Nevel and Demeyer, 1977; Chen and Wolin, 1979; Hanson and Klopfenstein, 1979; Poos *et al.*, 1979; Whetstone *et al.*, 1981; Russell and Martin, 1984; Newbold *et al.*, 1990; Wallace *et al.*, 1990; Chen and Russell, 1991) have indicated that lower ammonia concentrations are due to decreased proteolysis, degradation of peptides, and deamination of amino acids in the rumen. Ionophores appear to affect ruminal degradation of peptides and deamination of amino acids to a greater extent than proteolysis (Van Nevel and Demeyer, 1977; Wallace *et al.*, 1981; Whetstone *et al.*, 1981; Newbold *et al.*, 1990). The inability of ionophores to inhibit proteolysis is consistent with the observation that many proteolytic bacteria are resistant to ionophores (Chen and Wolin, 1979). Wallace *et al.* (1990) reported that the postprandial peak concentration of free peptides in the rumen was more than two-fold greater in ionophore-fed (monensin or tetronasin) sheep than in control sheep and persisted longer, thus increasing peptide flow from the rumen into the abomasum (Chen and Russell, 1991). Yang and Russell (1993) reported that monensin increased amino acid nitrogen passage from the rumen, and the quantity passing from the rumen was dependent on the protein source. Deamination of amino acids in the rumen is a nutritionally wasteful process, because the rate of ammonia production exceeds the rate of utilization (Tamminga, 1979).

The most active ammonia-producing ruminal bacteria were thought to be carbohydrate-fermenting species, principally *Prevotella ruminicola* (Bladen *et al.*, 1961). Being Gram-negative bacteria, these are not susceptible to ionophores. Therefore, the effect of ionophores on ammonia production in the rumen could not be explained, suggesting that the active amino acid-fermenting bacteria had not yet been isolated. Using an enrichment procedure, Russell and his associates (Russell and Chen, 1988; Chen and Russell, 1991) isolated three species of Gram-positive bacteria that were sensitive to monensin, not proteolytic, but had a specific activity of ammonia production which was about 20-fold greater than that of previously known rumen bacterial species. These bacteria were identified recently as *Peptostreptococcus anaerobius*, *Clostridium sticklandii*, and *Clostridium aminophilum* (Paster *et al.*, 1993). They appear to exist in significant numbers in the rumen (10^7-10^8 per ml of rumen fluid, representing <5% of the total bacterial population) but have not been isolated extensively. Decreased peptide degradation and amino acid deamination by ionophores is attributed to inhibition of these ammonia-producing bacteria (Yang and Russell, 1993). Ionophores also may affect peptide degradation or amino acid fermentation by monensin-resistant, Gram negative bacteria and possibly interfere with peptide uptake or alter the metabolic activity of bacteria such as *P. ruminicola* (Newbold and Wallace, 1989).

Ionophores have been shown to decrease ruminal urease activity (Starnes *et al.*, 1984). The lower urease activity may have resulted from selection against ureolytic bacteria or from inhibition of nickel transport into ureolytic bacteria. Because urea hydrolysis by urease occurs at a faster rate than ammonia assimilation by ruminal bacteria, the effect of ionophores on urease activity would have a beneficial effect on urea utilization in ruminants.

The net effect of ionophores on the nitrogen economy of the animal will depend upon the specific dietary situation. The greatest response would be expected when dietary protein is not excessive and is supplied in a soluble form likely to be fermented rapidly in the rumen (Hanson and Klopfenstein, 1979).

Reduction of ruminal disorders. Altered ruminal fermentation associated with ionophore feeding has been shown to reduce the incidence and severity of certain diseases of ruminants, such as acidosis, bloat, and acute bovine pulmonary edema and emphysema. Cereal grain is the major component of feedlot diets, and situations that lead to rapid fermentation of starch also lead to increased accumulation of organic acids in the rumen. Lactic acidosis is initiated by the rapid proliferation of lactic acid-producing bacteria (*Streptococcus bovis* and *Lactobacillus* spp.) in the rumen, resulting in the rate of lactic acid production exceeding the rate of utilization. The excessive production and accumulation of L(+) and D(-) lactic acids lead to ruminal acidosis, which consequently destroys the normal microbial population of the rumen and produces potentially toxic metabolites. The ionophore antibiotics possess ideal characteristics for preventing lactic acidosis. Because of their selectivity toward Gram-positive bacteria, the major lactic acid-producing rumen bacteria (*S. bovis* and *Lactobacillus* spp.) are inhibited, but Gram-negative lactic acid-fermenting bacteria are unaffected (Dennis *et al.*, 1981). Cattle subjected to experimental acidosis and treated with ionophore antibiotics maintain higher ruminal pH and lower lactate concentration than controls (Nagaraja *et al.*, 1985). Subacute or subclinical acidosis, which is characterized by less severe ruminal acidity, occurs when VFA are the predominant organic acids and this may be a more common form of acidosis in grain-fed ruminants. Ionophore antibiotics also provide protection against subacute acidosis by maintaining a favorable ruminal pH (Burrin and Britton, 1986). Maintenance of favorable ruminal fermentation also impacts on the feed intake of the animal. Monensin has been shown to decrease the mean variance in daily feed intake, particularly during the period of adaptation to a high grain diet (Burrin *et al.*, 1988). The influence on feed intake variability should potentially be additive to the ruminal benefits.

Frothy bloat, characterized by excessive foaming of ruminal contents, is another common digestive disorder of ruminants. Frothy bloat can be caused by legumes like alfalfa or clover (pasture bloat) and high-grain diets (grain or feedlot bloat). Froth is caused by a combination of feed and microbial factors (Clarke and Reid, 1973). The major microbial factor includes production of excessive microbial polysaccharides or slime that contribute to increased viscosity of rumen fluid, which, coupled with increased gas production, causes frothy bloat. Ionophore antibiotics generally do not eliminate the bloat problem completely but cause a significant reduction in incidence (Sakauchi and Hoshino, 1981; Bartley *et al.*, 1983). The reductions in microbial slime and gas production are attributed to antibacterial and antiprotozoal effects of monensin and other ionophores (Katz *et al.*, 1986). Not all ionophore antibiotics are equally effective in preventing bloat (Bartley *et al.*, 1983).

Acute bovine pulmonary edema and emphysema (ABPE) typically occurs in cattle moved from dry, sparse grazing to lush, green pastures. The biochemical pathogenesis of ABPE involves 3-methylindole, a ruminal fermentation product of tryptophan. The disease has been reproduced by oral administration of tryptophan or 3-methylindole or by intravenous administration of 3-methylindole, but not by intravenous administration of tryptophan (Breeze and Carlson, 1982), suggesting that ruminal fermentation of tryptophan is essential. Monensin and lasalocid offer protection against ABPE by decreasing tryptophan degradation and, therefore, ruminal 3-methylindole production (Nocerini *et al.*, 1985).

Other ruminal effects. Monensin has been shown to decrease rumen turnover rate of solids and liquids and, consequently, increase rumen fill (Lemenager *et al.*, 1978; Allen and Harrison, 1979). The decreased turnover may be independent of the effect of monensin on feed intake and, therefore, probably is a cause of decreased feed intake in forage-fed animals

(Lemenager *et al.*, 1978). The decreased turnover may increase the amount of organic matter fermented in the rumen, thereby compensating for reduced microbial activity. Monensin also has been shown to decrease motility of the rumen (Deswysen *et al.*, 1987), thereby providing a physiological basis for the increased ruminal fill and reduced feed intake .

Antimicrobial activity of ionophores

Generally, ionophore antibiotics are highly effective against Gram-positive bacteria but exhibit little or no activity against Gram-negative bacteria (Chen and Wolin, 1979; Watanabe *et al.*, 1981). Differences in the sensitivity of bacteria based on the Gram reaction suggest that cell envelope structure plays a role in ionophore susceptibility. Gram-negative bacteria possess an outer membrane that contains protein channels (porins) with a size exclusion limit of approximately 600 daltons. Most ionophores are larger than 600 daltons (Table 1) and, hence, would not pass through the porins. Also, the lipid layer in the outer membrane may act as a hydrophobic barrier, trapping ionophores before they reach the inner cell membrane. Gram-positive bacteria do not have an outer membrane to confer protection and, hence, are much more susceptible to the action of ionophores. However, the presence of an outer membrane is not an absolute criterion for resistance, because some Gram-negative bacteria become susceptible to high concentrations of ionophores (Nagaraja and Taylor, 1987).

Chen and Wolin (1979) were the first investigators to study the effects of lasalocid and monensin on pure cultures of rumen bacteria and to relate susceptibility and resistance to alterations in ruminal fermentation products. A number of other investigators have confirmed the antibacterial spectra of ionophore antibiotics, particularly in relation to cell wall structure and fermentation products (Dennis *et al.*, 1981; Henderson *et al.*, 1981; Dawson and Boling, 1987; Nagaraja and Taylor, 1987; Newbold *et al.*, 1988). In general, ionophore antibiotics are inhibitory to Gram-positive bacteria, such as *Eubacterium, Lactobacillus* and *Streptococcus,* and to those bacteria that often stain Gram-negative but have Gram-positive cell wall structure such as *Butyrivibrio, Lachnospira,* and *Ruminococcus*. Gram-negative bacteria, including *Anaerovibrio, Fibrobacter, Megasphaera, Prevotella, Ruminobacter, Selenomonas, Succinimonas, Succinivibrio,* and *Veillonella* species, are resistant to ionophores. Generally, ruminal bacteria sensitive to ionophores produce lactate, butyrate, formate, or hydrogen and bacteria resistant to ionophores produce succinate or propionate as fermentation products (Table 5; Chen and Wolin, 1979; Nagaraja and Taylor, 1987).

Mechanism of ionophore inhibition of ruminal bacteria. Although a considerable amount of information exists concerning the resistance and susceptibility of individual species of ruminal bacteria, the mode of action of ionophores in inhibiting bacterial growth has received little attention. Ionophores are generally bacteriostatic and not bacteriocidal (Nagaraja and Taylor, 1987). The mechanism of bacteriostatic activity of ionophores is related to their ability to alter the flow of cations across the cell membrane. Because monensin is a sodium/proton antiporter, Bergen and Bates (1984) suggested that it would cause entry of protons into ruminal bacteria in exchange for sodium. Later work of Russell (1987) demonstrated that the direction of sodium movement was opposite to this. When *S. bovis*, a Gram-positive ruminal bacterium, was treated with monensin, a decrease in intracellular potassium concentration and influx of protons resulting in lower intracellular pH were observed (Fig. 2). Once intracellular pH was acidic, monensin catalyzed an efflux of protons in exchange for sodium. The inhibition of *S. bovis* was attributed to futile cycling of ions across the cell membrane resulting in loss of intracellular potassium, a reversal of intracellular transmembrane ΔpH,

Table 5.   Susceptibility and resistance of ruminal bacteria to lasalocid or monensin.

Major fermentation products, genus and species	Gram reaction	Cell wall type	Minimum inhibitory concentration (µg ml^{-1})[a]	
			Lasalocid	Monensin
Hydrogen and formic acid producers				
Lachnospira multiparus	-	+	+(.38)[b]	+(.38)
Ruminococcus albus	-	+	+(.38)	+(.38)
Ruminococcus flavefaciens	-	+	+(.38)	+(.38)
Butyric acid producers				
Butyrivibrio fibrisolvens	-	+	+(.38)	+(.38)
Eubacterium cellulosolvens	+	+	+[c](.38)	+(.38)
Eubacterium ruminantium	+	+	+(.38-1.5)	+(.38-1.5)
Lactic acid producers				
Lactobacillus ruminis	+	+	+(1.5)	+(1.5-3.0)
Lactobacillus vitulinis	+	+	+(.38-1.5)	+(.38-1.5)
Streptococcus bovis	+	+	+(.38-.75)	+(.38-12.0)
Ammonia producers				
Clostridium aminophilum	+			+(<5.0)
Clostridium sticklandii	+			+(<5.0)
Peptostreptococcus anaerobius	+			+(<5.0)
Succinic acid and propionic acid producers				
Anaerovibrio lipolytica	-	-	-(>48.0)	-(>48.0)
Fibrobacter succinogenes	-	-	-(>20.0)	-(>20.0)
Megasphaera elsdenii	-	-	-(>48.0)	-(>48.0)
Prevotella ruminicola	-	-	-(>48.0)	-(>48.0)
Ruminobacter amylophilus	-	-	-(>48.0)	-(>48.0)
Selenomonas ruminantium	-	-	-(>48.0)	-(>48.0)
Succinimonas amylolytica	-	-	-(>48.0)	-(>48.0)
Succinivibrio dextrinosolvens	-	-	-(>48.0)	-(>48.0)
Methane producers				
Methanobrevibacter ruminantium	-	-	-(>20.0)	-(>40.0)
Methanobacterium formicum	-	-	-(>20.0)	-(>40.0)
Methanosarcina barkeri	-	-	-(>20.0)	-(>40.0)

[a] Adapted from Chen and Wolin (1979), Dennis *et al.* (1981), Russell *et al.* (1988), Chen and Russell (1989).
[b] +, susceptible; -, resistant; values in parentheses are minimum inhibitory concentrations in µg ml^{-1}.

accumulation of intracellular sodium and depletion of ATP (Table 6; Russell, 1987; Strobel *et al.*, 1989). The decline of ATP could have been caused by membrane-bound ATPases which used the ATP to counteract the influx of protons and sodium. This postulated mechanism of inhibition is supported by the evidence that antimicrobial activity of ionophores may be reversed in the presence of high potassium concentration (Dawson and Boling, 1987).

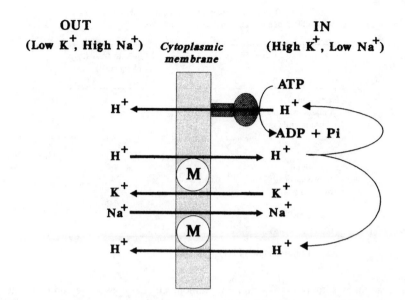

Figure 2. Schematic diagram showing hypothetical effects of monensin (M) on ion flux in *Streptococcus bovis* (Russell and Strobel, 1989).

Ruminal protozoa and fungi. Ionophore antibiotics are also inhibitory to ruminal ciliates (Dennis *et al.*, 1986; Newbold *et al.*, 1988) and anaerobic fungi (Newbold *et al.*, 1988; Marounek and Hodrova, 1989; Stewart and Richardson, 1989). Generally, holotrichid ciliates (*Dasytricha, Isotricha* and *Charonina*) are resistant, whereas entodiniomorphs (*Entodinium, Diplodinium* and *Ophryoscolex*) are sensitive to ionophore antibiotics (Dennis *et al.*, 1986). Protozoal inhibition by ionophore antibiotics is only transient, because continued feeding results in the return of the ciliate population to the pre-antibiotic-feeding level (Sakauchi and Hoshino, 1981; Dennis *et al.*, 1986), suggesting selection of a resistant population of ciliates in the rumen. *In vitro* studies have shown that fungi are sensitive to ionophore antibiotics (Newbold *et al.*, 1988; Marounek and Hodrova, 1989; Stewart and Richardson, 1989). However, the response of the fungal population in the rumen to dietary ionophores has not been consistent (Elliott *et al.*, 1987; Grenet *et al.*, 1989).

Antimicrobial activity and ionophore potency. The potency of antibiotics generally is described by the minimum inhibitory concentration (MIC). The MIC determination is usually done with unadapted bacteria in batch culture at optimal growth conditions. There is evidence that exposure to a low level of ionophore selects for resistant populations (Chen and Wolin, 1979), suggesting that the MIC for ruminal bacteria from cattle fed ionophores could be different from the MIC for bacteria from cattle fed control diets. The antimicrobial activity of ionophores also is influenced by cation concentrations in the medium (Dawson and Boling, 1987). Culturel pH could also affect ionophore activity on rumen bacteria. Lasalocid and monensin were more inhibitory to *S. bovis* at pH 5.7 than at pH 6.7 (Chow and Russell, 1990).

Table 6.   Effect of monensin on intracellular pH and cation and ATP concentrations in *Streptococcus bovis*.

Variable	Control	Monensin-treated $(5\ \mu g\ ml^{-1})$
Extracellular		
Potassium (mM)	9	9
Sodium (mM)	89	93
pH	6.65	6.65
Intracellular		
Potassium (mM)	613	134
Sodium (mM)	237	543
pH	7.08	6.20
ATP (mM)	5.1	1.5

From Strobel *et al.* (1989).

Certain ionophore antibiotics like narasin, salinomycin, tetronasin are more potent than lasalocid or monensin, based on performance response and alterations in rumen fermentation characteristics (Nagaraja *et al.*, 1987; Newbold *et al.*, 1988; Russell and Strobel, 1989). However, MICs of these new ionophores (except tetronasin; Newbold *et al.*, 1988) to ruminal bacteria are similar to that of lasalocid or monensin, suggesting that MIC is not a good indicator of the potency of ionophores in altering ruminal fermentation characteristics (Nagaraja and Taylor, 1987).

Antimicrobial activity and alterations in rumen fermentation.   The idea that the action of ionophores is primarily due to inhibition of Gram-positive bacteria is supported by the observation that ionophores and certain nonionophore antibiotics that inhibit cell wall synthesis (avoparcin, bacitracin) of Gram-positive bacteria have remarkably similar effects on fermentation end products (Froetschel *et al.*, 1983; Russell and Strobel, 1988). Alterations in rumen fermentation associated with ionophore feeding generally are attributed to a shift in microbial population resulting from elimination or decline in populations sensitive to ionophores and selection of populations resistant to ionophores. Ionophore-resistant bacteria are present in greater numbers in the rumen of animals fed ionophore-supplemented diets (Dawson and Boling 1983; Olyumeyan *et al.*, 1986). However, increased proportions of ionophore-resistant bacteria are not always associated with altered fermentation products (Dawson and Boling, 1983).

The significance of the antiprotozoal and antifungal activities of ionophore antibiotics in terms of ruminal fermentation is not clear. Although ciliate protozoa constitute an important fraction of the total microbial population in the rumen, they are not indispensable for feed digestion. Ruminal fungi possess major activities, such as fiber and protein degradation, but their quantitative significance to the total microbial activity in the rumen is not known. Possibly, the alterations in rumen fermentation seen with ionophore feeding are partly due to elimination or reduction of fungi and ciliates and their associated methanogenic bacteria, leading to change in hydrogen flow pattern (Elliot *et al.*, 1987; Stewart and Richardson, 1989).

Postruminal effects of ionophores

Because most ionophores are small molecular weight compounds, they are capable of being absorbed from the gut. In the case of monensin, up to 50% is absorbed (Donoho, 1984), metabolized, excreted in the bile, and eliminated in the feces. The effect of ionophores on hindgut fermentation appears to be minimal (Yokoyama *et al.*, 1985). Ionophores affect cell membranes of eukaryotic cells and subcellular organelles such as mitochondria. Therefore, the influence of monensin or other ionophores on nutrient absorption and tissue metabolism cannot be ruled out. Intravenous administration of 18 or 40 mg of monensin altered concentrations of free fatty acids, glucose, potassium, magnesium, phosphorus, insulin, and luteinizing hormone (Armstrong and Spears, 1988), thus providing evidence for an effect of ionophore on tissue metabolism independent of alterations in ruminal microbial metabolism. Some of the metabolic effects observed with ionophore feeding may be related to rumen fermentation changes. Increased propionate or amino acid availability could account for elevated blood glucose concentration. However, an increase in blood glucose independent of ruminal changes has been observed with monensin infused intravenously (Armstrong and Spears, 1988) or post-ruminally (Rogers *et al.*, 1991). The mechanism by which monensin acts post-ruminally is difficult to explain. It may act directly on the pancreas, perhaps affecting insulin secretion (Galitzer *et al.*, 1986). Wahle and Livesay (1985) reported an increased propionate oxidation by liver slices with monensin supplementation. Benz *et al.* (1989) observed changes in blood levels of intermediary metabolites of carbohydrate metabolism. An increased urea flux was observed with monensin, possibly because of a decrease in ruminal urease activity (Harmon and Avery, 1987).

Ionophore and mineral interaction

Ionophore antibiotics bind to numerous mono- and divalent cations, thus facilitating the passage of metal ions across lipid membranes. Transport of cations also may be influenced by an ionophore that does not specifically bind that ion, because an alteration in one ion gradient can affect indirectly the transport of other ions. Because the body depends on timely release and sequestering of ions, any disruption in ion flux could directly or indirectly alter host physiology. Ionophores potentially could alter host mineral metabolism by affecting ion bioavailability in feeds and water, uptake and transport of ions across biological membranes and tissues, distribution and storage of ions in tissues and bones, specific mineral-mineral interactions, and homeostatic and regulatory mechanisms governing intake and excretion of ions (Elsasser, 1984).

A number of studies have indicated that feeding ionophores affects the absorption and retention of certain minerals (Starnes *et al.*, 1984; Kirk *et al.*, 1985 a, b; Greene *et al.*, 1986). However, results have not been consistent, suggesting that the effect of ionophores on mineral metabolism is affected by dietary, environmental and physiological factors.

Ionophore and dietary fat interaction

Ionophores are lipophilic, and therefore the inclusion of fat in the diet may alter ruminal distribution and/or access of ionophores to microbes. Also, ionophores and fats have similar antimicrobial effects and affect similar populations of microbes; Gram-positive bacteria and ciliate protozoa are particularly sensitive. The mechanism of antimicrobial action in both cases involves an alteration in cellular membrane permeability. Fats, like ionophores, increase the molar proportion of propionate and lower methane production, thereby improving ruminal fermentation efficiency (Van Nevel and Demeyer, 1989). Although the individual effects of supplemental fat and ionophores have been researched extensively, not much information exists about their associative effects. Brethour (1984) reported improvements in feed efficiency and rate of gain when lasalocid or a commercial fat blend was fed separately, but not in combination. However, Zinn (1988) reported no interaction between monensin and animal fat on the performance of cattle fed a diet of steam-rolled barley, but observed significant interactions between supplemental fat and monensin on ruminal fermentation end products. Both supplemental fat and monensin decreased acetate and increased propionate but feeding them in combination gave no additive improvement over that observed when they were fed individually (Zinn, 1988). Brandt (1992) reported a significant interaction between ionophores (monensin and lasalocid) and supplemental fat in affecting feedlot cattle performance. The reduction in feed intake and improvement in feed efficiency observed with supplemental fat and monensin when fed separately were not additive when they were fed in combination. Apparently, supplemental fat increases the threshold level of ionophore response. Therefore, additional research is needed to understand the associative effects of supplemental fat and ionophores.

Ionophore feeding in calves

Because the primary mode of action of ionophores is to alter ruminal fermentation characteristics, the question arises whether ionophores could elicit growth response in calves during the first few months of life, before the rumen function is fully developed. Undoubtedly, ionophore supplementation has a favorable influence on the performance of young calves through the control of coccidiosis, one of the important and widespread parasitic diseases of ruminants. In the USA, most young cattle are infected with coccidia sometime during their first year of life, and it is most frequently observed in feedlot calves. Lower performance can occur when no overt signs of the disease are exhibited. Ionophore antibiotics are effective coccidiostats, and lasalocid and monensin are approved for the prevention of coccidiosis. Coccidia damage the absorptive surface of the intestine, leading to lower rates of gain and feed efficiency. A number of studies have documented the effectiveness of ionophores against both natural and induced coccidial infections in calves and lambs (Table 7; Bergstrom and Maki, 1974; Stromberg *et al.*, 1982; Watkins *et al.*, 1986).

Growth promotion by dietary ionophores has been observed in calves with no evidence of coccidiosis (Ilan *et al.*, 1981; El-Jack *et al.*, 1986; Fallon *et al.*, 1986; Anderson *et al.*, 1988; Elcher-Pruiett *et al.*, 1992). Ilan *et al.* (1981) showed that monensin (35 mg kg^{-1}) inclusion in a concentrate diet increased live weight gain and feed efficiency. Anderson *et al.* (1988) reported that lasalocid-fed calves had a greater feed intake and weight gain than calves fed no lasalocid. Any nutritional management that stimulates dry feed consumption leading to early weaning of calves is beneficial because of decreased labor and feed costs. Early weaning and increased dry feed intake promote rapid development of the ruminal tissues and microbial activity. The beneficial growth response is attributed mainly to favorable alterations in ruminal fermentation (Anderson *et al.*, 1988) and possibly to a post-ruminal physiological effect.

Table 7. Effect of monensin on calves challenged with coccidial oocysts [a].

Item	Monensin (mg/kg body weight)			
	0	0.4	0.8	1.2
No. of calves	31	31	31	30
Daily feed intake (kg DM)	2.51	2.53	2.73	3.00[c]
Daily weight gain (kg)	0.59	0.72[b]	0.88[d]	0.89[d]
Total oocysts (10^6 per g feces)	86.7	42.3	26.7	18.1
Mortality (%)	16	0	0	0

[a] On the third day after the start of monensin feeding, calves were inoculated with at least 200,000 sporulated *Eimeria bovis* or *E. zuernii* oocysts (Watkins *et al.*, 1986).
[b,c,d] Different from control at $P<0.1$, 0.05, or 0.01, respectively.

NONIONOPHORE ANTIBIOTICS

The nonionophore antibiotics approved for use in ruminant diets represent a diverse group differing in chemistry, primary antibacterial spectrum, mode of action of bacterial inhibition, molecular weight, and ability to be absorbed from the gut (Table 8). Antibiotics that are not absorbed from the gut or poorly absorbed at the low dosage used are more acceptable as feed additives, because of the absence of residues in milk and meat and because there is no need for a withdrawal period before slaughter. The molecular weight of the antibiotic may be relevant to the extent of its absorption from the gut. Thus, the antibiotics avoparcin, bacitracin, flavomycin, and neomycin have molecular weights in excess of 1000, and hence no residues appear in the tissue even when fed at high levels. On the other hand, the tetracyclines, with molecular weights of approximately 500, are absorbed; they leave detectable residues, and hence require withdrawal periods before slaughter (Hudd, 1983).

Growth-promotion response

Antibiotics are included at subtherapeutic concentrations principally for two reasons: firstly, they decrease the amount of feed needed, increase the rate of weight gain, and therefore improve feed conversion or efficiency; secondly, they are prophylactic against a specific organism or group of organisms. It is difficult to rate the antibiotics on the basis of potency (with respect to growth promotion) because of varying conditions under which ruminants are raised (diet, environment and management practices) and also because of the varying doses that have been used. The growth promotion response with antibiotics in ruminants has been much more varied than in chickens or pigs. As in simple-stomached animals, antibiotics in ruminants have worked best under conditions of stress and poor management. These conditions include subclinical infections, poor husbandry conditions, suboptimal nutrition (deviations from normal diets, poor quality diets or nutrient-deficient diets), environmental stresses (shipping, overcrowding, temperature), unthrifty animals and younger animals. The use of antibiotics for growth promotion involves the continuous use at low levels (2 to 50 g per tonne of feed). As a preventative measure against specific diseases, antibiotic concentrations in feeds are increased to higher levels (50 to 200 g per tonne). The greater

Table 8. Characteristics of nonionophore antibiotics used in ruminants.

Antibiotics	Producing organism	Chemistry	Primary antibacterial spectrum	Mode of action of bacterial inhibition	Molecular weight	Absorption from the gut
Avoparcin	*Streptomyces candidus*	Glycopeptide	Narrow (Gram positive)	Cell wall synthesis	1500	No
Bacitracins	*Bacillus subtilis*	Polypeptide	Narrow (Gram positive)	Cell wall synthesis	1488	No
Chlortetracycline	*Streptomyces aureofaciens*	Tetracyclines	Broad (Gram positive and negative)	Protein synthesis	479	Yes
Flavomycin (Bambermycin)	*Streptomyces bambergiensis*	Phosphorus containing glycopeptide	Narrow (Gram positive)	Cell wall synthesis	1700	No
Neomycin	*Streptomyces fradiae*	Aminoglycoside	Narrow (Gram positive)	Protein synthesis	909	No
Oxytetracycline	*Streptomyces rimosus*	Tetracyclines	Broad (Gram positive and negative)	Protein synthesis	499	Yes
Spiramycin	*Streptomyces ambofaciens*	Macrolide	Narrow (Gram positive)	Protein synthesis	842-898	Yes
Tylosin	*Streptomyces fradiae*	Macrolide	Narrow (Gram positive)	Protein synthesis	915	Yes
Virginiamycin	*Streptomyces virginiae*	Peptolide and macrocyclic lactone	Narrow (Gram positive)	Protein synthesis	525 and 823	Yes

dosages are used when an infectious disease is spreading in a herd or during periods of stress. The prophylactic levels of antibiotics are generally decreased to a lower level and in some instances withdrawn completely after the threat of the disease is over or the effects of stress have subsided. Table 9 illustrates the approved usage of antibiotics in various classes of ruminants in the US and EC. However, not all antibiotics are approved for use in both continents. For example, the tetracyclines are widely used in the US, but are not permitted for use in the EC because of their therapeutic importance in human and veterinary medicine. Avoparcin on the other hand does not have FDA approval for use ruminants.

Table 9. Antibiotics (nonionophore) used alone or in combination in ruminant feeds.

Antibiotics	Feedlot cattle	Dairy cows	Calves	Sheep
	Usage in			
Avoparcin[a]	F, G	F, G		F, G
Bacitracin (Methylene disalicylate)	L			
Bacitracin (Zinc)	F, G, M	M		
Chlortetracycline	F, G, L, M	M	F, G, M	F, G, M
Flavomycin (Bambermycin)	F, G			
Neomycin[b]			M	
Oxytetracycline	B, F, G, L, M	B, M	F, G, M	F, G, M
Spiramycin[a]			M	
Tylosin	L			
Virginiamycin	F, G		M	

[a] Not approved in US.
[b] Usually used in combination.
B, bloat prevention; F, feed efficiency; G, growth promotion; L, liver abscess control;
M, medicinal (prevention of bacterial diseases).

Use in calves and dairy cattle. The feeding of antibiotics to dairy cattle appears to be justified only in the diets of young dairy calves or those under 16 to 20 weeks of age. Although a number of studies have shown that dietary antibiotic is tolerated in the diet of mature cattle the feeding does not appear to afford any economic advantage. Also, the possibility of contamination of the milk has precluded much serious interest in the use of antibiotics for lactating dairy cattle.

The use of antibiotics in calves, particularly in the preruminant calf, is primarily for the control of common calfhood digestive and respiratory ailments. The need for antibiotics is greater in certain environmental (high evidence of *E. coli* infection) or nutritional (colostrum is unavailable) conditions. Numerous investigations have shown benefits from feeding antibiotics to young calves: increased growth rate, increased feed consumption, decreased scours and calf mortality, increased feed efficiency and general improvement in the condition and well being of the calf are reported (Table 10; Lassiter, 1955; Wallace, 1970).

Table 10. Effect of feeding chlortetracycline (CTC) on incidence of scours, mortality, and weight gain in calves[a].

Treatment	Scours (%)	Mortality (%)	Weight gain (kg) (0 - 16 weeks)	
			Holstein	Jersey
Control	66.7	44.4	47.6	38.5
CTC, 50 mg per day	14.3[b]	14.3[b]	59.5[b]	44.0[b]

[a] From Rusoff *et al.*, 1959.
[b] Different from control, P<0.05

Increased feed intake in a preruminant calf would be beneficial in stimulating the development and early onset of microbial fermentation in the rumen. In the USA, chlortetracycline and oxytetracycline are the most commonly used antibiotics in calf diets. In Europe, because of public health concern, antibiotics like flavomycin, spiramycin, and virginiamycin have replaced the use of tetracyclines. However, information on growth promotion with these antibiotics in calf diets is limited. Antibiotics have also been investigated as a supplements for lamb diets. Feed antibiotics appear to be effective in promoting gains and efficiency of feed utilization in finishing lambs and may also be partially effective in the prevention of enterotoxemia (Wallace, 1970).

Use in beef cattle. A number of experiments have been reported on the effect of antibiotics on beef cattle from birth to market weight. Most studies indicated that chlortetracycline, oxytetracycline and to some extent zinc bacitracin are the most effective nonionophore antibiotics for improving the performance of beef cattle. It appears that most useful applications of antibiotics for beef cattle involve stress situations such as diseases, shipping and diet adjustment. Antibiotics, particularly chlortetracycline and oxytetracycline, are often included in receiving rations for prevention of bacterial pneumonia and shipping fever complex (Table 11).

Mudd and Smith (1982) summarized the results of about 30 trials conducted in Europe and in the USA on the use of avoparcin as a growth promoter in beef cattle. Avoparcin at doses ranging from 15 to 60 mg per kg of feed improved daily gain and feed to gain ratio by averages of 5.4% and 10.6%, respectively. Virginiamycin in doses ranging from 20 to 50 mg per kg of feed improved daily gain and feed efficiency in cattle and sheep (Parigi-Bini, 1969; Hedde *et al.*, 1984; Rowe *et al.*, 1991). Antibiotics like flavomycin and virginiamycin are beneficial in optimizing forage utilization in protein- or starch-based supplementation programs in grazing animals (Rowe *et al.*, 1991).

Table 11.   Value of supplemental chlortetracycline in cattle after transit.

Item	Perry *et al.* (1971)		Perry *et al.* (1986)		
	0	350 mg for 28 d	0	350 mg for 56 d	1g for 14 d
No. of animals	52	72	95	95	96
Initial weight (kg)	208	199	194	190	195
28 d weight gain (kg)	237	238	-	-	-
56 d weight gain (kg)	-	-	251	253	256
Daily gain (kg)	1.19	1.38	1.02[a]	1.11[b]	1.09[ab]
Feed efficiency (kg feed per kg gain)	5.53	4.43	5.21[a]	4.99[ab]	5.03[ab]

[a,b] Values in the same row that do not have a common superscript differ ($P<0.05$).

Mode of action

The precise mechanism of action of antibiotics in improving growth and enhancing feed efficiency is not fully understood. However, it has long been accepted that the growth response is due primarily to actions on the microbial flora of the gut.   The most convincing evidence in support of this observation is the lack of improved growth under germ-free conditions (Jukes and Williams, 1953). It would be logical to expect that the overall effect of the antibiotic as a growth promoter in ruminants is likely to be a composite of the effect on the ruminal fermentation and that arising from any effect of the antibiotic in the small and possibly large intestine. In order to have a postruminal effect, at least a proportion of the antibiotic included daily in the feed must survive the rumen environment. Bradley *et al.* (1979) reported only 54 to 56% of oxytetracycline dosed orally was recovered in the abomasum, suggesting possible degradation and/or absorption. In sheep fed a pelleted diet containing 45 mg avoparcin per kg of feed, appreciable amounts of the antibiotic were detected entering and leaving the small intestine (MacGregor, 1984).

At least four general modes of action have been postulated to account for growth promotion by antibiotics:

- metabolic effect - the antibiotics directly influence the rate or pattern of metabolic processes of the animal
- nutrient sparing effect - the antibiotics alter the bacterial population resulting in a conservation of nutrients
- control of subclinical disease - the antibiotics suppress bacteria causing clinical or subclinical infections
- modification of ruminal fermentation - the antibiotics alter rumen microbial population to improve fermentation efficiency.

The first three suggestions have largely followed from studies done in chickens and pigs (Wallace, 1970; Hays, 1978). Similar detailed studies have not been done with ruminants and it would be reasonable to assume that the postulated modes of action would be applicable to ruminants also.

Metabolic effect. Because the tissue concentration of the antibiotics in animals fed at growth promoting levels would be low, the metabolic effects that would account for growth promotion may be minimal. In non-ruminant animals, one of the most distinctive features of feeding antibiotics is a thinning of the gut wall associated with changes in ultrastructure and enzyme activities of epithelial cells. Information on similar effects in gut tissues of ruminants is extremely limited. Rusoff *et al*. (1954) reported a decrease in the thickness of duodenal and jejunal sections of the intestinal wall in chlortetracycline-supplemented calves. Antibiotics in ruminant feeds can influence the rate of cell turnover in the small intestine and the rate of glucose uptake by isolated brush border vesicles (Parker, 1990). Thinning of the intestinal wall may enhance nutrient absorption and lower the metabolic energy cost. Gut tissues (ruminal and post-ruminal) are extremely active sites of metabolism, and therefore one of the major energy demanding organs of the body in ruminants (Britton and Krehbiel, 1993). Avoparcin (45 mg per kg of feed) increased absorption of amino acid nitrogen from the small intestine independent of any effect the antibiotic exerts in the rumen (MacGregor and Armstrong, 1984). This may account for increased milk production in dairy cows fed avoparcin despite no change in ruminal VFA metabolism (Abubaker *et al*., 1988).

Nutrient-sparing effect. It is well recognized the intestinal microorganisms synthesize nutrients such as amino acids and vitamins that are essential for the host. However, other intestinal microorganisms not only compete with the host for nutrients but may alter the nutrients entering the intestine and hence interfere with the nutrient supply to the host animal (Wallace, 1970; Visek, 1978; Coates, 1980; O'Connor, 1980). Thus, deamination of amino acids or hydrogenation of unsaturated fatty acids by microbial metabolism, if extensive, may decrease the supply of essential amino acids or fatty acids to the host (O'Connor, 1980). Another important aspect of intestinal microbial metabolism relates to production of toxic metabolites from substrates in digesta. Decarboxylation of amino acids produces pharmacologically active or toxic amines. Bile acids and sterols are modified extensively by microbial action, and some of the metabolites can be toxic to the host (Savage, 1986).

A number of studies have been conducted in non-ruminants to assess the influence of antibiotics on intestinal microorganisms and to relate changes in microbial population to the growth-promoting effect of antibiotics (Coates, 1980). However, virtually nothing is known concerning the microbial changes and significance of proposed mechanisms of the nutrient-sparing effect in the ruminant animal. Miller *et al*. (1986) investigated the influence of chlortetracycline feeding on ruminal B-vitamin production and intestinal absorption in steers. Chlortetracycline at 70 mg per head per day decreased apparent absorption of thiamin and niacin, possibly because of decreased destruction by intestinal bacteria. However, at a high dose (1 g per head per day), chlortetracycline increased duodenal thiamin apparently because of inhibition of thiaminase activity in the rumen (Miller *et al*., 1986).

One of the characteristic features of ruminants is the extensive recycling of nitrogen, primarily as urea. In high forage-fed animals, a major part of recycled urea enters the gastro-intestinal tract post-ruminally. The high concentration of ammonia, released by the action of intestinal bacterial urease on urea is potentially harmful to cell metabolism at the site of absorption.

The ammonia concentration in the intestinal lumen is higher than the concentration required to kill cells, alter nucleic acid synthesis, depress immune response, and increase bacterial and viral infections (Visek, 1978). Suppression of bacterial ammonia production in the small intestine may therefore be one of the mechanisms by which antibiotics stimulate growth (Visek, 1978).

Disease-control effect. Early in the history of antibiotic usage, it was recognized that the response to antibiotic feeding was inversely proportional to the general well being of the animal. Healthy, disease-free animals kept in clean and sterile quarters generally do not respond to feeding of antibiotics. In ruminants, subtherapeutic doses of antibiotics are used for the prevention of bacterial diarrhea, bacterial pneumonia and shipping fever, anaplasmosis, foot rot, vibrionic abortion, bacterial enteritis, and liver abscesses.

Unequivocal evidence that growth promotion by antibiotics is partly attributable to disease prevention is available from studies of liver abscesses in cattle fed high-grain diets. Liver abscesses in cattle are part of a disease complex in which abscess formation is secondary to the primary infection in the rumen wall. Ruminal acidosis resulting from feeding of highly fermentable grain predisposes the animal to invasion by opportunistic bacteria. *Fusobacterium necrophorum*, a normal inhabitant of the rumen, is the primary causative agent (Lechtenberg *et al.*, 1988). Liver abscesses in feedlot cattle are of serious economic concern in the feedlot industry in the USA. It is not uncommon to find 25 to 30% abscessed livers in cattle at slaughter. In addition to condemnation of livers, reduced weight gain and feed efficiency contribute to the economic loss. Liver function is vital to body metabolism, and it could be assumed logically that destruction of a large portion of the liver tissue by abscesses would cause it to function with less efficiency. Bacitracin dimethylene salicylate, chlortetracycline, oxytetracycline, and tylosin have been approved for control of liver abscesses in the USA. Tylosin has proven to be more efficacious than other antibiotics (Table 12), which is reflected in its widespread use in the feedlot industry. Tylosin is fed routinely in combination with monensin. Although tylosin, a macrolide, is primarily effective against Gram-positive bacteria, it is inhibitory to *F. necrophorum* (Lechtenberg and Nagaraja, 1989). It is believed that the mode of action of tylosin is to reduce the ruminal population of *F. necrophorum*. A number of studies have shown that tylosin inclusion in the feed reduces the incidence of liver abscesses with a consequent improvement in animal performance.

Ruminal fermentation effects. Inclusion of antibiotics in ruminant diets is bound to have some effect on the rumen microbial population and fermentation. Hungate *et al.* (1955) used manometric measurements of fermentative activity to suggest that chlortetracycline feeding altered the composition of the rumen microbial population. Subsequent studies provided more direct evidence that the microbial population is affected. However, many studies have failed to demonstrate significant changes in the microbial population (Lassiter, 1955).

Although the term 'antibiotic' has tended to become synonymous with 'antibacterial', many have activity against other living organisms, including protozoa and fungi. Protozoal populations generally are not affected, although oxytetracycline and virginiamycin have been shown to decrease ciliate population in the rumen (O'Connor *et al.*, 1970; Van Nevel *et al.*, 1984). Some have noted increased protozoal numbers in the rumen of sheep fed chlortetracycline (Klopfenstein *et al.*, 1964; Purser *et al.*, 1985). The reason for the increased protozoal numbers is not clear, but an increase in retention time of solids (because of

Table 12. Effect of tylosin and chlortetracycline on the incidence of liver abscesses in feedlot cattle.

Item	Control	Tylosin[a]	Chlortetracycline[a]
No. of cattle	600	594	606
Incidence of liver abscesses (%)	56.2	18.6	44.2
Improvement over control (%)		21	67
Average daily gain (kg)	1.10	1.19	1.14
Improvement over control (%)		+5.8	+3.3
Feed/gain ratio	8.21	7.87	8.14
Improvement over control (%)		-4.2	-0.8

[a] 75 mg tylosin or 70 mg chlortetracycline per head per day. From Brown *et al.* (1975).

depressed fiber degradation) and a decrease in rumen liquid volume could be factors. The nonionophore antibiotics have no activity against ruminal fungi (Marounek and Hodrova, 1989).

Antibiotic susceptibilities of ruminal bacteria have been determined (El Akkad and Hobson, 1966; Fulghum *et al.*, 1968; Wang *et al.*, 1969; Nagaraja and Taylor, 1987). Most feed-additive antibiotics have their antibacterial activity directed against Gram-positive bacteria, but some Gram-negative bacteria are also susceptible (Table 13). The tetracyclines are inhibitory to both Gram-positive and Gram-negative bacteria. Therefore, it is not surprising that the ruminal digestibility of feedstuffs and fermentation products such as VFA, acetate to propionate ratio, methane and ammonia are changed (Table 14). Alterations in acetate to propionate ratio have not been consistent (Mitchell *et al.*, 1969; O'Connor *et al.*, 1970). Baldwin *et al.* (1982) reported that chlortetracycline and oxytetracycline at concentrations of 2.5 μg ml^{-1} inhibited cellulose digestion by 17 to 35% and VFA production by 18 to 26%. For similar inhibitory effects, bacitracin was required in concentrations of 25 μg ml^{-1}. Tylosin at 1 μg ml^{-1} inhibited cellulose digestion and VFA production by about 80% and 50%, respectively. The detrimental influences on VFA production, fiber digestibility, and bacterial protein production may limit the effective use of some antibiotics. However, in certain situations, the inhibitory influences on microbial activity may be beneficial. The overall decrease in microbial activity has been the premise for the use of antibiotics to control the rate of fermentation in the rumen of animals fed starch-rich (Bullen and Scarisbrick, 1957) or bloat-provocative diets (Clarke and Reid, 1973) and in pre-ruminant calves (Mann *et al.*, 1954). Ruminants not accustomed to high-grain diets suffer from ruminal acidosis because of increased lactic acid production. Antibiotics selective against Gram-positive, lactate-producing bacteria have value in mitigating lactic acidosis (Beede and Farlin, 1977; Nagaraja *et al.*, 1987). The antibloat effect of antibiotics may be caused primarily by a decreased rate of gas production. Mann *et al.* (1954) observed that chlortetracycline-fed calves had less acidic rumens resulting in a pH value more desirable for rumen microbial establishment at an earlier age than calves not fed chlortetracycline. Many antibiotics decrease degradation of amino-N, thereby permitting ruminal escape of dietary protein (Hogan and Weston, 1969; Broderick and Balthrop, 1979). Also, another beneficial effect of antibiotics may be the reduction in ruminal methane production. As with the ionophores, the reduction does not appear to be due to an inhibitory effect on methanogens but rather to reduction in availability

Table 13. Susceptibility and resistance of ruminal microbes to antimicrobial feed additives.

Microbes	Avoparcin	Bacitracin	Chlortetra-cycline	Neomycin	Oxytetra-cycline	Tylosin	Virginiamycin
Fiber digesters							
Butyrivibrio fibrisolvens	+(<10)	+(1)	+(100)	-	+(1)	+(.75)	+(6)
Eubacterium cellulosolvens	+(3)	ND	ND	ND	ND	+(1.5)	+(1.5)
Fibrobacter succinogenes	+(32)	+(100)	+(1)	+(100)	+(10)	-(>48)	-(>48)
Lachnospira multiparus	+(<10)	+(10)	+(10)	-	+(1)	+(3)	+(.75)
Prevotella ruminicola	-(>50)	+(10)	+(10)	-	+(10)	-(>48)	-(>48)
Ruminococcus albus	+(.75)	+(100)	+(100)	+(100)	+(1)	+(.38)	+(.38)
Ruminococcus flavefaciens	+(.75)	+(.1)	ND	+(.1)	+(.1)	+(.38)	+(.75)
Starch and sugar fermenters							
Eubacterium ruminantium	+(.75)	+(10)	+(100)	-	+(1)	+(6)	+(1.5)
Ruminobacter amylophilus	-(>48)	-	+(100)	-	+(10)	-(>48)	-(>48)
Selenomonas ruminantium	-(>48)		+(100)	-	+(10)	-(>48)	-(>48)
Streptococcus bovis	+(5-12)	+(100)	+(100)	-	+(10)	+(12)	+(.75-3.0)
Succinimonas amylolytica	+(48)	+(10)	+(100)	-	+(10)	-(>48)	-(>48)
Succinivibrio dextrinosolvens	+(48)	+(100)	+(1)	-	+(10)	-(>48)	-(>48)
Treponema spp.	+(.75)	-	+(100)	+(200)	+(100)	+(.38)	+(12)
Lactate fermenters							
Megasphaera elsdenii	-(>50)	+(10)	+(10)	-	+(10)	-(>48)	-(>48)
Selenomonas lactilytica	-(>48)	ND	ND	ND	ND	-(>48)	-(>48)
Anaerovibrio lipolytica	-(>50)	ND	ND	ND	ND	-(>48)	-(>48)
Methanogens							
Methanobrevibacter ruminantium	-	ND	-	-	-	ND	ND
Fungi							
Neocallimastix frontalis	-(>50)	-(>50)	-(>50)	ND	ND	-(>50)	-(>50)
Piromonas communis	-(>50)	-(>50)	-(>50)	ND	ND	-(>50)	+(43)
Sphaeromonas communis	-(>50)	-(>50)	-(>50)	ND	ND	-(>50)	-(>50)

[a] Adapted from El Akkad and Hobson (1966), Fulghum et al. (1968), Wang et al. (1969), Stewart et al. (1983), Nagaraja and Taylor (1987) and Marounek and Hodrova (1989). +, susceptible; -, resistant; values in parenthesis are minimum inhibitory concentration in $\mu g\ ml^{-1}$.

Table 14. Effect of antimicrobial feed additives on ruminal metabolic reactions.

Feed additives	Fiber degradation	VFA Total	VFA A:P ratio	Lactate production	Methane production	Amino-N degradation	Ammonia concentration
Avoparcin	0	0	↓	↓	↓	↓	↓
Bacitracin	↓	↓	0	↓	↓	↓	↓
Chlortetracycline	↓	↓	↑	↑	↓	↓	↓
Neomycin	ND	0	0	ND	ND	ND	0
Oxytetracycline	↓	↓	↑	0	ND	ND	0
Spiramycin	ND	↓	↑	ND	ND	ND	ND
Tylosin	↓	↓	↑	↓	↓	ND	ND
Virginiamycin	ND	↓	↓	↓	↓	0	↓

↓, decrease; ↑, increase; 0, no effect; ND, not determined.
Adapted from Klopfenstein et al. (1964), Purser et al. (1965), Hogan and Weston (1969), Mitchell et al. (1969), Beede and Farlin (1977), Baldwin et al. (1982), Froetschel et al. (1983), MacGregor and Armstrong (1983), Nagaraja et al. (1987), Russell and Strobel (1988) and Van Nevel and Demeyer (1989).

of methane precursors (Hungate *et al.*, 1955; Zinn, 1992). Most studies dealing with the effect of antibiotics like bacitracin and tetracyclines have employed *in vitro* or short-term *in vivo* feeding of antibiotics. Because ruminal bacteria become adapted, results obtained from such procedures may be misleading.

Avoparcin, a glycopeptide antibiotic, has effects on ruminal fermentation comparable to those of ionophores. It increases the molar proportion of propionate (Cuthbert *et al.*, 1984), possibly because of a higher production rate (Froetschel *et al.*, 1983), decreases degradation of several feed proteins and amino acids (Jouany and Thivend, 1986), and partially inhibits methane production (MacGregor and Armstrong, 1983). Avoparcin is inhibitory to most Gram-positive organisms, including the cellulolytic *Ruminococcus* and *Butyrivibrio* spp. (Table 13). However, the antibiotic had no effect on fiber-degrading activities of mixed rumen bacteria *in vitro* (Stewart *et al.*, 1983).

CONCLUSIONS

Growth promoting dietary antibiotics have been used extensively in the past four decades and have played a vital role in improving intensive livestock production in many countries. Although hundreds of antibiotics have been tested for growth-promotion effects, only a few have achieved widespread success. There is little reason to doubt that the practice will continue in the foreseeable future. The positive effects of antibiotic supplementation in ruminant diets have been acknowledged universally. Essentially, these compounds enhance performance in terms of increased weight gain and/or feed efficiency and also maintain health in the face of stress and challenges associated with intensive livestock production.

Antibiotics (ionophores and nonionophores) enhance growth performance of ruminants by many mechanisms. Ionophores act primarily by modifying ruminal fermentation to increase energetic efficiency and flow of nutrients into the lower gut. Growth-promotion effects obtained with the nonionophore antibiotics, with the exception of avoparcin, tylosin and virginiamycin, are primarily exerted post-ruminally. However, more research clearly is needed to understand their mechanism of action before the full potential of antibiotics as feed supplements for ruminants can be realized. Undoubtedly, the complexity of the ruminal ecosystem has hindered progress in our thorough understanding of the overall mechanisms of action for growth-promoting antibiotics in ruminants.

REFERENCES

Abubaker, M.M., Rowlinson, P. and Armstrong, D.G. 1988. The influence of dietary inclusion of the antibiotic avoparcin on the lactation performance of dairy cows. *Anim. Prod.* **46**, 483-484.

Agtarap, A., Chamberlin, J.W., Pinkerton, M. and Steinrauf, L. 1967. The structure of monensin acid: a new biologically active compound. *J. Amer. Chem. Soc.* **89**, 5737-5739.

Allen, J.D. and Harrison, D.G. 1979. The effect of dietary addition of monensin upon digestion in the stomachs of sheep. *Proc. Nutr. Soc.* **38**, 32A.

Anderson, K.L., Nagaraja, T.G., Morrill, J.L., Reddy, P.G., Avery, T.B. and Anderson, N.V. 1988. Performance and ruminal changes of early-weaned calves fed lasalocid. *J. Anim. Sci.* **66**, 806-813.

Armstrong, J.D. and Spears, J.W. 1988. Intravenous administration of ionophores in ruminants: effects on metabolism independent of the rumen. *J. Anim. Sci.* **66**, 1807-1817.

Baile, C.A., McLaughlin, C.L., Potter, E.L. and Chalupa, W. 1979. Feeding behavior changes of cattle during introduction of monensin with roughage or concentrate diets. *J. Anim. Sci.* **48**, 1501-1508.

Baldwin, K.A., Bitman, J. and Thompson, M.J. 1982. Comparison of N,N-dimethyldodecanamine with antibiotics on *in vitro* cellulose digestion and volatile fatty acid production by ruminal microorganisms. *J. Anim. Sci.* **55**, 673-679.

Bartley, E.E., Fountaine, F.C. and Atkinson, F.W. 1950. The effects of an APF concentrate containing aureomycin on the growth and well being of young calves. *J. Anim. Sci.* **9**, 646-647.

Bartley, E.E., Nagaraja, T.G., Pressman, E.S., Dayton, A.D., Katz, M.P. and Fina, L.R. 1983. Effects of lasalocid or monensin on legume or grain (feedlot) bloat. *J. Anim. Sci.* **56**, 1400-1406.

Beede, D.K. and Farlin, S.D. 1977. Effects of antibiotics on apparent lactate and volatile fatty acid production: *in vitro* rumen fermentation studies. *J. Anim. Sci.* **45**, 385-392.

Benz, D. A., Byers, F.M., Schelling, G.T., Green, L.W., Lunt, D.K. and Smith, S.B. 1989. Ionophores alter hepatic concentrations of intermediary carbohydrate metabolites in steers. *J. Anim. Sci.* **67**, 2393-2399.

Bergen, W.G. and Bates, D.B. 1984. Ionophores: their effect on production efficiency and mode of action. *J. Anim. Sci.* **58**, 1465-1483.

Bergstrom, R.C. and Maki, L.R. 1974. Effect of monensin in young crossbred lambs with naturally occurring coccidiosis. *J. Amer. Vet. Med. Assoc.* **165**, 288-289.

Bladen, H.A., Bryant, M.P. and Doetsch, R.N. 1961. A study of bacterial species from the rumen which produce ammonia from protein hydrolyzate. *Appl. Microbiol.* **9**, 175-180.

Bradley, B.D., Alderson, N.E., Knight, W.M., Colaianne, J.J. and Bryant, H.H. 1979. Oxytetracycline absorption and excretion in wethers. *J. Anim. Sci.* **48**, 1464-1469.

Brandt, R.T. 1992. Fat in diets for feedlot cattle. In *Southwest Nutrition and Management Conference*, pp 27-42. Univ. of Arizona, Tucson, Arizona, US.

Breeze, R.G. and Carlson, J.R. 1982. Chemical induced lung injury in domestic animals. *Adv. Vet. Sci. Comp. Med.* **26**, 201-231.

Brethour, J.R. 1984. Adding fat to milo-based steer finishing rations. Rep. Prog. 452, Agric. Exp. Sta., p. 15. Kansas State Univ. Manhattan, Kansas.

Britton, R.J. and Krehbiel, C. 1993. Nutrient metabolism by gut tissues. *J. Dairy Sci.* **76**, 2125 -2131.

Broderick, G.A. and Balthrop, J.E. 1979. Chemical inhibition of amino acid deamination by ruminal microbes *in vitro*. *J. Anim. Sci.* **49**, 1101-1111.

Brown, H., Bing, R.F., Grueter, H.P., McAskill, J.W., Cooley, C.O. and Rathmacher, R.P. 1975. Tylosin and chlortetracycline for the prevention of liver abscesses, improved weight gains and feed efficiency in feedlot cattle. *J. Anim. Sci.* **40**, 207-213.

Bullen, J.J. and Scarisbrick, R. 1957. Enterotoxemia in sheep: experimental reproduction of the disease. *J. Path. Bacteriol.* **73**, 495-506.

Burrin, D.G. and Britton, R.A. 1986. Response to monensin in cattle during subacute acidosis. *J. Anim. Sci.* **63**, 888-893.

Burrin, D.G., Stock, R.A. and Britton, R.A. 1988. Monensin level during grain adaptation and finishing performance in cattle. *J. Anim. Sci.* **66**, 513-521.

Chalupa, W. 1984. Manipulation of rumen fermentation. In *Recent Advances in Animal Nutrition* (W. Haresign and D.J.A. Cole, eds) pp. 143-150. Butterworths, Boston, MA, US.

Chen, G. and Russell, J.B. 1989. More monensin-sensitive, ammonia-producing bacteria from the rumen. *Appl. Environ. Microbiol.* **55**, 1052-1057.

Chen, G. and Russell, J.B. 1991. Effect of monensin and a protonophore on protein degradation, peptide accumulation, and deamination by mixed ruminal microorganisms *in vitro. J. Anim. Sci.* **69**, 2196-2203.

Chen, M. and Wolin, M.J. 1979. Effect of monensin and lasalocid sodium on the growth of methanogenic and rumen saccharolytic bacteria. *Appl. Environ. Microbiol.* **38**, 72-77.

Chow, J.M. and Russell, J.B. 1990. Effect of ionophores and pH on growth of *Streptococcus bovis* in batch and continuous culture. *Appl. Environ. Microbiol.* **56**, 1588-1593.

Clarke, R.T.J. and Reid, C.S.W. 1973. Foamy bloat of cattle. A review. *J. Dairy Sci.* **57**, 753 -785.

Coates, M.E. 1980. The gut microflora and growth. In *Growth in Animals* (T.L.J. Lawrence, ed.) pp. 175-188. Butterworths, Boston, MA.

Cuthbert, N.H., Thiekett, W.S. and Smith, H. 1984. The efficacy of dietary avoparcin for improving the performance of growing-finishing beef cattle. *Anim. Prod.* **39**, 195-200.

Daniels, L., Sporling, R. and Sprott, G.D. 1984. The bioenergetics of methanogenesis. *Biochim. Biophys. Acta* **708**, 113-163.

Dawson, K.A. and Boling, J.A. 1983. Monensin-resistant bacteria in the rumens of calves on monensin-containing and unmedicated diets. *Appl. Environ. Microbiol.* **46**, 160-164.

Dawson, K.A. and Boling, J.A. 1987. Effects of potassium ion concentration on the antimicrobial activities of ionophores against ruminal anaerobes. *Appl. Environ. Microbiol.* **53**, 2863-2367.

Dellinger, C.A. and Ferry, J.G. 1984. Effect of monensin on growth and methanogenesis of *Methanobacterium formicium. Appl. Environ. Microbiol.* **48**, 680-682.

Dennis, S.M., Nagaraja, T.G. and Bartley, E.E. 1981. Effects of lasalocid or monensin on lactate producing or using rumen bacteria. *J. Anim. Sci.* **52**, 418-426.

Dennis, S.M., Nagaraja, T.G. and Dayton, A.D. 1986. Effect of lasalocid, monensin, and thiopeptin on rumen protozoa. *Res. Vet. Sci.* **41**, 251-256.

Deswysen, A.G., Ellis, W.C., Pond, K.P., Jenkins, W.L. and Connelly, J. 1987. Effects of monensin on voluntary intake, eating and ruminating behavior and rumen motility of heifers fed corn silage. *J. Anim. Sci.* **64**, 827-834.

Dinius, D.A., Simpson, M.E., and Marsh, P.B. 1976. Effect of monensin fed with forage on digestion and the ruminal ecosystem of steers. *J. Anim. Sci.* **42**, 229-234.

Donoho, A.L. 1984. Biochemical studies on the fate of monensin in animals and in the environment. *J. Anim. Sci.* **58**, 1528-1539.

Eicher-Pruiett, S.D., Morrill, J.L., Nagaraja, T.G., Higgins, J.J ., Anderson, N.V. and Reddy, P.G. 1992. Response of young dairy calves with lasalocid delivery varied in food sources. *J. Dairy Sci.* **75**, 857-862.

El Akkad, I. and Hobson, P.N. 1966. Effect of antibiotics on some rumen and intestinal bacteria. *Nature* **209**, 1046-1047.

El-Jack, E.M., Fallon, R.J. and Harte, F.J. 1986. Effect of avoparcin, flavomycin, and monensin inclusion in a calf concentrate diet on calf performance. *Irish J. Agric. Res.* **25**, 197-204.

Elliott, R., Ash, A.J., Calderon-Cortes, F., Norton, B.W., and Bauchop, T. 1987. The influence of anaerobic fungi on rumen volatile fatty acid concentrations *in vivo. J. Agric. Sci.* **109**, 13-17.

Elsasser, T.H. 1984. Potential interactions of ionophore drugs with divalent cations and their function in the animal body. *J. Anim. Sci.* **59**, 845-853.

Fallon, R.J., El-Jack, E.M., Harte, F.J. and Drenna, M.J. 1986. Effects on calf performance of including flavomycin and salinomycin alone and combined in a calf concentrate diet. *Irish J. Agric. Res.* **25**, 205-212.

Froetschel, M.A., Croom, W.J.Jr., Gaskins, H.R., Leonard, E.S. and Whitcare, M.D. 1983. Effects of avoparcin on ruminal propionate production and amino acid degradation in sheep fed high and low fiber diets. *J. Nutr.* **113**, 1355-1362.

Fulghum, R.S., Baldwin, B.B and Williams, P.P. 1968. Antibiotic susceptibility of anaerobic bacteria. *Appl. Microbiol.* **16**, 301-307.

Galitzer, S.J., Kruckenberg, S.M. and Kidd, J.R. 1986. Pathologic changes associated with experimental lasalocid and monensin toxicosis in cattle. *Amer. J. Vet. Res.* **47**, 2624 - 2626.

Goodrich, R.D., Garrett, J.E., Gast, D.R., Kirick, M.A., Larson, D.A. and Meiske, J.C. 1984. Influence of monensin on the performance of cattle. *J. Anim. Sci.* **58**, 1484-1498.

Greene, L.W., Schelling, G.T. and Byers, F.M. 1986. Effect of dietary monensin and potassium on apparent absorption of magnesium and other macroelements in sheep. *J. Anim. Sci.* **63**, 1960-1967.

Grenet, E., Fonty, G., Jamot, J. and Bonnemy, F. 1989. Influence of diet and monensin on development of anaerobic fungi in the rumen, duodenum, cecum and feces of cows. *Appl. Environ. Microbiol.* **55**, 2360-2364.

Hanson, T.L. and Klopfenstein, T.J. 1979. Monensin, protein source and protein levels for growing steers. *J. Anim. Sci.* **48**, 474-479.

Harmon, D.L. and Avery, T.B. 1987. Effects of dietary monensin and sodium propionate on net nutrient flux in steers fed a high-concentrate diet. *J. Anim. Sci.* **65**, 1610-1616.

Hawkridge, J. 1980. Monensin-dose response relationship under European conditions. European Congress for Improved Beef Productivity, session III, pp. 1-8.

Hays, V.W. 1978. The role of antibiotics in efficient livestock production. In *Nutrition and Drug Interrelations* (J.N. Hathcock and J. Coon, eds) pp. 545-575. Academic Press, New York.

Hedde, R. D. 1984. Nutritional aspect of virginiamycin in feeds. In *Antimicrobials and Agriculture* (M. Woodbine, ed.) pp. 359-368. Butterworths, Boston, MA, US.

Henderson, C., Stewart, C.S. and Nekrep, F.V. 1981. The effect of monensin on pure and mixed cultures of rumen bacteria. *J. Appl. Bacteriol.* **51**, 159-169.

Hogan, J.P. and Weston, R.H. 1969. The effect of antibiotics on ammonia accumulation and protein digestion in the rumen. *Aust. J. Agric. Res.* **20**, 339-346.

Hudd, D.L. 1983. The addition of antibiotics to feedingstuffs. In *Pharmacological Basis of Large Animal Medicine* (J.A. Bogan, P. Lees and A.T. Yoxall, eds) pp. 107-128, Blackwell Scientific Publ., Boston, MA, US.

Hungate, R.E., Fletcher, D.W., and Dyer, I.A. 1955. Effects of chlortetracycline feeding on bovine rumen microorganisms. *J. Anim. Sci.* **14**, 997-1002.

Ilan, D., Ben-Aster, A., Holzer, Z., Nir, I. and Lery, D. 1981. Effect of monensin supplementation on growth, feed digestibility and utilization in young calves. *Anim. Prod.* **32**, 125-131.

Jarrell, K.F. and Sprott, G.D. 1983. The effects of ionophores and metabolic inhibitors on methanogenesis and energy-related properties of *Methanobacterium bryantii*. *Arch. Biochem. Biophys.* **225**, 33-41.

Jouany, J.P. and. Thivend, P. 1986. *In vitro* effects of avoparcin on protein degradability and rumen fermentation. *Anim. Feed Sci. Technol.* **15**, 215-229.

Jukes, T.H. and Williams, W.L. 1953. Nutritional effects of antibiotics. *Pharmacol. Rev.* **5**, 381-420.

Katz, M.P., Nagaraja, T.G. and Fina, L.R. 1986. Ruminal changes in monensin- and lasalocid-fed cattle grazing bloat-provocative alfalfa pasture. *J. Anim. Sci.* **63**, 1246-1257.

Kirk, D.J., Greene, L.W., Schelling, G.T. and Byers, F.M. 1985a. Effects of monensin on monovalent ion metabolism and tissue concentrations in lambs. *J. Anim. Sci.* **60**, 1479-1484.

Kirk, D.J., Greene, L.W., Schelling, G.T. and Byers, F.M. 1985b. Effects of monensin on Mg, Ca, P and Zn metabolism and tissue concentrations in lambs. *J. Anim. Sci.* **60**, 1485-1490.

Klopfenstein, T.J., Purser, D.B. and Tyznik, W.J. 1964. Influence of aureomycin on rumen metabolism. *J. Anim. Sci.* **23**, 490-495.

Lassiter, C.A. 1955. Antibiotics as growth stimulants for dairy cattle: a review. *J. Dairy Sci.* **36**, 1102-1137.

Lechtenberg, K. L. and Nagaraja, T.G. 1989. Antimicrobial sensitivity of *Fusobacterium necrophorum* isolates from bovine hepatic abscesses. *J. Anim. Sci.* **67**, 544. (Abstract).

Lechtenberg, K.L., Nagaraja, T.G., Leipold, H.W. and Chengappa, M.M. 1988. Bacteriologic and histologic studies of hepatic abscesses in cattle. *Amer. J. Vet. Res.* **49**, 58-62.

Lemenager, R.P., Owens, F.N., Shockey, B.J., Lusby, K.S. and Tokusck, R. 1978. Monensin effects on rumen turnover rate, twenty four hour VFA pattern, nitrogen components and cellulose disappearance. *J. Anim. Sci.* **47**, 255-261.

Loosli, J.K. and Wallace, H.D. 1950. Influence of APF and aureomycin on the growth of dairy calves. *Proc. Soc. Exp. Biol. Med.* **75**, 531-533.

MacGregor, R.C. and Armstrong, D.G. 1983. The effect of avoparcin on rumen fermentation *in vitro*. *Proc. Nutr. Soc.* **43**, 21A.

MacGregor, R.C. and Armstrong, D.G. 1984. The feed antibiotic avoparcin and net uptake of amino acids from the small intestine of sheep. *Can. J. Anim. Sci.* **64** (Suppl.), 134-135.

Mann, S.O., Masson, F.M. and Oxford, A.E. 1954. Effect of feeding aureomycin upon the establishment of their normal rumen microflora and microfauna. *Br. J. Nutr.* **8**, 246-252.

Marounek, M. and Hodrova, B. 1989. Susceptibility and resistance of anaerobic fungi to antimicrobial feed additives. *Lett. Appl. Microbiol.* **9**, 173-175.

Miller, B.L., Meiske, J.C. and Goodrich, R.D. 1986. Effects of dietary additives on B-vitamin production and absorption in steers. *J. Anim. Sci.* **62**, 484-496.

Mitchell, G.E., Little, C.O., Kennedy, L.G. and Karr, M.R. 1969. Ruminal volatile fatty acid concentrations in steers fed antibiotics. *J. Anim. Sci.* **29**, 509-511.

Mudd, A.J. and Smith, H. 1982. The use of avoparcin as a growth promotor for beef cattle in Europe. *Anim. Prod.* **48**, 376 (Abstract).

Nagaraja, T.G., Avery, T.B., Galitzer, S.J., and Harmon, D.L. 1985. Effect of ionophore antibiotics on experimentally induced lactic acidosis in cattle. *Amer. J. Vet. Res.* **46**, 2444-2452.

Nagaraja, T.G. and Taylor, M.B. 1987. Susceptibility and resistance of ruminal bacteria to antimicrobial feed additives. *Appl. Environ. Microbiol.* **53**, 1620-1625.

Nagaraja, T.G., Taylor, M.B., Harmon, D.L. and Boyer, J.E. 1987. *In vitro* lactic acid inhibition and alterations in volatile fatty acid production by antimicrobial feed additives. *J. Anim. Sci.* **65**, 1064-1076.

Newbold, C.J. and Wallace, R.J. 1989. Changes in the rumen bacterium, *Bacteroides ruminicola*, grown in the presence of the ionophore, tetronasin. *Australian-Asian J. Anim. Sci.* **2**, 452-453

Newbold, C.J., Wallace, R.J., Watt, N.D. and Richardson, A.J. 1988. Effect of the novel ionophore tetronasin (ICI 139603) on ruminal microorganisms. *Appl. Environ. Microbiol.* **54**, 544-547.

Newbold, C.J., Wallace, R.J. and McKain, N. 1990. Effects of the ionophore tetronasin on nitrogen metabolism by ruminal microorganisms *in vitro*. *J. Anim. Sci.* **68**, 1103-1109.

Nocerini, M.R., Honeyfield, D.C., Carlson, J.R. and Breeze, R.G. 1985. Reduction of 3-methylindole production and prevention of acute bovine pulmonary edema and emphysema with lasalocid. *J. Anim. Sci.* **60**, 232-238.

O'Connor, J.J. 1980. Mechanisms of growth promoters in single stomach animals. In: *Growth in Animals* (T.L.J. Lawrence, ed.) pp 207-227. Butterworths, London, UK.

O'Connor, J.J., Myers, G.S., Mapleden, D.C. and Vander Noot, G.W. 1970. Chemical additives in rumen fermentations: *in vitro* effects of various drugs on rumen volatile fatty acids and protozoa. *J. Anim. Sci.* **30**, 812-818.

Olyumeyan, D.B., Nagaraja, T.G., Miller, G.W., Frey, R.A. and Boyer, J.E. 1986. Rumen microbial changes in cattle fed diets with or without salinomycin. *Appl. Environ. Microbiol.* **51**, 340-345.

Ørskov, E.R., MacLeod, N.A. and Nakashima, Y. 1991. Effect of different volatile fatty acids mixtures on energy metabolism in cattle. *J. Anim. Sci.* **69**, 3389-3397.

Oscar, T.P., Spears, J.W. and Shih, J.C.H. 1987. Performance, methanogenesis and nitrogen metabolism of finishing steers fed monensin and nickel. *J. Anim. Sci.* **64**, 887-896.

Parigi-Bini, R. 1979. Researches on virginiamycin supplementation of feeds used in intensive cattle management. In *Performance in Animal Production* (G. Piana and G. Piva, eds) pp. 237-250. Smith Kline, Milan, Italy.

Parker, D.S. 1990. Manipulation of the functional activity of the gut by dietary and other means (antibiotics/probiotics) in ruminants. *J. Nutr.* **120**, 639-648.

Paster, B.J., Russell, J.B., Yang, C.M.J., Chow, J.M., Woes, C.R. and Tanner, R. 1993. Phylogeny of the ammonia producing ruminal bacteria *Peptostreptococcus anaerobius, Clostridium sticklandii,* and *Clostridium aminophilum* sp. nov. *Int. J. Syst. Bacteriol.* **43**, 107-110.

Perry, T.W., Beeson, W.M., Mohler, M.T. and. Harrington, R.B. 1971. Value of chlortetracycline and sulfamethazine for conditioning feeder cattle after transit. *J. Anim. Sci.* **32**, 137-140.

Perry, T.W., Riley, J.G., Mohler, M.T. and Pope, R.B. 1986. Use of chlortetracycline for treatment of new feedlot cattle. *J. Anim. Sci.* **62**, 1215-1219.

Poos, M.I., Hanson, T.L. and Klopfenstein, T.J. 1979. Monensin effects on diet digestibility, ruminal protein bypass and microbial protein synthesis. *J. Anim. Sci.* **48**, 1516-1524.

Prange, R.W., Davis, C.L. and Clark, J.H. 1978. Propionate production in the rumen of Holstein steers fed either a control or monensin supplemented diet. *J. Anim. Sci.* **46**, 1120-1124.

Purser, D.B., Klopfenstein, T.J. and Cline, J.H. 1965. Influence of tylosin and aureomycin upon rumen metabolism and the microbial populations. *J. Anim. Sci.* **24**, 1039-1044.

Raun, A.P. 1990. Ionophores - a case study in additive development. *Feed Manag.* **41**, 63.

Raun, A.P., Cooley, C.O., Potter, E.L., Rathmacher, R. P. and Richardson, L.F. 1976. Effect of monensin on feed efficiency of feedlot cattle. *J. Anim. Sci.* **43**, 670-677.

Richardson, L.F, Raun, A.P., Potter, E.L., Cooley, C.O. and Rathmacher, R.P. 1976. Effect of monensin on rumen fermentation *in vitro* and *in vivo*. *J. Anim. Sci.* **43**, 657-664.

Rogers, J.A. and Davis, C.L. 1982. Rumen volatile fatty acid production and nutrient utilization in steers fed a supplemented with sodium bicarbonate and monensin. *J. Dairy Sci.* **65**, 944-952.

Rogers, M., Jouany, J.P., Thivend, P. and Fontnot, J.P. 1991. Comparative effects of feeding and duodenal infusion of monensin on digestion in sheep. *Can. J. Anim. Sci.* **71**, 1125-1133.

Rowe, J.B., Murray, P.J. and Godfrey, S.I. 1991. Manipulation of fermentation and digestion to optimize the use of forage resources for ruminant production. In *Isotope and Related Techniques in Animal Production and Health,* pp. 83-99. International Atomic Energy Agency, Vienna, Austria.

Rumpler, W.V., Johnson, D.E. and Bates, D.B. 1986. The effect of high dietary cation concentration on methanogenesis by steers fed diets with and without ionophores. *J. Anim. Sci.* **62**, 1737-1741.

Rusoff, L.L., Cummings, A.H., Stone, E.J. and Johnston, J.E. 1959. Effect of high-level administration of chlortetracycline at birth on the health and growth of young dairy calves. *J. Dairy Sci.* **42**, 856-862.

Rusoff, L.L., Landogora, F.T. and Hester, H.H. 1954. Effect of aureomycin on certain blood constituents, body temperature, weights of organs and tissues and thickness of small intestines. *J. Dairy Sci.* **37**, 654. (Abstract).

Russell, J.B. 1987. A proposed model of monensin action in inhibiting rumen bacterial growth: effects on ion flux and proton motive force. *J. Anim. Sci.* **64**, 1519-1525.

Russell, J.B. and Martin, S.A. 1984. Effects of various methane inhibitors on the fermentation of amino acids by mixed rumen microorganisms *in vitro*. *J. Anim. Sci.* **59**, 1329-1338.

Russell, J.B. and Strobel, H.J. 1988. Effect of additives on *in vitro* ruminal fermentation: a comparison of monensin and bacitracin, another gram positive antibiotic. *J. Anim. Sci.* **66**, 552-558.

Russell, J.B. and Strobel, H.J. 1989. Effect of ionophores on ruminal fermentation. *Appl. Environ. Microbiol.* **55**, 1-6.

Russell, J.B., Strobel, H.J. and Chen, G. 1988. The enrichment and isolation of a ruminal bacterium with a very high specific activity of ammonia production. *Appl. Environ. Microbiol.* **54**, 872-877.

Sakauchi, R. and Hoshino, S. 1981. Effects of monensin on ruminal fluid viscosity, pH, volatile fatty acids and ammonia levels, and microbial activity and population in healthy and bloated feedlot steers. *Z. Tierphysiol. Tierernahrag. u. Futtermittelkde.* **46**, 21-33.

Savage, D.C. 1986. Gastrointestinal microflora in mammalian nutrition. *Ann. Rev. Nutr.* **6**, 155-178.

Schelling, G.T. 1984. Monensin mode of action in the rumen. *J. Anim. Sci.* **58**, 1518-1527.

Shumard, R.F. and Callender, M.E. 1968. Monensin, a new biologically active compound VI. Anti-coccidial activity. *Antimicrob. Agents. Chemother.* 369-377.

Slyter, L.L. 1979. Monensin and dichloracetamide influences on methane and volatile fatty acid production by rumen bacteria *in vivo*. *Appl. Environ. Microbiol.* **37**, 283-288.

Spires, H.R. and Algeo, J.W. 1983. Laidlomycin butyrate - an ionophore with enhanced intraruminal activity. *J. Anim. Sci.* **57**, 1553-1560.

Starnes, S.R., Spears, J.W., Froetschel, M.A. and Croom, W.J. 1984. Influence of monensin and lasalocid on mineral metabolism and ruminal urease activity in steers. *J. Nutr.* **114**, 518-525.

Stewart, C.S., Crossley, M.V. and Garrow, S.H. 1983. The effect of avoparcin on laboratory cultures of rumen bacteria. *Eur. J. Appl. Microbiol. Biotechnol.* **17**, 292-297.

Stewart, C.S. and Richardson, A.J. 1989. Enhanced resistance of anaerobic rumen fungi to the ionophores monensin and lasalocid in the presence of methanogenic bacteria. *J. Appl. Bacteriol.* **66**, 85-93.

Strobel, H.J., Chow, J.M. and Russell, J.B. 1989. Ruminal ionophores: Manipulating fermentation and control of acidosis. In *Cornell Nutr. Conf. Proc.*, pp. 16-21. Cornell University, Ithaca, New York, US.

Stromberg, B.E., Schlotthauer, J.C., Armstrong, B.D., Brandt, W.E. and Liss, C. 1982. Efficacy of lasalocid sodium in the control of coccidiosis (Eimeria bovis and Eimeria zuernii) in calves. *Amer. J. Vet. Res.* **43**, 583-585.

Stuart, R.L. 1982. Comparison of Bovatec to Rumensin to feedlot cattle. In *Bovatec Symposium Proceedings* (R.L. Stuart and C.R. Zimmerman, eds), pp 85 -106. Hoffmann-La Roche Inc., Nutley, NJ, US.

Tamminga, S. 1979. Protein degradation in the forestomachs of ruminants. *J. Anim. Sci.* **49**, 1615-1627.

Van Nevel, C.J. and Demeyer, D.I. 1977. Effect of monensin on rumen metabolism *in vitro*. *Appl. Environ. Microbiol.* **34**, 251-257.

Van Nevel, C.J., Demeyer, D.I. and Hendrickx, H.K. 1984. Effect of virginiamycin on carbohydrate and protein metabolism in the rumen *in vitro*. *Arch. Tierernahr., Berlin* **2**, 149-155.

Van Maanen, R.W., Harbein, J.H., McGilliard, A.D. and Young, J.W. 1978. Effects of monensin on *in vitro* rumen propionate production and blood glucose kinetics in cattle. *J. Nutr.* **108**, 1002-1007.

Visek, W.J. 1978. The mode of growth promotion by antibiotics. *J. Anim. Sci.* **46**, 1447-1464.

Wahle, K.W.J. and Livesay, C.T. 1985. The effect of monensin supplementation of dried grass or barley diets on aspects of propionate metabolism, insulin secretion and lipogenesis in the sheep. *J. Sci. Food Agric.* **36**, 1227-1236.

Wallace, H.D. 1970. Biological responses to antibacterial feed additives in diets of meat producing animals. *J. Anim. Sci.* **31**, 1118-1126.

Wallace, R.J., Czerkawski, J.W. and Breckenridge, G. 1981. Effect of monensin on the fermentation of basal rations in the rumen simulation technique (Rusitec). *Br. J. Nutr.* **114**, 101-105.

Wallace, R.J., Newbold, C.J. and McKain, N. 1990. Influence of ionophores and energy inhibitors on peptide metabolism by rumen bacteria. *J. Agric. Sci. Camb.* **115**, 285-290.

Wang, C.L., Baldwin, B.B., Fulghum, R.S. and Williams, P.P. 1969. Quantitative antibiotic sensitivities of ruminal bacteria. *Appl. Microbiol.* **18**, 677-679.

Watanabe, K., Watanabe, J., Kuramitsu, S. and Maruyama, H.B. 1981. Comparison of the activity of ionophores with other antibacterial agents against anaerobes. *Antimicrob. Agents Chemother.* **19**, 519-525.

Watkins, L.E., Wray, M.I., Basson, R.P., Feller, D.L., Olson, R.D., Fitzgerald, P.R., Stromberg, B.E. and Davis, G.W. 1986. The prophylactic effects of rumensin fed to cattle inoculated with coccidia oocysts. *Agr. Practice* **7**, 18-20.

Westley, J.W. 1983. Notation and classification. In *Polyether Antibiotics* (J.W. Westley, ed.) vol. 1, pp 1-20. Marcel Dekker, Inc., New York.

Whetstone, H.D., Davis, C.L. and Bryant, M.P. 1981. Effect of monensin on breakdown of protein by ruminal microorganisms *in vitro*. *J. Anim. Sci.* **53**, 803-809.

Wilkinson, J.I.D., Appleby, W.G.C., Shaw, C.J., Lebas, G. and Pflug, R. 1980. The use of monensin in European pasture cattle. *Anim. Prod.* **31**, 159-162.

Yang, C.M.J. and Russell, J.B. 1993. Effect of monensin on the specific activity of ammonia production and disappearance of amino nitrogen from the rumen. *Appl. Environ. Microbiol.* **59**, 3250-3254.

Yokoyama, M.T., Johnson, K.A., Dickerson, P.S. and Bergen, W.G. 1985. Effect of dietary monensin on the cecal fermentation of steers. *J. Anim. Sci.* **61**, 469 (Abstract).

Zinn, R.A. 1988. Comparative feeding value of supplemental fat in finishing diets for feedlot steers supplemented with and without monensin. *J. Anim. Sci.* **66**, 213-227.

Zinn, R.A. 1992. Influence of oral antibiotics on digestive function in holstein steers fed a 71% concentrate diet. *J. Anim. Sci.* **70**, 213-217.

10 Microbial probiotics for pigs and poultry

Stanislava Stavric and Ervin T. Kornegay[1]

Bureau of Microbial Hazards, Food Directorate, Health Canada, Ottawa, Ontario K1A OL2, Canada, and [1]Dept. of Animal Sciences, Virginia Polytechnic Institute and State University, Blacksburg, Virginia 24061-0306, US

INTRODUCTION

The use of probiotics in pig and poultry production has seen renewed interest as public concern about antibacterial growth promoting agents has increased. This interest stems from a desire to enhance the development of a more favorable microflora by using probiotics, especially during periods of stress, thereby reducing the need for, and the use of, antibacterial agents. Intensive rearing conditions for livestock are thought to contribute towards a delay or a disturbance in the development of normal intestinal microflora. Young chicks hatched in commercial hatcheries, for example, have never been exposed to bacteria from the mother hen while young pigs weaned from the mother sow are exposed to stress and microbial challenges when moved into nursery facilities. Proposed production benefits of probiotics include enhanced survival of newborns, reduction or prevention of diarrhea, increased growth rate, improved feed efficiency, and enhanced immune response.

The idea that bacterial cultures could benefit human health came from Metchnikoff (1908), who attributed the longevity of Bulgarians to daily consumption of yogurt. He believed that "beneficial organisms" (lactobacilli) could balance the intestinal environment, prevent the growth of pathogenic bacteria and as a consequence improve health and prolong life. One yogurt organism, *Lactobacillus acidophilus,* was widely used during the first half of the twentieth century, before the introduction of sulfanilamides, to control outbreaks of diarrhea in children (Winkelstein, 1956) and was subsequently shown to have antibacterial activity (Vincent *et al.*, 1959). The administration of "beneficial organisms" to animals started in the 1920s and the name "probiotics" was introduced by Parker (1974) when the production of bacterial feed supplements began on a commercial scale (Fuller, 1992a). Variable beneficial responses have been reported for the use of probiotics in pig and poultry production and several mechanisms have been suggested to explain these effects. However, the mode of action is still not understood.

The concept of probiotics has scientific merit, but the perceived beneficial value is not based on well-controlled research studies (Pollmann, 1992; Barrow, 1992). There appears some justification for treating animals of poor health with probiotics, but in healthy or gnotobiotic animals it has been more difficult to show consistent benefits. Only in cases where animals are under stress and their intestinal microflora has been disrupted or its development delayed has the response been more favourable. For example, in poultry reared commercially, a consistent benefit has been shown from introducing adult-type microflora in order to make chicks more resistant to *Salmonella* spp. (Stavric and D'Aoust, 1993).

The aim of this chapter is to summarise and to give a brief overview of different aspects of probiotic usage in pigs and poultry. Emphasis will be given to research completed recently and to publications which have become available since 1990. A comprehensive book covering the scientific basis for probiotics was recently published (Fuller, 1992a). In addition, there are numerous reviews (Jernigan *et al.*, 1985; Fox, 1988; Fuller, 1989; Kozasa, 1989; Lloyd-Evans, 1989; Sissons, 1989; Tournut, 1989; Raibaud and Raynaud, 1990; Vanbelle *et al.*, 1990; Juven *et al.*, 1991; Veldman, 1992; Chesson, 1993; Gedek, 1993), book chapters (Fuller, 1992a,b,c; Havenaar and Huis in't Veld, 1992; Ballongue, 1993; Nousiainen and Setälä, 1993) and proceedings (Pollmann, 1992; Huis in't Veld and Havenaar, 1993) dealing with different aspects of these rapidly developing products. These reviews, chapters and proceedings provided valuable information for this chapter.

DEVELOPMENT OF INTESTINAL MICROFLORA IN PIGS AND POULTRY AND ITS ROLE IN ANIMAL HEALTH

The digestive tract of the newborn pig is usually sterile but rapidly develops a microflora characteristic of the species as it is exposed to a traditional commercial environment (Fuller, 1989). Similarly, essentially sterile at the time of hatching, the intestinal tract of poultry becomes rapidly colonized by microorganisms from the environment (Jayne-Williams and Fuller, 1971). Within a few hours, lactobacilli appear in the crop and persist there throughout life (Fuller and Brooker, 1974), while in the lower intestinal tract (duodenum to cecum), *Enterococcus faecalis* is the predominant species and is accompanied by enterobacteria. By the third day, lactobacilli appear in the intestine and form a major part of the cecal flora together with clostridia, coliforms and fecal enterococci, but it takes several weeks for the complete establishment of an adult-type microflora (Smith, 1965; Barnes *et al.*, 1980). The development of a stable microflora helps the animal resist infections, particularly in the gastrointestinal tract (Fuller, 1989). This phenomenon has been referred to as bacterial antagonism (Freter, 1956); bacterial interference (Dubos, 1963); the barrier effect (Ducluzeau et al., 1970); colonization resistance (Van Der Waaij *et al.*, 1971); and competitive exclusion (Lloyd *et al.*, 1977).

Many different types of anaerobic bacteria (numbering about 10^9 to 10^{11} bacteria g^{-1} of intestinal material) are present in a normal digestive tract of non-ruminant animals. According to Gedek (1989), the principal species can be classified into three different groups, the main flora, the satellite flora and the residual flora. The main group, which makes up more than 90% of the total, is mostly obligate anaerobes (bifidobacteria, lactobacilli, and bacteroidaceae). The satellite or accompanying group (less than 1% facultative anaerobes) is made up primarily of *Escherichia coli,* and enterococci. The residual group (less than 0.01%) includes organisms from the genera *Clostridium, Proteus, Staphylococcus, Pseudomonas,* yeasts of the *Candida* species and other pathogenic and non-pathogenic species of bacteria. However, the normal microflora of different animal species is not identical and each part of the intestinal tract has a unique collection of microorganisms (Savage, 1987).

The genera and species of bacteria are dependent on the physiological conditions present in that particular area and are regulated by allogenic (exerted by the environment) and autogenic (generated within the ecosystem) factors (Savage, 1987). Although little is known about autogenic factors, it is thought that competition between microbial species for space and nutrients is of major importance. Many of these microbes elicit a physiological effect within the host, which, if disrupted, can result in or predispose animals to disease. Evidence of this comes from experiments in which germ-free or conventional mice, hamsters and chickens treated with antibiotic were much more sensitive to infection with *Salmonella, E. coli* or *Clostridium difficile* than were non-treated animals (Bonhoff *et al.*, 1954; Smith *et al.*, 1985;

Borriello, 1990; Hentges, 1992). The development of a stable, protective microflora is important for the health and well-being of the animal. Despite accumulated knowledge of intestinal microflora and gastrointestinal function, many of the operating mechanisms and factors influencing the microbial population in the gut remain unknown (Savage, 1987; Freter, 1988; Rolfe, 1991). However, excessive hygiene, antibiotic therapy and stress were suggested as important factors which can disrupt the development of a protective, stable microflora in the gut (Fuller, 1989).

PROBIOTICS

Definition

Parker (1974) may have been the first to use the term probiotic to describe "organisms and substances which contribute to intestinal microbial balance". Twenty years later "probiotic" has become a world-wide generic title, encompassing almost any living or dead microorganisms or fermentation by-products administered to animals (Fox, 1988). The term probiotic originated from two Greek words meaning "for life" and is contrasted with the term antibiotic which means "against life" (Lyons, 1987). Because the definition proposed by Parker (1974) was too imprecise and could even include antibiotics, Fuller (1989) proposed to define probiotic as "a live microbial feed supplement which beneficially affects the host animal by improving its intestinal microbial balance". This revised definition emphasized the importance of live organisms as an essential component of an effective probiotic and removed the confusion created by the use of the word "substances". Subsequently Pollmann (1992) suggested that probiotics could be classified into two major types: viable microbial cultures and microbial fermentation products.

The United States Food and Drug Administration (FDA) requires manufacturers to use the term direct-fed microbial (DFM) instead of probiotics. The FDA defines DFM as "a source of live (viable) naturally-occurring microorganisms" (Pendelton, 1992). At present, microorganisms which are being used as DFM fall into the category classified by FDA and the Association of American Feed Control Officials (AAFCO) as generally recognized as safe (GRAS) ingredients. The GRAS status is defined as food and feed additives that have been designated as safe for consumption having been judged by a panel of expert pharmacologists and toxicologists who considered the available data, including technical experience of their common usage in human food (Pollman, 1986). In Canada, the term "viable microbial products" has been adapted for probiotics designed for administration to farm animals. These are regulated by the Departments of Agriculture and Health (AC), as feeds or drugs, according to their claim of action (AC, 1990). At a recent meeting of the European Community-Food Linked Agro Industrial Research group (EC-FLAIR, 1993), it was concluded that the term probiotic was confusing and should be replaced with the term ecological health control products (EHCP). This seems unlikely to attract support and the term probiotic remains in general use for any product containing viable microorganisms.

In this chapter the term "probiotic" will be used to represent a single or mixed culture of live microorganisms which, applied to animals or man, affect the host beneficially by improving the properties of the indigenous microflora (Havenaar and Huis in't Veld, 1992).

Composition of products used

The most commonly used probiotics are lactic acid producing bacteria, which have a long tradition of use in the food industry and have been accepted as being safe by health regulatory agencies. The number of strains in a preparation can vary from one to eight (Fuller, 1989). A single strain is most often used, with two or more strains belonging to different genera being occasionally used (Raibaud and Raynaud, 1990). The exception is preparations used for the control of *Salmonella* in poultry which contain a large number of strains (Mead, 1991; Stavric, 1992). The claim for multiple-strain preparations is that they are active against a wider range of conditions and in a wider range of animal species.

Bacterial spores, which reportedly resist stomach acidity and germinate in the upper gut where they become active, have also been employed. These include strains from the genus *Bacillus* and, less commonly, a particular strain of *Clostridium butyricum* (Han *et al.*, 1984; Kozasa, 1989; Lloyd-Evans, 1989; Tournut, 1989; Vanbelle *et al.*, 1990; Koide, 1992; Tobey, 1992).

Commercial preparations consisting of strains from the following genera are being used for various animals including pigs and poultry in the USA, Canada and Europe - *Bifidobacterium, Lactobacillus, Streptococcus, Bacillus, Bacteroides, Pediococcus, Leuconostoc* and *Propionibacterium* (Lloyd-Evans, 1989; Tobey, 1992). A strain of *Clostridium* is additionally used in Japan and, in some EC countries, mixtures of undefined intestinal bacteria under the trade names Broilact® and Aviguard® are used for the prevention of *Salmonella* colonization in poultry (Stavric and D'Aoust, 1993).

Some 42 different microorganisms are considered GRAS and can be used as DFM (AAFCO, 1993), but most commonly used are species of lactobacilli (*L. bulgaricus, L. acidophilus, L. casei, L. helveticus, L. lactis, L. salivarius, L. plantarum*) in addition to *Streptococcus thermophilus, Enterococcus faecium, Ent. faecalis, Bifidobacterium* spp. and *E. coli* (Fuller, 1989). With the exception of *L. bulgaricus* and *S. thermophilus*, which are yogurt starter organisms, all are intestinal strains. *Bacillus subtilis* is also used as one of the components in some products, but according to Fuller (1989) it is difficult to understand how it can be active in the gut since it is a strict aerobe.

Probiotics for poultry have been generally divided according to their site of colonization and proposed mode of action: the lactobacilli for their colonization of the crop and effect on nutritional and performance parameters, and mixtures of undefined or defined intestinal cultures for their action in the cecum against pathogens which are passed into the human food chain (Barrow, 1992). These include mono- and multigeneric preparations (up to 65 strains) which are being used in experiments for control of *Salmonella* in poultry (Impey *et al.*, 1982; Mead, 1991; Stavric, 1992; Corrier *et al.*, 1993).

Selection criteria for probiotic cultures

Very little is known about how the microorganisms in probiotics associate with gut mucosa, how they exert their beneficial physiological effect or how they antagonize unwanted microorganisms in the gut (Freter, 1992). Therefore, the set of proposed criteria for an effective probiotic is very arbitrary. Havenaar *et al.* (1992) presented a comprehensive review and discussion of general criteria that can be used for the selection of microbial strains (bacteria, fungi and yeasts) for probiotic use. These general criteria (origin of the strain, viability, processing and storage, resistance to *in vivo* and *in vitro* conditions, adherence and colonization and antimicrobial activity) are concerned with aspects of biological safety, production and processing, the method of administering the probiotic, and the location on/in the body where the microorganisms of the probiotic must be active.

According to Fuller (1992a), an effective probiotic should be capable of being prepared as a viable product on an industrial scale, remain stable and viable for long periods under storage and field conditions, have the ability to survive (not necessarily grow) in the intestine, and produce a beneficial effect in the host animal. Even though there is no definitive evidence for the mode of action of probiotics, Chesson (1993) indicates that it appears desirable that strains used should be of gut origin (or able to tolerate conditions encountered in the digestive tract), have strong adherent qualities independent of metabolic activity or viability, have a capacity to revitalize rapidly under gut conditions after lyophilization, be capable of producing compounds antagonistic to pathogens, and have a capacity to stimulate the cell-mediated immune response.

Criteria by which intestinal isolates should be selected for controlling *Salmonella* in poultry also are not defined. The most effective preparations are anaerobically grown fecal or cecal contents of healthy adult birds (CE culture) whose bacterial composition is not defined. However, the regulatory agencies in most countries do not allow the use of undefined preparations in commercial poultry production (Stavric and D'Aoust, 1993). Attempts have, therefore, been made to isolate and identify strains from cecal microflora and prepare mixtures of defined cultures. Isolates have been selected empirically since no information is available on the desired properties of protective microorganisms (Mead and Impey, 1987). Some research workers selected isolates based on the bacterial composition of the cecum to include representatives of all major groups of cecal bacteria (Impey *et al.*, 1982; Stavric *et al.*, 1985). Others have chosen only lactobacilli because of their capacity to adhere to the epithelial cells of the crop (Nurmi *et al.*, 1983). Most recently, cecal isolates which replicate in an acid environment, have constant generation times, utilize lactose, and produce specific short chain volatile fatty acids (VFA), have been used in mixture(s) whose efficacy was dependent on the presence of lactose in the chicks' diet (Corrier *et al.*, 1990, 1993).

The above selection criteria are not easily met. Only some of the properties (e.g. resistance to low pH, bile, intestinal juices or antibiotics and viability during production and storage) can be measured by *in vitro* assays (Alm *et al.*, 1989). The majority could be verified only with *in vivo* experimentation. *In vivo* tests are necessary for determination of the most desirable characteristics, such as the ability to colonize the intestine, inhibit or eliminate a pathogen, or improve animal performance (Freter, 1992; Havenaar *et al.*, 1992; Stavric, 1992).

The bacteriostatic or bacteriocidal activity of lactobacilli measured *in vitro* (e.g. production of bacteriocin-like compounds) does not permit extrapolation on the behavior of these strains *in vivo* (Chateau *et al.*, 1993). The exception is lactobacilli whose adhesion in *in vitro* systems could in some instances be used to predict adhesion in animals (Conway, 1989). Lactobacilli isolated from animals other than birds failed to adhere to chicken crop cells *in vitro* (Fuller, 1973). However, a close correlation between attachment *in vitro* and colonization of germ-free chickens was obtained with several avian strains, indicating host specificity (Fuller, 1978). In contrast, adherence of porcine lactobacilli *in vitro* was not useful in predicting their colonization in piglets (Pedersen and Tannock, 1989).

To make the selection process even more complicated, some of the required properties can change upon storage and by laboratory manipulations. Loss of the adhesive property or capacity to produce bacteriocin-like compounds has been found with lactobacilli (Conway, 1989). Similarly, mixtures of defined cultures can lose their effectiveness for reducing *Salmonella* in chicks, the magnitude of the loss being dependent on storage time and frequency of transfer (Gleeson *et al.*, 1989; Stavric, 1992).

Since probiotics are used for therapeutic and/or growth promoting purposes, the dosage and the frequency of administration vary. For prophylactic action in newborn animals or for prevention of diarrhea in weanling piglets, high doses (10^9 colony forming units [cfu]) are administered for at least three to five consecutive days (Tournut, 1989). An exception is the prevention of colonization with *Salmonella* in poultry, where administration is done only once either in the hatchery or in the first drinking water (Pivnick and Nurmi, 1982). For growth promotion, a minimum effective dosage of approximately 10^6 to 10^7 cfu g^{-1} of feed are administered daily for at least one to two months (Tournut, 1989).

Viability of organisms during production, application and storage

Despite the fact that the viability of microorganisms is one of the most easily measurable characteristics, data indicate that this criterion has not always been met (Havenaar *et al.*, 1992). Examination of fifteen feed supplements marketed by eight manufacturers as containing *L. acidophilus* revealed that three of the products contained no lactobacilli, eight had lactobacilli other than the declared strain, and only one contained *L. acidophilus* in low numbers (Gilliland, 1981).

Stability of *Lactobacillus* preparations is influenced by the storage environment (heat and humidity), length of storage, and certain drugs that might be used in the feed (Pollmann and Bandyk, 1984). Feed manufacture and storage conditions also can affect viability. The viability of the microorganisms (other than bacterial spores) can be decreased by temperatures associated with pelleting feeds (60 to 80°C). The stability of *Lactobacillus* preparations was prolonged when stored under refrigeration, but was decreased when stored at room temperature in the pig nursery (Pollman and Bandyk, 1984). Havenaar *et al.* (1992) recommended that storage conditions and expiration date be stated on packaging, and that the viability of probiotic strains under different storage conditions (e.g. temperature, relative humidity) should be monitored. However, in the view of Chesson (1993), it has yet to be demonstrated conclusively that viability is an essential or even a desirable characteristic of a probiotic since few of many modes of action postulated for such products are necessarily dependent on the presence of growing or metabolically active cells.

MODE OF ACTION

Numerous authors have speculated on the mode of action of probiotics, but there is little definitive evidence to support any of the proposed mechanisms. Fuller (1992b) suggested that the mechanism of the probiotic effect may:
  • Competition for adhesion receptors on the gut epithelium (Jonsson and Conway, 1992)
  • Competition for nutrients (Freter, 1992)
  • Production of antibacterial substances (Hentges, 1992)
  • Stimulation of immunity (Perdigon and Alvarez, 1992).

However, complex interactions are likely to occur in practice.

Competition for adhesion receptors on intestinal mucosa

Evidence that the indigenous gastrointestinal microflora has the ability to inhibit colonization of invading microorganisms comes from studies in poultry and germ-free or antibiotic-treated experimental animals (Hentges, 1992). The classical example is young chicks from commercial hatcheries, in which development of a native microflora is delayed. Introduction of a gut microflora from adult healthy birds into newly hatched chicks made them resistant to infection when subsequently challenged with food poisoning salmonellae (Nurmi and Rantala, 1973). This inhibition process is known as the "Nurmi concept" or "competitive exclusion" (CE) (Pivnick and Nurmi, 1982). Similar effects obtained by the introduction of native microflora for controlling other pathogens (e.g. *E. coli, C. difficile*) in animals or humans have been dubbed "colonization resistance" or "barrier effect to colonization" (Borriello, 1990; Vanbelle *et al.*, 1990; Hentges, 1992).

Although the mechanism(s) of protection has not been elucidated, those most often cited in CE are competition between existing microflora and pathogen for adherence on intestinal mucosa and the production of volatile fatty acids (VFA) (Pivnick and Nurmi, 1982). Indirect evidence for such competition was derived from studies where homogenates of washed ceca, collected from chicks treated with native microflora, had markedly lower numbers of *Salmonella* or *E. coli* than non-treated chicks, and the protective flora was cecal wall associated (Soerjadi *et al.*, 1982; Stavric *et al.*, 1987). Similarly, homogenates of washed intestinal tissue collected from piglets treated with *L. lactis* had a higher number of attached lactobacilli and lower *E. coli* counts than scouring or non-treated control pigs (Muralidhara *et al.*, 1977).

Competition for nutrients

The hypothesis of competition for nutrients in the intestinal lumen between resident and invading bacteria was derived from observations that bacteria in a continuous-flow culture compete for nutrients. However, not enough data is available to provide evidence for such competition operating in the intestine (Freter, 1992; Hentges, 1992). It was pointed out by Jonsson and Conway (1992) that *in vivo* colonization of a site in the gastrointestinal mucosa involves many more aspects than simply adhesion to the epithelium. Lactic acid bacteria growing at the site of colonization may utilize nutrients that would otherwise be available for pathogens and/or produce metabolites that inhibit the growth of pathogens.

Production of antibacterial compounds

Inhibitory compounds produced by *Lactobacillus* spp. include well characterized bacteriocins (e.g nisin, reuterin, acidolin, bulgaricin), bacteriocin-like substances and other antagonists such as hydrogen peroxide and certain organic acids (Juven *et al.*, 1991). Although viable lactobacilli were generally not effective in reducing *Salmonella* colonization in poultry, the compounds they produce were active *in vitro* against a broad spectrum of bacterial species (Havenaar *et al.*, 1992; Juven *et al.*, 1991). The inhibitory spectrum varied; some bacteriocins inhibited only Gram-positive bacteria, while acidolin inhibited some Gram-positive and Gram-negative species and reuterin inhibited all bacteria, yeast and fungi tested (Havenaar *et al.*,

1992). However, the role of such antagonistic compounds in the intestine is largely unknown, because there have been no complementary *in vivo* and *in vitro* studies confirming the production of the growth inhibitory effects *in vivo* (Conway, 1989).

The exceptions are organic acids (lactic, acetic, butyric and propionic), produced by facultative and obligate anaerobes which, in their undissociated form, are known to decrease intestinal pH.   Lactic and acetic acid-producing bacteria (strains of *Lactobacillus, Enterococcus* and *Bifidobacterium*) have been most commonly used as probiotics.   More recently *Veillonella* spp., which produce acetic and propionic acids, have shown some promise in their use against pathogens (Szylit *et al.*, 1988; Hinton *et al.*, 1991). VFA are produced in the ceca of chicks by about the second week after hatching (Pivnick and Nurmi, 1982). The undissociated form of VFA shows the greatest antibacterial activity and the degree of dissociation is related to environmental pH (Bonhoff *et al.*, 1964; Meynell, 1963). Indirect evidence for involvement of VFA in the reduction of pathogens comes from studies where lactobacilli administered to chicks lowered the pH of the upper portion of the chicks' intestine and suppressed colonization of *E. coli* in the crop (Fuller, 1977). A similar effect was obtained by supplementing lactose in a chick diet, where a reduction of *Salmonella* was accompanied by an increase in the production of VFA and a decrease in the cecal pH (Morishita *et al.*, 1982). Since chicks lack lactase activity, some of the lactose provided in a diet could reach the cecum and provide a substrate for microorganisms (Mead, 1989). Conversely, in streptomycin-treated mice, an increase in the multiplication of *Salmonella* was accompanied by a decrease in VFA and an increase in Eh and pH (Meynell, 1963). The restoration of resistance against enterotoxigenic *E. coli* (ETEC) and *Shigella sonnei* in streptomycin-treated mice after antibiotic withdrawal was accompanied by an increase in total VFA (Pongpech and Hentges, 1989).

Since the protective effect against *Salmonella* in chicks obtained by the introduction of an adult cecal flora occurs within one hour, Pivnick and Nurmi (1982) argued that VFA could not be involved because they could not be produced so rapidly.   More recent studies, however, indicate that VFA may play a role in protection. The effect of cecal flora, cultured in lactose-based broths, against *Salmonella* was enhanced by adding lactose to chick diets. The reduction in cecal colonization was accompanied by an increase in the concentration of VFA and a decrease in the cecal pH (Corrier *et al.*, 1990, 1993).   Anaerobic CE cultures containing bacteria which produced significant amounts of propionic acid were more effective in reducing colonization than those where propionic acid production was not increased (Hinton *et al.*, 1991).

Activation of the immune response

The digestive tract immunity during the neonatal period differs in pigs and poultry. During the first weeks of life the piglet is protected by maternal antibodies and non-immunological factors. Stimulation of the development of the piglet's active immune system and its ability to respond to a microbial challenge has been of great interest, but the mode of action and effectiveness of various factors, including probiotics and their metabolic products, is not clearly understood. Sasaki *et al.* (1987) reported a higher number of IgA-bearing cells in the lamina propria of the middle jejunum and in the ileum, and a lower number of *E. coli* in various portions of the small intestine of pigs at five to six weeks of age. These pigs had previously been dosed orally after birth with peptidoglycan derived from *Bif. thermophilum* and weaned at four weeks. However, a *Lactobacillus* sp. fermentation product added to the creep feed two weeks before weaning and in the starter feed for four weeks after weaning increased serum IgG levels but did not influence serum IgA levels compared with control pigs (Lessard and Brisson, 1987). In contrast, feeding of *Bif. globosum* A to pigs for five weeks after weaning at four weeks of age did not consistently influence the humoral immune response to sheep red blood cells or ovalbumin and did not influence the reaction to an intradermal injection of a phytohemagglutinin (Apgar *et al.*, 1993). Similarly, *Ent. faecium* treatment of weaned pigs did not influence their cell-mediated immune response (Kluber *et al.*, 1985).

Immune protection in poultry is concentrated in the egg yolk, which discharges its antibodies directly into the intestinal lumen and assures protection of the young bird against infections during the first four days after hatching (Schat and Myers, 1991). Although there is some evidence that cell-mediated immunity plays a major role in coccidial resistance (Lillehoj, 1993), the role of the immune response in controlling components of the intestinal flora in poultry is largely unknown (Barrow, 1992). Maternal antibody IgG passively acquired in the developing chicken apparently does not offer significant protection against *Salmonella* (Spencer, 1992). Also, the immune mechanism appeared to have little influence on early intestinal colonization. The observation that conventional animals equipped with complete microflora had higher immunoglobulin levels and phagocytic activity than their germ-free counterparts suggested that probiotics could enhance immunity (Nousiainen and Setälä, 1993). Actual activation of the mucosal intestinal immunity in mice was obtained against enteropathogens with lactobacilli (Perdigon *et al.*, 1993) and in germ-free piglets (Pollmann *et al.*, 1980).

EFFECT OF PROBIOTICS ON THE GASTROINTESTINAL TRACT AND ANIMAL PERFORMANCE

Gut microflora

Manipulation of the gastrointestinal microflora has frequently been suggested as a method of preventing diarrhea and improving the health of young pigs. However, attempts to change the microflora or reduce scouring by the administration of probiotics to pigs have produced variable results. Eigel (1989) reported that diarrhea mediated by an oral challenge with ETEC could be reduced if pigs were dosed with lactic acid bacteria prior to the ETEC challenge. However, there was little difference in the number of anaerobic bacteria, lactic acid bacteria, *E. coli,* and the ratio of lactic acid bacteria to *E. coli* in the various segments of the gastrointestinal tract. More than half of all isolates picked from the *pars esophagus*, small intestine and cecum of weaned pigs treated with lactic acid bacteria and challenged with ETEC were identical to the lactic acid bacteria in the treatment.

It was suggested that the protection provided by lactic acid bacteria against ETEC induced diarrhea may be related to the ability of the lactic acid bacteria to colonize the *pars esophagus* and then to provide a continuous supply of these bacteria to the small intestine, cecum and colon (Eigel, 1989). This also could be achieved by a continuous supply of lactic acid bacteria in the diet, either supplied from a commercial probiotic or from intestinal homogenates from suckling and recently weaned pigs (Eigel, 1989). All of the evidence accumulated to date suggests that constant reinoculation is required to maintain proper numbers of probiotic microbials in the digestive tract (Chesson, 1993).

Huis in't Veld and Havenaar (1993) reported that numbers of lactobacilli declined dramatically immediately after weaning pigs at 28 days of age. This was accompanied by a concurrent increase in the numbers of E. coli far above the numbers of lactobacilli. This change in microflora could lead to an overgrowth of enteropathogenic E. coli (EEC) resulting in diarrhea. Huis in't Veld and Havenaar (1993) found that such a change in microflora could be prevented by treating the pigs five days before weaning until five days after weaning with three carefully selected Lactobacillus strains (2 - 4 x 10^6 cfu g^{-1} feed) isolated from healthy pigs and concluded that the composition of the gastrointestinal microflora could be influenced by external conditions such as weaning and by probiotic products. Muralidhara et al. (1977) also found that feeding a concentrate of a human isolate of L. lactis and colostrum to piglets during the first 48 h after birth was effective in preventing diarrhea and high mortality before and after a challenge with EEC (serotype 09:K:NM) at 72 h after birth. Pigs that received only lactobacilli did not scour before the EEC challenge and many lactobacilli were present in tissues from the small intestine. However, 72 h after EEC challenge these latter pigs revealed symptoms of diarrhea, and both coliforms and lactobacilli were observed in the small intestine tissue.

A substantial amount of evidence exists concerning the efficacy of CE bacterial cultures for reduction of food-poisoning Salmonella in poultry (Mead and Impey, 1987; Stavric and D'Aoust, 1993). Undefined CE cultures derived from chicken intestinal flora consistently protected chicks and turkey poults against challenges with up to 10^6 cfu of different serotypes of Salmonella (Stavric and D'Aoust, 1993). Protection was also obtained in several species of Salmonella-infected mature birds that had been treated with antibiotics prior to CE treatment (Mead, 1991). The efficacy of CE culture against repeated challenges of naturally occurring Salmonella in commercial poultry production has not been consistent. However, a substantial reduction of Salmonella has been observed in most field trials, particularly when there was strict adherence to hygiene measures (Stavric and D'Aoust, 1993).

Defined cultures derived from adult-type chicken microflora have proven to be less effective. Single strains of Lactobacillus, Streptococcus, Bifidobacterium or Bacteroides generally failed to reduce Salmonella colonization in poultry (Stavric, 1992). Similarly, probiotic preparations containing strains of Bacillus, Lactobacillus or Enterococcus (Hinton and Mead, 1991), monogeneric multistrain preparations of Lactobacillus spp., Bifidobacterium spp. or mixtures of the two (Stavric et al., 1992), or Bacillus spores (Guillot et al., 1990; Guillot and Yvore, 1993) failed to protect birds. Larger mixtures, however, containing 28 to 65 strains from up to ten genera were comparable in efficacy to undefined CE culture in protecting chicks against 10^3 - 10^4 cfu challenges in the laboratory experiments. The extent of protection was dependent on challenge dose, method of administration, mode of growth of isolates and the length of storage of isolates (Impey et al., 1982; Stavric et al., 1985; Gleeson et al., 1989). These chicken-derived defined mixtures failed to protect turkey poults in a limited number of field trials (Mead and Impey, 1985).

Scouring

The effectiveness of probiotic administration for preventing or reducing scouring in pre- and post-weaned pigs is also variable. Post-weaning scours in pigs weaned between four and five weeks of age were reduced when a non-viable Lactobacillus sp. fermentation product was fed (Hale and Newton, 1979). In agreement, the incidence of scouring was lower for pigs treated with *Ent. faecium* (Cernelle 68) before and after weaning than for controls (Maeng *et al.*, 1989). Eigel (1989) similarly reported that administration of three oral doses (about 10^{11} cfu per dose) of a commercial lactic acid bacteria product or a laboratory isolated strain of lactic acid bacteria (from the pig) prior to a challenge with ETEC protected weanling pigs (19 to 23 d of age) against diarrheal disease. Nine of 21 pigs developed diarrhea in the lactic acid treatment compared with 18 of 22 for non-treated pigs.

In contrast, feeding *Ent. faecium* (M-74, 6 x 10^6 cfu g^{-1} diet) did not decrease diarrhea in pigs weaned at 28 days of age, or reduce the total number of days diarrhea occurred, or shorten convalescent time (Wu *et al.*, 1987). Similarly, a mixture of *L. acidophilus*, yeast extract, an organic acid and a sweetener added to the water of pigs weaned at four weeks did not improve performance or decrease scouring when pigs were concurrently receiving unmedicated feed and consuming water with elevated mineral levels (McLeese *et al.*, 1992). These authors suggests that the disruptive effect of poor quality drinking water cannot be ameliorated by the use of *Lactobacillus* sp. cultures or organic acids. The addition of a *Bacillus* sp. ("*B. toyoi*") (1 x 10^9 cfu g^{-1}), *Lactobacillus* spp. (7.5 x 10^7 cfu g^{-1}) or *Ent. faecium* (5.5 x 10^8 cfu g^{-1}) to the diet of pigs weaned at four weeks of age and orally infected with *E. coli* (0141:K85ab) did not improve fecal consistency, prevent mortality, or shift the percentage of pigs excreting hemolytic *E. coli* (De Cupere *et al.*, 1992).

Using pigs weaned at 24 d of age and challenged with ETEC, Havenaar and Huis in't Veld (1993) reported that intestinal disturbances of challenged pigs were similar among probiotic treatments (*Ent. faecium* or *Bacillus* spores) and were not different from challenged controls. Also, the number of hemolytic and non-hemolytic *E. coli* in contents and on the mucosa of the small intestine did not differ between challenged controls and probiotic groups. Only non-challenged controls had a lower number of *E. coli* on the mucosa, and consequently no intestinal disturbance was observed. In four trials, the effectiveness of *Bif. globosum* A (5.0 x 10^4 to 7.5 x 10^8 cfu day^{-1}) was evaluated using weanling pigs. Only mild scouring was observed during the first ten days after weaning, and the feeding of bifidobacteria did not affect scour scores (Apgar *et al.*, 1993). During the course of these trials, both lower and higher scour scores were observed for the pigs fed the various levels of bifidobacteria than for the controls, with no consistent pattern evident.

Growth rate and feed conversion

Pigs. A larger proportion of studies has been conducted with young, and generally newly weaned, pigs because of the potential for reducing the poor performance that usually follows weaning. Pollmann (1986, 1992) suggested that despite extensive usage of probiotics since the 1900's, documented evidence of their therapeutic and nutritional value in swine production was still inconclusive and that it appeared that many of the presently available commercial probiotic products had limited value in environments where satisfactory pig health conditions existed. The data collected to date on adding probiotics during late gestation and lactation appear promising, especially for sows that had not received an *E. coli* vaccine.

The results of 26 trials using young pigs given non-viable and viable *Lactobacillus* strains (mainly *L. acidophilus*) or viable *Ent. faecium* were summarized by Nousiainen and Setälä (1993). When compared with controls, positive growth responses were obtained for 16 trials (only significant, P < 0.05, in two trials), and negative growth responses were obtained in nine trials (only significant, P < 0.05, in two trials). Probiotics improved feed efficiency in eight trials, and decreased feed efficiency in nine trials. Nousiainen and Setälä (1993) further reported the results of seven trials conducted on commercial farms in which host-specific strains of *L. fermentum* and *Ent. faecium* were fed alone or in combination with lactulose and lactitol. The probiotic treatments improved growth in five of the seven trials with an overall average improvement of 5.5% and a slight decrease in mortality was recorded (7.7 vs 9.9%). The authors suggested that the mixed probiotic was superior to simple ones. In another three trials, average daily gain was only increased during weeks three to five for pigs fed a medium level (5 x 10^5 cfu per dose) of *Bif. globosum* A (Apgar *et al.*, 1993).

The use of *Bacillus* spp. in the form of viable endospores preparations that have a greater stability than vegetative cultures has been reported in pig and sow diets (Kozasa, 1986; Pollmann, 1992). It is proposed that they decrease the number of pathogenic *E. coli* and may decrease ammonia production in the gastrointestinal tract. The results of six trials using *B. subtilis* in starter diets showed inconsistent benefits when no major post-weaning diarrhea was evident (Pollmann, 1992). However, when Toyocerin[®] (active ingredient "*B. toyoi*") was fed alone, it was as effective as Toyocerin[®] in combination with Zn-bacitracin, virginiamycin or tylosin for improving weight gain and feed efficiency of weanling pigs (Kozasa, 1986). Two *Bacillus* products fed to weanling pigs produced somewhat similar performance and did not differ from the controls (Lindemann, 1993). In contrast, no improvement in weight gain for weanling pigs challenged with ETEC and fed diets containing Toyocerin[®], *Lactobacillus* spp, or *Ent. faecium* as compared with control pigs was reported by others (De Cupere *et al.*, 1992).

Findings with growing-finishing pigs are less encouraging than those with weanling pigs. Older pigs are more resistant to intestinal disorders, have improved immunity and may digest the feed more efficiently than young pigs (Nousiainen and Setälä, 1993). Of seven trials reported in the 1970's and early 1980's and summarized by Pollmann (1986), only two trials showed a positive response with the addition of probiotics (mixed *Lactobacillus* spp. or *Ent. faecium*), and one trial showed a negative response. Several other studies in which there was no response to the addition of lactobacilli or enterococci have been recently reviewed (Nousiainen and Setälä, 1993; Pollmann, 1992). However, Kozasa (1986) reported that the weight gain of grower-finisher pigs was improved 10 to 18% when Toyocerin[®] was included in the diet. This response was of the same magnitude as that obtained with flavophospholipol, tylosin, virginiamycin, and Zn-bacitracin. The improved gain resulted from increased feed intake and improved feed efficiency. The overall inconsistency of these findings is, perhaps, not surprising since it is recognized that the general response of grower-finisher pigs is much less than that of starter pigs (Fox, 1988; Vanbelle *et al.*, 1990).

Poultry. Most studies on the efficacy of probiotics in poultry production have been done with *L. acidophilus* and have been reviewed extensively (Jernigan *et al.*, 1985; Miles and Bootwalla, 1991; Barrow, 1992). Comparison of results from different studies is difficult since the majority were not evaluated statistically and many were published only in abstract form (Barrow, 1992). In addition, experimental protocols (identity and dose of *Lactobacillus* strains, method of administration, duration of treatment, diet, housing, age of birds, duration of experiments etc.) varied. Differences in the concentration of probiotics incorporated into feeds varied ten-fold (0.02% to 0.2%) and, in water, by about two log units (10^7 to 10^9 cfu per chick) and the actual concentration of the probiotics in feed usually was not confirmed by microbiological assay. In several studies, the identity of probiotics was listed only as "direct-fed microbials " or by trade name (McNaughton *et al.*, 1992; Black *et al.*, 1993).

Reports on the efficacy of probiotic products circulated by probiotic suppliers may not be based on scientifically designed and statistically controlled work and often are not easy to obtain (Lloyd-Evans, 1989).

A few small-scale studies with broilers have shown that *Lactobacillus* treatment can increase daily weight gain. In these studies, feed consumption was either increased or decreased resulting in a reduced (Tortuero, 1973) or improved feed conversion index (Couch, 1978). In other studies, no effect on the growth rate or feed efficiency was evident (Dilworth and Day, 1978; Fethiere and Miles, 1987; Bolder *et al.*, 1993). Under commercial conditions broilers showed either an improved weight gain and feed efficiency (Arends, 1981), or no effect (Burkett *et al.*, 1977). With turkeys, an increase in body weight was obtained at 12 weeks, but not at 16 weeks, with the commercial preparation Probios® (Francis *et al.*, 1978). In a large field study with turkeys, improved feed efficiency and body weight gain were found with commercial products based on *L. reuteri* (Casas *et al.*, 1993).

The data are even less conclusive with laying hens. Lactobacilli either resulted in an improvement in egg production and feed efficiency (Krueger *et al.*, 1977; Nahashon *et al.*, 1993), or had no effect (Charles and Duke, 1978). It is interesting to note that a study carried out in three different locations across the US using the same preparation and experimental protocol did not yield uniform results (Miles *et al.*, 1981). Increased egg production was evident in Florida and Arizona, but not in South Dakota, while feed efficiency was improved only in Arizona.

Results with other probiotics are also inconclusive. Improved body weight gain and feed efficiency in broilers were obtained with a preparation containing *Bif. bifidum, L. acidophilus, Pediococcus acidilactici* and *Ent. faecium* administered in the diet or occasionally in the drinking water (Mazurkiewicz *et al.*, 1992), and with spores of *Bacillus* (Paciflor® or Toyocerin®) fed to gnotobiotic or to conventional chicks, respectively (Guillot *et al.*, 1990; Nguyen et al., 1988). Spores of *Cl. butyricum* ID fed to broilers through eight weeks of age also significantly increased body weight gain but, in this case, feed utilization was not changed (Han *et al.*, 1984). Conversely, the administration of nine commercial probiotics containing organisms from the genera *Streptococcus, Lactobacillus* and *Saccharomyces* or spores of *Bacillus* sp. to broilers through the feed or drinking water during a four-week period did not result in observable effects on body weight or on the composition of the cecal microflora (Bolder *et al.*, 1993). Layers showed no increase in egg production when fed a preparation of *L. acidophilus, Saccharomyces cerevisae, Ent. faecium* and *Kluveromyces fragilis* (Ibanez, 1990). Competitive exclusion products appear to have little or no effect on feed conversion and weight gain of poultry (Goren *et al.*, 1988; Schneitz *et al.*, 1991). Lactobacilli are also said to be of value during stressful conditions of poultry rearing, such as new housing, cold weather, poor diet, heat stress and crowding (Tortuero, 1973; Dilworth and Day, 1978; Suzuki *et al.*, 1989; Edens *et al.*, 1991). However, scientific data to substantiate such claims are limited (Barrow, 1992).

Reproductive performance in pigs

Feeding *B. subtilis* to sows for two weeks before farrowing and during lactation increased survival rate of pigs at weaning (Trotter, 1984; Noland, 1985; Peo, 1986; Danielson, 1988), although this is not always the case (LaForge and Pollman, 1984). Pollmann (1992) suggested that sows which had previously received *E. coli* vaccine might not respond to the feeding of a probiotic. Reported results of a two-year study showed that survival rate of pigs was increased and weaning to first estrus interval was decreased when Toyocerin® was fed to sows before farrowing and during lactation (Gedek, 1989). The addition of a mixture of *B. subtilis* and *Bacillus licheniformis* to sow and piglet feed had no effect on sow reproductive efficiency but improved growth rate 14% and feed utilization 7% with piglets (Bonomi, 1992). Phelps (1987) reported a 6.3% increase in the survival rate from birth to weaning following the administration of *L. acidophilus* at birth. Results of feeding probiotics to sows and newborn pigs are generally less variable and more positive than those for weanling, growing and finishing pigs, especially in situations where health problems are present.

Digestion

Only a limited number of reports have evaluated the influence of probiotic feeding on nutrient digestibility and retention and these findings generally are inconsistent. Hale and Newton (1979) reported that N retention and digestion of dry matter were similar for growing pigs fed a basal corn-soybean meal diet or one supplemented with 0.72 ml kg^{-1} of a non-viable lactobacillus fermentation product. Enhanced N retention as a percent of N intake (46.1 vs 48.7 and 48.2%, respectively for control, 10^9 and 10^{10} cfu kg^{-1} of feed) was reported for growing pigs fed Paciflor® (containing spores of *Bacillus* strain CIP 5832) (Scheuermann, 1993). Hale and Newton (1979) reported N retention (N balance as a percent of N intake) of 47.8 and 47.0%, respectively for control and pigs fed the lactobacillus product. The improvement in N utilization reported by Scheuermann (1993) was due primarily to reduced urinary N excretion, since apparent digestibility coefficients for N were similar for the control and treatment groups (81.1 vs 83.0 and 81.4%, respectively). Blood ammonia (13.5 to 20.1%) and urea (5.5 to 17.0%) concentrations were reduced by Paciflor®, supporting improved N utilization, but the metabolizable energy was not affected by the treatments. Maxwell *et al.* (1983) reported that apparent digestibility of dry matter and N was greater for 100 kg pigs fed either of two probiotic products (Feedmate 68® or Primalac®) compared with the controls; however, fecal ammonia, pH and urease activity were similar among treatments. Apparent digestion coefficients of dry matter and N obtained by Maxwell *et al.* (1983) for controls were much lower (65.4 and 67.7%, respectively) than reported by Hale and Newton (1979) (79.8 and 78.1%, respectively).

In a recent study, the addition of two *Bacillus* products separately (at a level of 0.5 g kg^{-1} to supply about 10^6 cfu g^{-1} of feed) in a corn-soybean meal finishing diet for pigs did not improve the digestibilities of dry matter, crude protein, ash, neutral detergent fiber and acid detergent fiber (Kornegay, 1993). Similarly, the addition of cellulase or *Bacillus* sp. (1.1 x 10^6 cfu kg^{-1} feed) to a sorghum-based diet for finishing pigs did not affect growth performance, carcass merit or nutrient utilization (Kim *et al.*, 1993) and, in cannulated pigs, did not affect pH, concentration of bacterial metabolites (lactic acid, ammonia, VFA) or the apparent digestibility of protein and organic matter (Spriet *et al.*, 1987).

FACTORS AFFECTING THE EFFICACY OF PROBIOTICS

Interaction with other additives, nutrients and types of ingredients

Probiotics are often considered as "natural" substitutes for feed antibiotics. Based on the results of some studies, it may be feasible to combine the probiotic and antibiotic treatments to obtain an additive advantage. Nousiainen and Setälä (1993) suggested that the natural microflora resists the invasion of both harmful and probiotic bacteria. Therefore, the probiotic bacteria may be established more easily in the gastrointestinal tract of target animals if the natural flora is weakened by the use of an antibacterial feed additive.

Kozasa (1986) suggested that Toyocerin® was usually as effective as several antibacterial feed additives when used in pigs and poultry diets. In the young pig, the probiotic was more effective when fed in combination with a variety of feed antibiotics. A combination of lincomycin and a *Lactobacillus* sp. was found to have an additive effect (Pollmann *et al.*, 1980). However, no interactive effects were observed for weanling pigs when a *Lactobacillus* sp. was fed in combination with virginiamycin (Harper *et al.*, 1983) or organic acids (Risley *et al.*, 1991). A somewhat different view was expressed by Rosen (1992). Based on a summary of 12 trials, it was suggested that antibiotics left pigs with no capacity to respond to probiotics. This led Chesson (1993) to suggest that additivity was unlikely since the consequences of probiotic and antibiotic additions to diets is essentially the same although the routes taken to achieve the effect are likely to be different.

On the basis of limited available data, Nousiainen and Setälä (1993) suggest that some non-absorbable sugar-lactic acid bacteria combinations provided an additional advantage in the treatment of young farm animals compared with the probiotic fed alone. Lactulose and lactitol have been used widely for this purpose. There is also growing interest in the use of oligosaccharides, primarily fructooligosaccharides (FOS), to encourage the overgrowth of selected autochthonous strains of bacteria, identified as having beneficial properties (see Chapter 11). Many naturally occurring oligosaccharides increase the number of bifidobacteria in the gastrointestinal tract. However, production or health benefits following addition of such oligosaccharides to diets have yet to be demonstrated conclusively in livestock (Chesson, 1993).

The addition of a commercial mixture of FOS to starter diets has been suggested to enhance the post-weaning performance of weanling pigs by increasing body weight gains, improving feed efficiency, and by preventing diarrhea (Hidaka *et al.*, 1986). However, Farnworth *et al.* (1992) reported that feeding starter diets containing 1.5% Jerusalem artichoke tuber flour (which contains fructooligosaccharides) or 1.5% FOS to pigs weaned at 28 days of age did not enhance feed intake, feed efficiency or body weight gain. Furthermore, VFA production and microbiological profile at the end of the four week trial were not significantly affected. In agreement, no improvement in performance of weanling pigs fed diets with 0.25 or 0.50% FOS was evident (Kornegay *et al.*, 1992). The basal diets used by Farnworth *et al.* (1992) and Kornegay *et al.* (1992) did not contain a probiotic.

The use of FOS in poultry appears more promising. Addition of FOS to broilers diets (0.25% and 0.50%) improved feed efficiency and reduced air sac lesions (Ammerman *et al.*, 1988). In agreement, Izat *et al.* (1990) reported improved body weight gain and a reduced level of salmonellae on processed carcasses when broilers were fed 0.375% FOS in their diet. Although Bailey *et al.* (1991) did not obtain a significant reduction of *Salmonella* spp. in broilers with the same or with higher levels (0.75%) of FOS when chicks were given partially protective CE culture and FOS, the protective activity of CE culture was significantly increased. Results of several field trials reported by Coors Biotech (Speights, 1990) showed improvement in body weight gain and feed efficiency in a majority of the trials. Air sac lesion scores and condemnations were reduced, and there was a trend for improved carcass yield.

Data concerning the influence of feed composition on probiotic action in poultry are limited. Chicks fed a *Lactobacillus* preparation in combination with sub-optimal amino acid levels (methionine, cysteine and lysine were restricted to 90% of the control) had a growth rate equal to that of chicks fed the control diet without the probiotic, but growth rate was not increased by adding the probiotic to control diets (Dilworth and Day, 1978). The addition of lactobacilli to a 17% protein diet resulted in larger eggs, but no change in egg size was observed when the probiotic was added to a 14% protein diet (Cerniglia *et al.*, 1983). Supplementation of whey in a diet of turkey poults enhanced the effect of *L. reuteri* by increasing body weight gain and resistance to salmonellae (Edens *et al.*, 1991). The addition of whey to withdrawal feed containing *L. acidophilus* and two strains of *Bifidobacterium* potentiated the increase in cecal weight, but had no effect on *Salmonella* infection in broilers (Bilgili and Moran, 1990).

The effect of antibiotics in comparison or in combination with probiotics varies depending on the nature of the antibiotic. In some cases, both antibiotics and probiotics fed separately to birds improved body weight gain and feed efficiency in broilers (Tortuero, 1973; McNaughton *et al.*, 1992) or improved egg weight in layers (Ibanez, 1990). When probiotic preparations containing *Cl. butyricum* ID in combination with Zn-bacitracin (Han *et al.*, 1984) or *Ent. faecium* M-74 with flavomycin (Roth and Kirchgeβner, 1986) were administered to broilers, the antibiotics did not interfere with the action of probiotics to improve weight gain. More recently, a study to evaluate the effect of three antibacterial products consisting of lincomycin, roxarsone and bacitracin and *Ent. faecium* M-74 on broilers was conducted. Antibacterial products alone or in combination with a probiotic significantly depressed feed conversion and body weight gain (Owings *et al.*, 1990). A probiotic containing *Bacillus* sp. did not interfere with the action of anticoccidial drugs in broilers (Saylor *et al.*, 1993). Interactions of some antibiotics, anticoccidials and carbohydrates with CE cultures have been reported. The effectiveness of CE treatments was dependent on the type of additive and the method of administration to the chicks (Stavric and D'Aoust, 1993).

Housing and environment

Stress can greatly affect the production of livestock. Broilers reared at temperature extremes exhibited changes in gut microflora and depressed body weight gain and feed efficiency. However, the effect on these parameters was not as great when the diet contained strains of *Lactobacillus* or *Bifidobacterium* (Suzuki *et al.*, 1989). A significant reduction in *Salmonella* contamination during transport of seven week-old broilers was achieved by incorporating a commercial *Lactobacillus* preparation in their feed and water for one week prior to the transport (Jones, 1992). The success of CE culture for reduction of salmonellae in commercial poultry also has been found to be critically dependent on the farm environment. Strict hygienic measures in poultry production, routinely used in the Scandinavian countries, could have contributed to the consistent efficacy of CE culture for elimination of *Salmonella* spp. in these countries (Wierup *et al.*, 1988). On the other hand, in trials where hygienic measures were not strictly followed, the competitive exclusion culture treatment was not as effective (Humbert *et al.*, 1992).

LACK OF UNIFORMITY OF RESULTS AND FUTURE PROSPECTS

The general conclusion of those reviewing results of probiotic feeding trials is that variable, inconsistent results have been and continue to be obtained when various probiotic products are fed to pigs and poultry (Sissons, 1989; Barrow, 1992; Fuller, 1992b; Jonsson and Conway, 1992; Pollmann, 1992; Nousiainen and Setälä, 1993). Several reasons have often been cited that might explain the variability of results:

- the health and nutritional status of the animal
- the presence of any kind of environmental stress
- genetic and strain differences of the animals
- the age and type of animal
- probiotic viability and stability
- the species specificity of problem (probiotic to host)
- dose level and frequency of feeding or administering
- drug and other interactions
- lack of systematic investigation by researchers.

Need for strict quality control and selection criteria for probiotics

Neither strict quality control systems nor basic selection criteria for probiotics are generally available. Although a number of criteria have been proposed there is no regulation in place to ensure existing and future product will comply to these specifications. Authorities throughout the world are working toward regulating these products, but there is no agreement between them about the definition of probiotics, whether they should be regarded as a veterinary medicine or feed additive and whether to adapt existing legislation or create new laws (Lloyd-Evans, 1989). Probiotics are often not of the quality, efficacy and perhaps safety which is demanded of other animal health or performance products (see Chapter 2). One of the major concerns is the lack of communication between research, industry and the regulators. The industry is of the opinion that they should be self-regulated, while regulators hold that efficacy must be proven in order for product to be registered (Chambers *et al.*, 1992). It appears that regulations controlling the production, packaging and distribution of these products are lenient and proposed selection criteria are usually not met by producers or researchers.

Requirements for standardized test protocols

A standardized protocol for testing the efficacy of probiotics in animals is generally not available. The exception is a recommended protocol for poultry which has been used by researchers to study CE products for reduced contamination with human enteropathogens (Mead *et al.*, 1989). Within this protocol, experimental conditions and expression of results are standardized, making it possible to compare results from different laboratories and to screen preparations before their use in large scale trials.

Since probiotics are used for different age and classes of animals, it appears that it will be difficult to develop a common protocol for all animal species. Even in the same test group the susceptibility of an animal to probiotics or pathogens could vary. Conway (1989) recommended that the number of animals be carefully considered so that statistically significant results could be obtained if differences exist. Also, experimental facilities and methods should be designed rigorously to eliminate the risk of inoculation of the control group. There is clearly a need to characterize the product used and dosage given as well as the animals used, environmental conditions, antibiotics, nutritional status, and other factors that could influence the results.

Need to elucidate the mechanism of probiotic action

The paucity of conclusive data on the claimed effects of probiotics clearly indicates the lack of understanding of their action. Also, the availability of clearly defined stable products which can be used to develop feeding and dosing schemes that are consistently effective are generally not available. Additional research is needed to elucidate the mechanism(s) by which probiotics act in the gastrointestinal system. Several interesting statements and speculations from recent reviews concerning probiotics illustrate their present status and future prospects. In the view of Tannock (1992), "there is a need to increase knowledge of the molecular biology of the bacteria that are indigenous to the digestive tract of vertebrate animals. When the colonization mechanisms of lactobacilli and the other lactic acid bacteria are identified, and the influences that their activities have on the host have been confidently established, it may be possible to exploit the microbes in animal husbandry." In general agreement, Fuller (1989) wrote, "What is needed at the moment is more information on the way that probiotic supplements act. When we have this sort of information it may be possible to improve the strain by genetic manipulation. In this way it would be possible to bring together the ability to survive in the gut with the ability to produce the metabolites which are responsible for the probiotic effect." Fuller (1993) further suggested that as more is known about the mode of action of probiotics and the metabolites responsible for the effects identified, it will be possible to develop non-viable, stimulatory compounds whose activity depends on the specific effect on the key probiotic microorganisms already present in the gastrointestinal tract in low numbers. It may also be possible to give an inoculation of the probiotic organism of choice and maintain it in the gastrointestinal tract by the continuous administration of the non-viable microbial stimulant or nutrient.

CONCLUSIONS

Development of a desirable and stable gastrointestinal microflora is generally accepted as essential for the health and productivity of pigs and poultry. Although the modes of action of probiotics are not well understood, it is generally accepted that probiotics exert their influence on the animal primarily through the microflora. Inconsistent research findings, however, continue to be reported for numerous probiotic products. The products contain a variety of microbial strains administered at varying dosing rates to pigs and poultry. Research findings suggest that probiotics are more effective in situations where the microflora of the animal is developing or its stability has been threatened.

The probiotic products and dosing rates that are used in reported research must be more clearly characterized, and also the animals' health and environmental conditions. Efforts to elucidate the mode(s) of action of probiotics need to be intensified. Selection criteria can be more carefully developed as the mechanism of action of probiotics is more clearly understood. Interactive effects of the various types of probiotics with numerous nutritional, environmental and health situations must be evaluated for the various ages and classes of pigs and poultry. More scientifically designed and statistically evaluated research is needed to provide more meaningful results. Furthermore, findings of these experiments must be confirmed by applied industry studies where environmental conditions may be more difficult to maintain. Finally, it would be helpful if an internationally acceptable definition for probiotics could be developed.

REFERENCES

AAFCO. 1993. Association of American Feed Control Officials. Official Publication.

AC. 1990. Agriculture Canada Trade Memorandum T-3-143 (December 1, 1990). Regulation of viable microbial products for oral administration to livestock, pp. 1-3. Agriculture Canada, Ottawa, Canada.

Alm, L., Leijonmarck, C.E. Persson, A.K. and Midtvedt, T. 1989. Survival of lactobacilli during digestion: an *in vitro* and *in vivo* study. In *The Regulatory and Protective Role of the Normal Microflora* (R. Grubb, T. Midtvedt and E. Norin, eds) pp. 293-297. M. Stockton Press. New York, US.

Ammerman, E., Quarles, C. and Twining, Jr., P.V. 1988. Broiler response to the addition of dietary fructooligosaccharides. *Poultry Sci.* **67** (Suppl. 1), 41.

Apgar, G.A., Kornegay, E.T., Lindemann, M.D. and Wood, C.M. 1993. The effect of feeding various levels of *Bifidobacterium globosum* A on the performance, gastrointestinal measurements, and immunity of weanling pigs and on the performance and carcass measurements of growing-finishing pigs. *J. Anim. Sci.* **71**, 2173-2179.

Arends, L.G. 1981. Influence of *Lactobacillus acidophilus* administered via the drinking water on broiler performance. *Poultry Sci.* **60**, 1619.

Bailey, J.S., Blankenship, L.C. and Cox, N.A. 1991. Effect of fructooligosaccharide on *Salmonella* colonization of the chicken intestine. *Poultry Sci.* **70**, 2433-2438.

Ballongue, J. 1993. Bifidobacteria and probiotic action. In *Lactic Acid Bacteria* (S. Salminen and A. von Wright, eds) pp. 357-428. Marcel Dekker, Inc., New York, US.

Barnes, E.M., Impey, C.S. and Cooper, D.M. 1980. Manipulation of the crop and intestinal flora of the newly hatched chick. *Amer. J. Clin. Nutr.* **33**, 2426-2433.

Barrow, P.A. 1992. Probiotics for chickens. In *Probiotics. The Scientific Basis* (R. Fuller, ed) pp. 225-257. Chapman & Hall, London, UK.

Bilgili, S.F. and Moran, E.T. 1990. Influence of whey and probiotic supplemented withdrawal feed on the retention of *Salmonella* intubated into market age broilers. *Poultry Sci.* **69**, 1670-1674.

Black, B.L., Jones, F.T., Qureski, M.A. and Brake, J. 1993. Effect of a direct fed microbial compound on the intestinal physiology and morphology of heat stressed broilers inoculated with *Salmonella typhimurium*. *Poultry Sci.* **72** (Suppl. 1), 136. (Abstract).

Bolder, N.M., van Lith, L.A.J.T., Putirulan, F.F. and Mulder, R.W.A.W. 1993. Influence of probiotic products administered through the feed or drinking water on weight and the intestinal microflora of broilers. In FLAIR No. 6 *Prevention and Control of Potentially Pathogenic Microorganisms in Poultry and Poultry Meat Processing. Proceedings, 12. Probiotics and Pathogenicity.* (J.F. Jensen, M.H. Hinton and R.W.A.W. Mulder, eds) pp. 115-122. COVP-DLO Het Spelderholt, DA Beekbergen, Netherlands.

Bonhoff, M., Drake, B.L. and Miller, C.P. 1954. Effect of streptomycin on susceptibility of intestinal tract to experimental *Salmonella* infection. *Proc. Soc. Exp. Biol. Med.* **86**, 132-137.

Bonhoff, M., Miller, C.P. and Martin, W.R. 1964. Resistance of the mouse's intestinal tract to experimental *Salmonella* infection. I. Factors which interfere with the initiation of infection by oral inoculation. *J. Exp. Med.* **120**, 805-816.

Bonomi, A. 1992. I probiotici in suinicoltura. Acquisizioni circa l'impiego del *Bacillus subtilis* e del *Bacillus licheniformis* (contributo sperimentale). *La Rivista della Societa Italiana di Scienza dell'Alimentazione* **21**, 481-499.

Borriello, S.P. 1990. The influence of the normal flora on *Clostridium difficile* colonisation of the gut. *Annals Med.* **22**, 61-67.

Burkett, R.F., Thayer, R.H. and Morrison, R.D. 1977. Supplementing market broiler rations with lactobacillus and live yeast cultures. *Animal Science Agricultural Research Report*, Oklahoma State University and USDA, US.

Casas, I.A., Edens, F.W., Dobrogosz, W.J. and Parkhurst, C.R. 1993. Performance of GAIAfeed® and GAIAspray®: A *Lactobacillus reuteri*-based probiotic for poultry. In FLAIR No. 6 *Prevention and Control of Potentially Pathogenic Microorganisms in Poultry and Poultry Meat Processing. Proceedings 12. Probiotics and Pathogenicity.* (J.F. Jensen, M.H. Hinton and R.W.A.W. Mulder, eds) pp. 63-71. COVP-DLO Het Spelderholt, D.A. Beekbergen, Netherlands.

Cerniglia, G.J., Goodling, A.C. and Herbert, J.A. 1983. The response of layers to feeding lactobacillus fermentation products. *Poultry Sci.* **62**, 1399. (Abstract).

Chambers, J.R., Trenholm, H.L., Foster, R.J. and Dauphin, F. 1992. Reports from roundtable discussion groups. Summary of group discussions. In *Proceedings of the International Roundtable on Animal Feed Biotechnology - Research and Scientific Regulation* (D.A. Leger and S.K. Ho, eds) pp. 215-221. Agriculture Canada, Ottawa, Canada.

Charles, O.W. and Duke, S. 1978. The response of laying hens to dietary fermentation products and probiotic-antibiotic combinations. *Poultry Sci.* **57**, 1125. (Abstract).

Chateau, N., Castellanos, I. and Deschamps, A.M. 1993. Distribution of pathogen inhibition in the *Lactobacillus* isolates of a commercial probiotic consortium. *J. Appl. Bacteriol.* **74**, 36-40.

Chesson, A. 1993. Probiotics and other intestinal mediators. In *Principles of Pig Science* (D.J.A. Cole, J. Wiseman and M.A. Varley, eds) pp. 197-214. Nottingham University Press, Loughborough, UK.

Conway, P. 1989. Lactobacilli: fact and fiction In *The Regulatory and Protective Role of the Normal Microflora* (R. Grubb, T. Midtvedt and E. Norin, eds) pp. 263 -281. M. Stockton Press, New York, US.

Corrier, D.E., Hinton, A., Ziprin, R.L., Beier, R.C. and DeLoach, J.R. 1990. Effect of dietary lactose on cecal pH, bacteriostatic volatile fatty acids and *Salmonella typhimurium* colonization of broiler chickens. *Avian Dis.* **34**, 617-625.

Corrier, D.E., Nisbet, D.J., Hollister, A.G., Scanlan, C.M., Hargis, B.M. and DeLoach, J.R. 1993. Development of defined cultures of indigenous cecal bacteria to control salmonellosis in broiler chicks. *Poultry Sci.* **72**, 1164-1168.

Couch, J.R. 1978. Poultry researchers outline benefits of bacteria, fungistatic compounds, other fecal additives. *Feedstuffs* April 3, p. 6.

Danielson, D.M. 1988. Role of *Bacillus subtilis* in prefarrowing, lactation, weaner and grower swine diets. *Nutr. Rep. Int.* **37**, 189-195.

De Cupere, F., Deprez, P., Demeulenaere, D. and Muylle, E. 1992. Evaluation of the effect of 3 probiotics on experimental *Escherichia coli* enterotoxaemia in weaned piglets. *J. Vet. Med. B* **39**, 277-284.

Dilworth, B.C. and Day, E.J. 1978. *Lactobacillus* cultures in broiler diets. *Poultry Sci.* **57**, 1101. (Abstract).

Dubos, R.J. 1963. Staphylococci and infection immunity. *Am. J. Dis. Child.* **105**, 643-645.

Ducluzeau, R., Bellier, M. and Raibaud, P. 1970. Transit digestif de divers inoculums bacteriens introduits 'per os' chez des souris axéniques et holoaxéniques (conventionnelles): effect antagoniste de la microflor du tractus gastro-intestinal. *Zbl. Bakt. I. Orig.* **213**, 533-548.

EC-FLAIR. 1993. Annex 2, Press release. In FLAIR No. 6 *Prevention and Control of Potentially Pathogenic Microorganisms in Poultry and Poultry Meat Processing. Proceedings, 12. Probiotics and Pathogenicity* (J.F. Jensen, M.H. Hinton, and R.W.A.W. Mulder, eds) pp. 129-130, COVP-DLO Het Spelderholt, D.A. Beekbergen, Netherlands.

Edens, F.W., Parkhurst, C.R. and Casas, I.A. 1991. *Lactobacillus reuteri* and whey reduce *Salmonella* colonization in the ceca of turkey poults. *Poultry Sci.* **70** (Suppl. 1), 158. (Abstract).

Eigel, W.N. 1989. Ability of probiotics to protect weanling pigs against challenge with enterotoxigenic *E. coli*. In *Proceedings Chr. Hansen Biosystems Technical Conf.*, pp. 10-19, San Antonio, Texas, US.

Farnworth, E.R., Modler, H.W., Jones, J.D., Cave, N., Yamazaki, H. and Rao, A.V. 1992. Feeding Jerusalem artichoke flour rich in fructooligosaccharides to weanling pigs. *Can. J. Anim. Sci.* **72**, 977-980.

Fethiere, R., and Miles, R.D. 1987. Intestinal tract weight of chicks fed an antibiotic and probiotic. *Nutr. Rep. Int.* **36**, 1305-1309.

Fox, S.M. 1988. Probiotics: intestinal inoculants for production animals. *Vet. Med.* **83**, 806-830.

Francis, C., Janky, D.M., Arafa, A.S. and Harms, R.H. 1978. Interrelationship of *Lactobacillus* and zinc bacitracin in the diets of turkey poults. *Poultry Sci.* **57**, 1687-1689.

Freter, R. 1956. Experimental enteric shigella and vibrio infection in mice and guinea pigs. *J. Exp. Med.* **104**, 411-418.

Freter, R. 1988. Mechanism of bacterial colonization of the mucosal surfaces of the gut. In *Virulence Mechanisms of Bacterial Pathogens* (J.A. Roth, ed) pp. 45-60. American Society for Microbiology, Washington, DC, US.

Freter, R. 1992. Factors affecting the microecology of the gut. In *Probiotics: The Scientific Basis* (R. Fuller, ed.) pp. 111-144. Chapman and Hall, London, UK.

Fuller, R. 1973. Ecological studies on the *Lactobacillus* flora associated with the crop epithelium of the fowl. *J. Appl. Bacteriol.* **36**, 131-139.

Fuller, R. 1977. The importance of lactobacilli in maintaining normal microbial balance in the crop. *Br. Poultry Sci.* **18**, 85-94.

Fuller, R. 1978. Epithelial attachment and other factors controlling the colonization of the intestine of the gnotobiotic chicken by lactobacilli. *J. Appl. Bacteriol.* **45**, 389-395.

Fuller, R. 1989. Probiotics in man and animals. *J. Appl. Bacteriol.* **66**, 365-378.

Fuller, R. 1992a. History and development of probiotics. In *Probiotics. The Scientific Basis.* (R. Fuller, ed) pp. 1-8. Chapman and Hall, London, UK.

Fuller, R. 1992b. Problems and prospects. In *Probiotics. The Scientific Basis.* (R. Fuller, ed) pp. 377-386, Chapman and Hall, London, UK.

Fuller, R. 1992c. The effect of probiotics on the gut micro-ecology of farm animals. In *The Lactic Acid Bacteria Vol. 1* (B.J.B. Wood, ed) pp. 171-192. Elsevier Applied Science, London, UK.

Fuller, R. 1993. The history and development of probiotics. In FLAIR No. 6. *Prevention and Control of Potentially Pathogenic Microorganisms in Poultry and Poultry Meat Processing. Proceedings, 12. Probiotics and Pathogenicity* (J.F. Jensen, M.H. Hinton, and R.W.A.W. Mulder, eds), COVP-DLO Het Spelderholt, D.A. Beekbergen, Netherlands.

Fuller, R. and Brooker, B.E. 1974. Lactobacilli which attach to the crop epithelium of the fowl. *Am. J. Clin. Nutr.* **27**, 1305-1312.

Gedek, von B.R. 1989. Intestinal flora and bioselfugulation. *Rev. Sci. Tech. Off. Int. Epiz.* **8**, 417-437.

Gedek von B.R. 1993. Probiotic agents for regulating intestinal flora. *Tierärztl. Umschau* **48**, 97-104.

Gilliland, S.E. 1981. Enumeration and identification of lactobacilli in feed supplements marketed as sources of *Lactobacillus acidopilus*. Animal Science Report. pp. 61-63. Oklahoma Agricultural Experimental Station, US.

Gleeson, T.M., Stavric, S. and Blanchfield, B. 1989. Protection of chicks against Salmonella infection with a mixture of pure cultures of intestinal bacteria. *Avian Dis.* **33**, 636-642.

Goren, E., de Jong, W.A., Doornenbal, P., Bolder, N.M., Mulder, R.W.A.W. and Jansen, A. 1988. Reduction of salmonella infection of broilers by spray application of intestinal microflora: a longitudinal study. *Veter. Quarterly* **10**, 249-255.

Guillot, J.F., Jule, S., and Yvore, P. 1990. Effect of a strain of *Bacillus* used as a probiotic against *Salmonella* carriage and experimental coccidiosis in chickens. *Microecol. Therapy* **20**, 19-22.

Guillot, J.F. and Yvore, P. 1993. Experimental studies of a *Bacillus* used as a probiotic against Salmonella carriage and coccidiosis in chickens. In FLAIR No. 6 *Prevention and Control of Potentially Pathogenic Microorganisms in Poultry and Poultry Meat Processing. Proceedings, 12. Probiotics and Pathogenicity* (J.F. Jensen, M.H. Hinton and R.W.A.W. Mulder, eds) pp. 107-

111. COVP-DLO Het Spelderholt, D.A. Beekbergen, Netherlands.

Hale, O.M. and Newton, G.L.   1979.   Effects of a nonviable lactobacillus species fermentation product on performance of pigs. *J. Anim. Sci.* **48**, 770-775.

Han, I.K., Lee, S.C., Lee, J.H., Kim, J.D. Jung, P.K. and Lee, J.C.   1984.   Studies on the growth promoting effects of probiotics II. The effects of *Clostridium butyricum* ID on the performance and the changes in the microbial flora of the feces and intestinal contents of the broiler chicks. *Korean J. Anim. Sci.* **26**, 158-165.

Harper, A.F., Kornegay, E.T., Bryant, K.L. and Thomas, H.R.   1983.   Efficacy of virginiamycin and a commercially-available lactobacillus probiotic in swine diets. *Anim. Feed Sci. Technol* **8**, 69-76.

Havenaar, R. and Huis in't Veld, J.H.J.   1992.   Probiotics: A general view. In *The Lactic Acid Bacteria Vol. 1.* (B.J.B. Wood, ed) pp. 151-170. Elsevier Applied Science, London, UK.

Havenaar, R. and Huis in't Veld, J.H.J.   1993.   *In vitro* and *in vivo* experiments with two commercial probiotic products containing *Enterococcus faecium* and *Bacillus toyoi*. In FLAIR No. 6 *Prevention and Control of Potentially Pathogenic Microorganisms in Poultry and Poultry Meat Processing. Proceedings, 12. Probiotics and Pathogenicity* (J.F. Jensen, M.H. Hinton, and R.W.A.W. Mulder, eds) pp. 53-62. COVP-DLO Het Spelderholt, D.A. Beekbergen, Netherlands.

Havenaar, R., Brink, B.T. and Huis in't Veld, J.H.J.   1992.   Selection of strains for probiotic use. In *Probiotics. The Scientific Basis* (R. Fuller, ed) pp. 209 -224. Chapman and Hall, London.

Hentges, D.J.   1992.   Gut flora in disease resistance. In *Probiotics The Scientific Basis* (R. Fuller, ed) pp. 87-110. Chapman and Hall, London, UK.

Hidaka, H., Eida, T., Takizawa, T., Tokunaga, T. and Tashiro, Y.   1986.   Effects of fructooligosaccharides on intestinal flora and human health. *Bifidobacteria Microflora* **5**, 37-50.

Hinton, M. and Mead, G.C.   1991.   *Salmonella* control in poultry: the need for the satisfactory evaluation of probiotics for this purpose. *Lett. Appl. Microbiol.* **13**, 49-50.

Hinton, A., Spates, G.E., Corrier, D.E., Hume, M.E., DeLoach, J.R. and Scanlan, C.M. 1991.   *In vitro* inhibition of the growth of *Salmonella typhimurium* and *Escherichia coli* O157:H7 by bacteria isolated from the cecal contents of adult chickens. *J. Food Prot.* **54**, 496-501.

Huis in't Veld, J.H.J. and Havenaar, R.   1993.   Selection criteria for microorganisms for probiotic use. In FLAIR No. 6 *Prevention and Control of Potentially Pathogenic Microorganisms in Poultry and Poultry Meat Processing. Proceedings, 12. Probiotics and Pathogenicity* (J.F. Jensen, M.H. Hinton, and R.W.A.W. Mulder, eds) pp 11-19. COVP-DLO Het Spelderholt, D.A. Beekbergen, Netherlands.

Humbert, F., Lalande, F., Salvat, G., Lahellec, C. and Colin, P.   1992.   Experimental field trial and some laboratories aspects of competitive exclusion (CE). In *Reports and Communications. Salmonella and Salmonellosis,* pp. 428-435. Ploufragan/Saint-Brieuc, France.

Ibanez, C.   1990.   The use of probiotics and zinc bacitracin in the diet of commercial layers. *Poultry Sci.* **69**, 65. (Abstract).

Impey, C.S., Mead, G.C. and George, S.M.   1982.   Competitive exclusion of salmonellas from chick caecum using a defined mixture of bacterial isolates from caecal microflora of an adult bird. *J. Hyg. Camb.* **89**, 479-490.

Izat, A.L., Skinner, J.T., Hierholzer, R.E., Kopek, J.M., Adams, M.H. and Waldroup, P.W.   1990.   Effects of fructooligosaccharide on performance of broilers and salmonellae contamination of broiler carcasses. *Poultry Sci.* **69**, 66. (Abstract).

Jayne-Williams, D.J. and Fuller, R.   1971.   The influence of the intestinal microflora on nutrition. In *Physiology and Biochemistry of the Domestic Fowl* (D.J. Bell and B.M. Freeman, eds) pp. 74-92. Academic Press, London, UK.

Jernigan, M.A., Miles, R.D. and Arafa, A.S.   1985.   Probiotics in poultry nutrition - A review. *World's Poultry Sci. J.* **41**, 99-107.

Jones, F.T.   1992.   Effect of Primalac® on *Salmonella* counts from experimentally inoculated processed broilers. *Poultry Sci.* **71**, 159.

Jonsson, E. and Conway P.   1992.   Probiotics for pigs. In *Probiotics. The Scientific Basis.* (R. Fuller, ed.), pp 260-316. Chapman and Hall, London, UK.

Juven, B.J., Meinersmann, R.J. and Stern, N.J. 1991. A review. Antagonistic effects of lactobacilli and pediococci to control intestinal colonization by human enteropathogens in live poultry. *J. Appl. Bacteriol.* **70**, 95-103.

Kim, I.H., Hancock, J.D., Hines, R.H. and Risley, C.R. 1993. Effects of cellulose and bacterial feed additives on the nutritional value of sorghum grain for finishing pigs. *Kansas State Agric. Exp. Stat. Res. Rep.* **695**, 144-147.

Kluber, E.F., Pollmann, D.S. and Blecha, F. 1985. Effect of feeding *Streptococcus faecium* to artificially reared pigs on growth, hematology and cell-mediated immunity. *Nutr. Rep. Int.* **32**, 57-65.

Koide, K. 1992. Animal feed biotechnology in Japan. In *Proceedings of the International Roundtable on Animal Feed Biotechnology-Research and Regulation* (D.A. Leger and S.K. Ho, eds) pp. 23-34. Agriculture Canada, Ottawa, Canada.

Kornegay, E.T. 1993. Influence of bacillus products on the nutrient digestibility of a corn-soybean meal diet fed to finishing swine. Internal Report, Dept. of Animal and Poultry Sciences, Virginia Tech, Blacksburg, VA, US.

Kornegay, E.T., Wood, C.M. and Eng, L.A. 1992. Effectiveness and safety of fructo-oligosaccharides for pigs. *J. Anim. Sci.* **70** (Suppl. 1), 19. (Abstract).

Kozasa, M. 1986. Toyocerin (*Bacillus toyoi*) as growth promotor for animal feeding. *Microb. Alim. Nutr.* **4**, 121-135.

Kozasa, M. 1989. Probiotics for animal use in Japan. *Rev. Sci. Tech. Off. Int. Epiz.* **8**, 517-531.

Krueger, W.F., Bradley, J.W. and Patterson, R.H. 1977. The interaction of gentian violet and lactobacillus organisms in the diet of Leghorn hens. *Poultry Sci.* **56**, 1729. (Abstract).

LaForge, R.R. and Pollmann, D.S. 1984. Effect of *Bacillus subtilis* on sow and baby pig performance and fecal populations. *J. Anim. Sci.* **59** (Suppl. 1), 248. (Abstract).

Lessard, M. and Brisson, G.J. 1987. Effect of a lactobacillus fermentation product on growth, immune response and fecal enzyme activity in weaned pigs. *Can. J. Anim. Sci.* **67**, 509-516.

Lillehoj, H.S. 1993. Avian gut-associated immune system: Implication in coccidial vaccine development. *Poultry Sci.* **72**, 1306-1311.

Lindemann, M.D. 1993. An evaluation of two *Bacillus* products (Biomate-2B and Pelletmate) in weanling pig diets. Internal Report, Dept. of Animal and Poultry Sciences, Virginia Tech, Blacksburg, VA, US.

Lloyd, A.B., Cumming, R.B. and Kent, R.D. 1977. Prevention of *Salmonella typhimurium* infection in poultry by pretreatment of chickens and poults with intestinal extracts. *Aust. Vet. J.* **53**, 82-87.

Lloyd-Evans, L.P.M. 1989. *Probiotics.* PJB Publications Ltd. Richmond, Surrey, UK.

Lyons, T.P. 1987. Probiotics: an alternative to antibiotics. *Pig News Info.* **8**, 157-164.

Maeng, W.J., Kim, C.M. and Shin, H.T. 1989. Effect of feeding lactic acid bacteria concentrate (LBC, *Streptococcus faecium*, Cernelle 68) on the growth rate and prevention of scouring in piglet. *Korean J. Anim. Sci.* **31**, 318-323.

Maxwell, C.V., Buchanan, D.S., Owens, F.N., Gilliland, S.E., Luce, W.G. and Vencl, R. 1983. Effect of probiotic supplementation on performance, fecal parameters and digestibility in growing-finishing swine. *Oklahoma Agric. Exp. Stat., Anim. Sci. Res. Rep.* **114**, 157-161.

Mazurkiewicz, M., Jamroz, D., Gawel, A., Wieliczko, A., Klimentowski, S. and Madej, J.A. 1992. The effect of probiotics Biogen D^W and Biogen D^P on productional effects and physiological parameters of slaughter chickens. *Medycyna Wet.* **48**, 368-371.

McLeese, J.M., Tremblay, M.L., Patience, J.F. and Christison, G.I. 1992. Water intake patterns in the weanling pig: effect of water quality, antibiotics and probiotics. *Anim. Prod.* **54**, 135-142.

McNaughton, J.L., Quarles, C.L. and Hinds, M.A. 1992. Direct-fed microbials in broiler rations: 1. Effect of application rate of a direct-fed microbial on broiler performance. *Poultry Sci.* **71** (Suppl. 1), 166. (Abstract).

Mead, G.C. 1989. Microbes of the avian cecum: types present and substrates utilized. *J. Exp. Zool.* Suppl. 3, 48-54.

Mead, G.C. 1991. Developments in competitive exclusion to control *Salmonella* carriage in poultry.

In *Colonization Control of Human Bacterial Enteropathogens in Poultry* (L.C. Blankenship, ed.) pp. 91-104. Academic Press, San Diego, US.

Mead, G.C. and Impey, C.S. 1985. Control of Salmonella colonization in poultry flocks by defined gut-flora treatment. In *Proceedings of the International Symposium on Salmonella* (G.H. Snoeyenbos, ed.) pp. 72-79. American Association of Avian Pathologists, University of Pennsylvania, US.

Mead, G.C., and Impey, C.S. 1987. The present status of the Nurmi Concept for reducing carriage of food-poisoning salmonellae and other pathogens in live poultry. In *Elimination of Pathogenic Organisms from Meat and Poultry* (F.J.M. Smulders, ed) pp. 57-77. Elsevier, Amsterdam, Netherlands.

Mead, G.C., Barrow, P.A., Hinton, M.H., Humbert, F., Impey, C.S., Lahellec, C., Mulder, R.W.A.W., Stavric, S. and Stern, N.J. 1989. Recommended assay for treatment of chicks to prevent *Salmonella* colonization by "competitive exclusion". *J. Food Prot.* **52**, 500-502.

Metchnikoff, E. 1908. *Prolongation of Life.* G.P. Putnam and Sons, New York, US.

Meynell, G.G. 1963. Antibacterial mechanisms of the mouse gut. II: The role of Eh and volatile fatty acids in the normal gut. *Br. J. Exp. Pathol.* **44**, 209-219.

Miles, R.D. and Bootwalla, S.M. 1991. Direct-fed microbials in animal production "avian". In *Direct-Fed Microbials in Animal Production. A Review of Literature.* pp. 117-146. NFIA, West Des Moines, Iowa, US.

Miles, R.D., Arafa, A.S., Harms, R.H., Carlson, C.W., Reid, B.L. and Crawford, J.S. 1981. Effects of a living nonfreeze-dried *Lactobacillus acidophilus* culture on performance, egg quality, and gut microflora in commercial layers. *Poultry Sci.* **60**, 993-1004.

Montes, A.J. and Pugh, D.G. 1993. The use of probiotics in food-animal practice. *Vet. Med.* **88**, 282-288.

Morishita, Y., Fuller, R. and Coates, M.E. 1982. Influence of dietary lactose on the gut flora of chicks. *Br. Poult. Sci.* **23**, 349-359.

Muralidhara, K.S., Sheggeby, G.G., Elliker, P.R., England, D.C. and Sandine, W.E. 1977. Effect of feeding lactobacilli on the coliform and lactobacillus flora of intestinal tissue and feces from piglets. *J. Food Prot.* **40**, 288-295.

Nahashon, S.N., Nakaue, H.S. and Mirosh, L.W. 1993. Effect of direct-fed microbials on nutrient retention and production parameters of single comb white Leghorn (SCWL) pullets. *Poultry Sci.* **72** (Suppl. 7), 87. (Abstract)

Nguyen, T.H., Eckenfelder, B. and Levesque, A. 1988. Growth promoting efficiency of two probiotics, TOYOCERIN® and PACIFLOR®, in broiler diets. *Arch. Geflugelk.* **52**, 240-245.

Noland, P.R. 1985. More pigs with Biomate FG. Bio-Gram Report. Ch. Hansen Laboratory, Inc., Milwaukee, Wisconsin, US.

Nousiainen, J. and Setälä, J. 1993. Lactic acid bacteria as animal probiotics. In *Lactic Acid Bacteria* (S. Salminen and A. von Wright, eds) pp 315-356. Marcel Dekker, New York, US.

Nurmi, E. and Rantala, M. 1973. New aspects of *Salmonella* infection in broiler production. *Nature* **241**, 210-211.

Nurmi, E., Schneitz, C.E. and Mäkelä, P.H. 1983. Process for the production of a bacterial preparation. Canadian Patent No. 1,151,066.

Owings, W.J., Reynolds, D.L., Hasiak, R.J. and Ferket, P.R. 1990. Influence of dietary supplementation with *Streptococcus faecium* M-74 on broiler body weight, feed conversion, carcass characteristics, and intestinal microbial colonization. *Poultry Sci.* **69**, 1257-1264.

Parker, R.B. 1974. Probiotics, the other half of the antibiotics story. *Anim. Nutr. Health* **29**, 4-8.

Pedersen, K. and Tannock, G.W. 1989. Colonization of the porcine gastrointestinal tract by lactobacilli. *Appl. Environ. Microbiol.* **55**, 279-283.

Pendelton, B. 1992. Challenges of regulation: United States industry perspective. In *Proceedings of the International Roundtable on Animal Feed Biotechnology - Research and Scientific Regulation* (D.A. Leger and S.K. Ho, eds) pp. 185-190. Agriculture Canada, Ottawa, Canada.

Peo, E.R. 1986. Alternatives to the use of antibiotics in swine production. 26th Ann. Nebraska SPF

Conf., Lincoln, NE, pp. 44-62.

Perdigon, G. and Alvarez, S. 1992. Bacterial interactions in the gut. In *Probiotics. The Scientific Basis.* (R. Fuller, ed), pp. 146-180, Chapman and Hall, London, UK.

Perdigon, G., Medici, M., Bibas Bonet De Jorrat, M.E., Valverde De Budeguer, M. and Pesce De Ruiz Holgado, A. 1993. Immunomodulating effects of lactic acid bacteria on mucosal and humoral immunity. *Int. J. Immunother.* **9**, 29-52.

Phelps, A. 1987. Probiotics boost baby piglet survival rate. *Feedstuffs* **59**, 24-27.

Pivnick, H. and Nurmi, E. 1982. The Nurmi concept and its role in the control of salmonellae in poultry. In *Developments in Food Microbiology-1* (R. Davies, ed.) pp. 41-70. Applied Science Publishers, Essex, UK.

Pollmann, D.S. 1986. Probiotics in pig diets. In *Recent Advances in Animal Nutrition* (W. Haresign and D,J.A. Cole, eds), pp. 193-205, Butterworth, London, UK.

Pollmann, D.S. 1992. Probiotics in swine diets. In *Proceedings of the International Roundtable on Animal Feed Biotechnology - Research and Scientific Regulation* (D.A. Leger and S.K. Ho eds) pp. 65-74. Agriculture Canada, Ottawa, Canada.

Pollmann, D.S. and Bandyk, C.A. 1984. Stability of viable *Lactobacillus* products. *Anim. Feed Sci. Technol.* **11**, 261-267.

Pollmann, D.S., Danielson, D.M., Wren, W.B., Peo, E.R. and Shahani, K.M. 1980. Influence of *Lactobacillus acidophilus* inoculum on gnotobiotic and conventional pigs. *J. Anim. Sci.* **51**, 629-637.

Pongpech, P. and Hentges, D.J. 1989. Inhibition of *Shigella sonnei* and enterotoxigenic *Escherichia coli* by volatile fatty acids in mice. *Microb. Ecol. Health Dis.* **2**, 153-161.

Raibaud, P. and Raynaud, J.P. 1990. Experimental data on the modes of action of probiotics. In *European Association for Animal Production Publ. No. 52. New Trends in Veal Calf Production* (J.H.M. Metz and C.M. Groenstein, eds) pp. 269-275. Pudoc, Wageningen, Netherlands.

Risley, C.R., Kornegay, E.T., Lindemann, M.D. and Weakland, S.M. 1991. Effects of organic acids with and without a microbial culture on performance and gastrointestinal tract measurements of weanling pigs. *Anim. Feed Sci. Tech.* **35**, 259-270.

Rolfe, R.D. 1991. Population dynamics of the gastrointestinal tract. In *Colonization Control of Human Bacterial Enteropathogens in Poultry* (L.C. Blankenship, ed) pp. 59 -77. Academic Press, San, Diego, US.

Rosen, G.D. 1992. Antibacterials in disease control and performance enhancement. *Feed Compounder* **12**, 22-27.

Roth, F.X. and Kirchgeβner, M. 1986. Nutritive effects of *Streptococcus faecium* (strain M-74) in broiler chicks. *Arch. Geflugelk.* **50**, 225-228.

Sasaki, T., Meade, Y. and Namioka, S. 1987. Immunopotentiation of the mucosa of the small intestine of weaning piglets by peptidoglycans. *Jpn. J. Vet Sci.* **49**, 235-243.

Savage, D.C. 1987. Factors influencing biocontrol of bacterial pathogens in the intestine. *Food Technol.* **41**, 82-87.

Saylor, W.W., Korver, D.R., Mullins, T.M. and Malone, G.W. 1993. Response of broiler chickens to a direct-fed microbial (*Bacillus* sp.) in the presence of anticoccidial drugs and coccidial infection. *Poultry Sci.* **72**, 58.

Schat, K.A. and Myers, T.J. 1991. Avian intestinal immunity. *Crit. Rev. Poultry Biol.* **3**, 19-34.

Scheuermann, S.E. 1993. Effect of the probiotic Paciflor (CIP 5832) on energy and protein metabolism in growing pigs. *Anim. Feed Sci. Tech.* **41**, 181-189.

Schneitz, C., Nuotio, L., Kiiskinen, T. and Nurmi, E. 1991. Pilot-scale testing of the competitive exclusion method in chickens. *Br. Poultry Sci.* **32**, 881-884.

Sissons, J.W. 1989. Potential of probiotic organisms to prevent diarrhea and promote digestion in farm animals - A review. *J. Sci. Food Agric.* **49**, 1-13.

Smith, H.W. 1965. The development of the flora of the alimentary tract in young animals. *J. Path. Bacteriol.* **90**, 495-513.

Smith, H.W., Barrow, P.A. and Tucker, J.F. 1985. The effect of oral antibiotic administration on the excretion of salmonellas by chickens. In *Proceedings of International Symposium on Salmonella* (G.H. Snoeyenbos, ed.) pp. 88-93. American Association of Avian Pathologists, University of Pennsylvania, US.

Soerjadi, A.S., Rufner, R., Snoeyenbos, G.H. and Weinack, O.M. 1982. Adherence of salmonellae and native gut microflora to the gastrointestinal mucosa of chicks. *Avian Dis.* **26**, 576-584.

Speights, R.M. 1990. Natural products for food and feed. FOS 50 Technical Bulletin, Coors BioTech, Inc., AgriProducts Div., Westminster, CO, US.

Spencer, J.L. 1992. Probiotics: Potential for reducing the *Salmonella* and *Campylobacter* carrier state in poultry - Part I *Salmonella*. In *Proceedings of the International Roundtable on Animal Feed Biotechnology - Research and Scientific Regulation* (D.A. Leger and S.K. Ho, eds) pp. 97-101. Agriculture Canada, Ottawa, Canada.

Spriet, S.M., Decuypere, J.A. and Henderickx, H.K. 1987. Effect of *Bacillus toyoi* (Toyocerin) on the gastrointestinal microflora, concentration of some bacterial metabolites, digestibility of the nutrients and the small intestinal mean retention time in pigs. *Med. Fac. Landbouww. Rijksuniv. Gent* **52**, 1673-83.

Stavric, S. 1992. Defined cultures and prospects. *Int. J. Food Microbiol.* **15**, 245-263.

Stavric, S. and D'Aoust, J.-Y. 1993. Undefined and defined bacterial preparations for the competitive exclusion of *Salmonella* in poultry- A review. *J. Food Prot.* **56**, 173-180.

Stavric, S., Gleeson, T.M., Blanchfield, B. and Pivnick, H. 1985. Competitive exclusion of *Salmonella* from newly hatched chicks by mixtures of pure bacterial cultures isolated from fecal and cecal contents of adult birds. *J. Food Prot.* **48**, 778-783.

Stavric, S., Gleeson, T.M., Blanchfield, B. and Pivnick, H. 1987. Role of adhering microflora in competitive exclusion of *Salmonella* from young chicks. *J. Food Prot.* **50**, 928-932.

Stavric, S., Gleeson, T.M., Buchanan, B. and Blanchfield, B. 1992. Experience on the use of probiotics for *Salmonella* control in poultry. *Lett. Appl. Microbiol.* **14**, 69-71.

Suzuki, K., Kodama, Y. and Mitsuoka, T. 1989. Stress and intestinal flora. *Bifidobacteria Microflora* **8**, 23-38.

Szylit, O., Dabard, J., Durand, M., Dumay, C., Bensaada, M., and Raibaud, P. 1988. Production of volatile fatty acids as a result of bacterial interactions in the cecum of gnotobiotic rats and chickens fed a lactose-containing diet. *Reprod. Nutr. Develop.* **28**, 1455-1464.

Tannock, G.W. 1992. The lactic microflora of pigs, mice and rats. In *The Lactic Bacteria. Vol. 1* (B.J.B. Wood, ed) pp. 21-48. Elsevier Applied Science, London, UK.

Tobey, J.F. 1992. A current perspective: the utilization of microbial fermentation products in feed and forage. In *Proceedings of the International Roundtable on Animal Feed Biotechnology - Research and Scientific Regulation* (D.A. Leger and S.K. Ho, eds) pp. 7-17. Agriculture Canada, Ottawa, Canada.

Tortuero, F. 1973. Influence of the implantation of *Lactobacillus acidophilus* in chicks on the growth, feed conversion, malabsorption of fats syndrome and intestinal flora. *Poultry Sci.* **52**, 197-203.

Tournut, J. 1989. Applications of probiotics to animal husbandry. *Rev. Sci. Tech. Off. Int. Epiz.* **8**, 551-566.

Trotter. 1984. Unpublished data cited by Pollmann (1986) and Peo (1986).

Van Der Waaij, D., Berghuis-de Vries, J.M., Lekkerkerk-Van der Wees, J.E.C. 1971. Colonization resistance of the digestive tract in conventional and antibiotic-treated mice. *J. Hyg.* **59**, 405-411.

Vanbelle, M., Teller, E. and Focant, M. 1990. Probiotics in animal nutrition: A review. *Arch. Anim. Nutr. Berlin.* **40**, 543-567.

Veldman, A. 1992. Probiotics. *Tijdschr. Diergeneeskd.* **117**, 345-348.

Vincent, J.G., Veomett, R.C. and Riley, R.F. 1959. Antibacterial activity associated with *Lactobacillus acidophilus*. *J. Bacteriol.* **78**, 477-484.

Wierup, M., Wold-Troell, M., Nurmi, E. and Häkkinen, M. 1988. Epidemiological evaluation of the *Salmonella*-controlling effect of a nationwide use of a competitive exclusion culture in poultry. *Poultry Sci.* **67**, 1026-1033.

Winkelstein, A. 1956. *L. acidophilus* tablets in the therapy of functional intestinal disorders. *Am. Practioner Dig. Treatment* **7**, 1637-1639.

Wu, M.C., Wung, L.C., Chen, S.Y. and Kuo, C.C. 1987. Study on the feeding value of *Streptococcus faecium* M-74 for Pigs: I. Large scale of feeding trial of *Streptococcus faecium* M-74 on the performance of weaning pigs. Research Report, Animal Industry Research Institute, Taiwan Sugar Corp., Chunan Miaoli, Taiwan, pp. 11-12.

11 Oligosaccharide feed additives

Pierre F. Monsan[1] and François Paul

BioEurope S.A., BP 4196, 31031 Toulouse Cedex, France

INTRODUCTION

An alternative approach to the use of microorganisms and antibiotics for manipulating the intestinal flora and metabolism of non-ruminant animals is the use of oligosaccharides. These oligosaccharides can be regarded as "soluble fibre". They have in common the property that they resist attack by the digestive enzymes of humans and animals and thus are not metabolized directly by the host. For this reason, they are able to reach the colon. Here they interact with the microbial flora, acting as specific growth substrates, and with the carbohydrate receptors present at the surface of either microbial or epithelial cells, affecting cell adhesion and immunomodulation. When used in limited amounts in feed (below 1%), oligosaccharides may result in an increase in weight gain and an improvement in the health status of the animal.

Oligosaccharides can be obtained by different routes (Morgan *et al.*, 1992; Chesson, 1993). These include:

- extraction from plant sources (fructooligosaccharides, α-galactooligosaccharides)
- controlled enzymatic hydrolysis of polysaccharides (fructooligosaccharides, xylooligosaccharides)
- enzymatic synthesis (fructooligosaccharides, α-glucooligosaccharides, β-glucooligosaccharides, β-galactooligosaccharides).

AVAILABLE OLIGOSACCHARIDES

Fructooligosaccharides

Fructooligosaccharides consist of a linear chain of β-D-fructofuranose units linked 1,2 by glycosidic bonds. Chains may terminate with a D-glucopyranose unit at the non-reducing end (sucrose moiety) (Fig. 1). They can be obtained from three different sources. They can be extracted from plants. Onions (Shiomi, 1978) and asparagus (Shiomi *et al.*, 1976), for example, contain particularly high amounts of fructooligosaccharides compared to other plant sources (Fishbein *et al.*, 1988). A second source is by controlled (limited) enzymatic hydrolysis of inulin polymers from chicory roots (Heinz and Vogel, 1991). An industrial production process using this method has been developed by Raffineries Tirlemontoises in Belgium. The third route is by enzymatic synthesis from sucrose using a fructosyltransferase (EC 2.4.1.100) from *Aspergillus niger* or *Aureobasidium pullulans* (Hidaka *et al.*, 1988; Hidaka and Hirayama, 1991) according to the reaction:

---

[1]Present address: Centre de Bioingénierie Gilbert Durand, INSA, Complexe Scientifique de Rangueil, 31077 Toulouse, France

$$\underset{\text{sucrose}}{\text{n G-F}} \xrightarrow{\textit{fructosyltransferase}} \underset{\text{Neosugar}^{\circledR}}{\text{G-F}_n} + (n\text{-}1)\text{G}$$

Neosugar$^{\circledR}$ is a mixture of glucose, sucrose and fructooligosaccharides (FOS) with a terminal glucose unit (Fig. 1). Glucose and sucrose can be removed from the reaction mixture by chromatography to obtain a product with increased FOS purity.

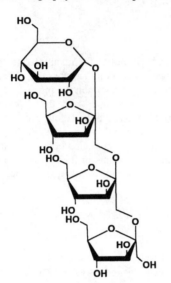

Figure 1. Structure of nystose - an α-1,2-linked fructofuranosyl tetrasaccharide with a terminal glucose unit.

α-Glucooligosaccharides

α-Glucooligosaccharides containing α-1,6 bonds (isomaltooligosaccharides) can be obtained from starch hydrolysates (maltose and maltodextrins) through the action of the α-transglucosidase (EC 2.4.1.24) from *Aspergillus* sp. (Roper and Koch, 1988). Maltose and maltodextrins act as both glucosyl donor and acceptor. This transglucosylation reaction has been developed to an industrial scale in Japan by Hayashibara (Yoneyama *et al.*, 1992).

An alternative route for isomaltooligosaccharide production, developed by the Showa Sangyo Co., uses glucoamylase (EC 3.2.1.3) combined with the action of pullulanase (EC 3.2.1.41). Both hydrolases are used for glucose production from starch hydrolysates, but also are able to catalyse the synthesis of α-glucooligosaccharides mainly linked 1,6 when used with concentrated carbohydrate solutions. This process was developed from the initial work of the National Food Research Laboratory of the Japanese Ministry for Agriculture, Forest and Fisheries (Amarakone *et al.*, 1984). Similar isomaltooligosaccharides are obtained by a transglucosylation reaction catalysed by a neopullulanase enzyme (EC 3.2.1.135) from *Bacillus stearothermophilus* modified by site-directed mutagenesis (Kuriki *et al.*, 1993).

α-Glucooligosaccharides can also be obtained using the acceptor-reaction catalyzed with dextransucrase (EC 2.4.1.5). This enzyme is an extracellular enzyme usually obtained from the soil bacterium *Leuconostoc mesenteroides*, but also from *Streptococcus* sp. It catalyzes the synthesis of high molecular weight glucans (dextrans) according to the reaction:

$$\text{n G-F} \quad \xrightarrow{\textit{dextransucrase}} \quad (G)_n \;+\; nF$$
$$\text{sucrose} \qquad\qquad\qquad\qquad \text{dextran} \quad \text{fructose}$$

The dextran oligomers produced have a linear chain of D-glucopyranosyl units linked α-1,6 with variable amounts of α-1,2 and α-1,3 and α-1,4-linked side chains, according to the origin of the dextransucrase (Jeanes *et al.*, 1954). Under the usual conditions of use, a high molecular weight polymer (10^6-10^7 Da) is obtained. This is the case, for example, with the enzyme from *L. mesenteroides* NRRL-512F which is used to produce dextran polymers of industrial interest (chromatography supports, photographic emulsions, iron carrier, blood plasma substitute). However, when efficient acceptors are added to the reaction mixture, dextransucrase catalyzes the synthesis of α-glucooligosaccharides (Koepsell *et al.*, 1953; Robyt and Ecklund, 1983; Paul *et al.*, 1986). Maltose and isomaltose are the most efficient acceptors in this reaction.

With the dextransucrase from *L. mesenteroides* NRRL B-1299 and maltose as acceptor, it has been possible to obtain α-glucooligosaccharides (GOS) which have one or more D-glucopyranosyl units linked via α-1,2 glycosidic bonds (Fig. 2) (Paul *et al.*, 1992; Remaud-Simeon *et al.*, 1994).

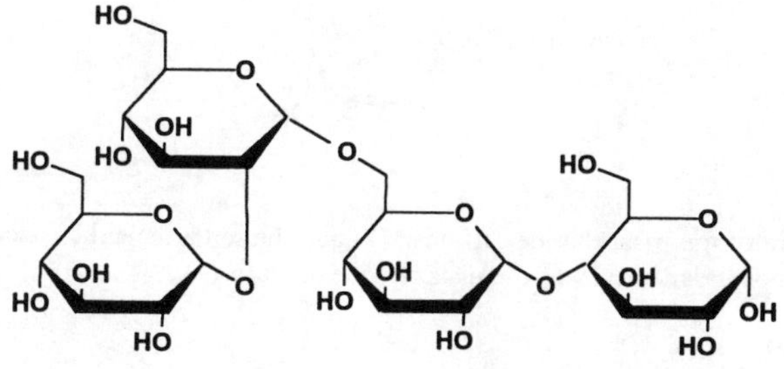

Figure 2. Structure of an α-linked glucopyranosyl tetrasaccharide (GOS).

α-Galactooligosaccharides

α-Galactosyl derivatives of sucrose are present in many legume seeds. Mono-, di- and tri-α-galactosylsucrose, known respectively as raffinose, stachyose (Fig. 3) and verbascose, are produced by extraction from plant sources, particularly soybean (Minami *et al.*, 1983). They are known, in part, to be responsible for flatulence and diarrhoea problems following consumption of beans, due to the lack of an α-galactosidase enzyme in the gastrointestinal tract of humans and animals.

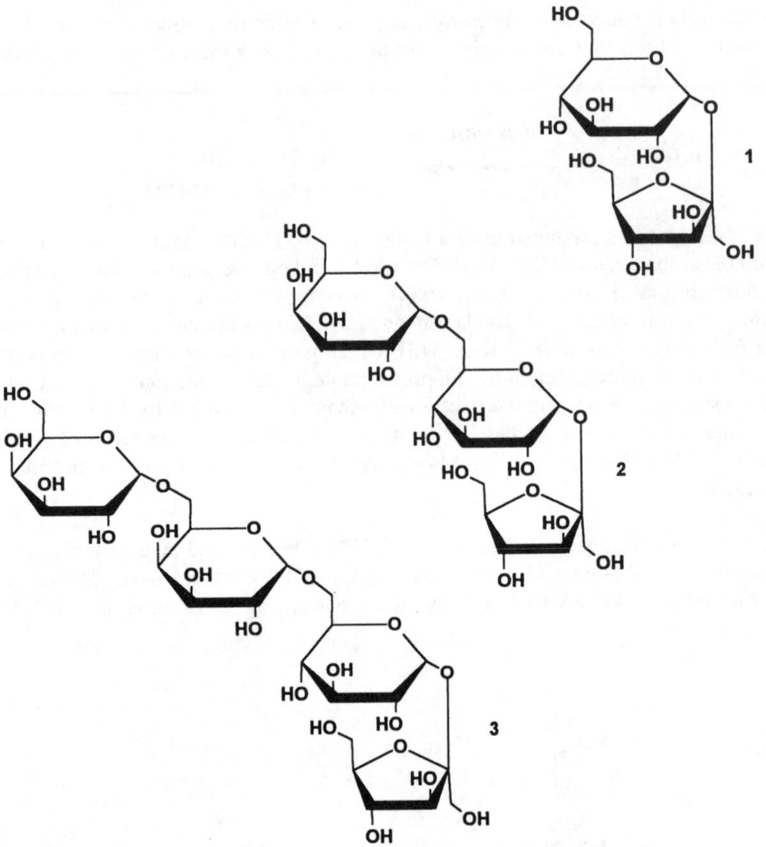

Figure 3. Structure of the trisaccharide raffinose (2) and the tetrasaccharide stachyose (3) - α-1,6-linked galactopyranosyl derivatives of the disaccharide sucrose (1).

β-Glycooligosaccharides

A variety of β-glycooligosaccharides can be obtained by enzymatic techniques (Fujii and Komoto, 1991), but these are not available in sufficient quantities and at a sufficiently low cost to allow their use as feed additives. Laboratory studies showed that they are as resistant to the action of host digestive enzymes as the previously described oligosaccharides.

β-Glucooligosaccharides are obtained when highly concentrated glucose solutions (70%, w/w) are submitted to the action of a β-glucosidase (EC 3.2.1.21) (Ajisaka *et al.*, 1987). This reaction yields a mixture of disaccharides and trisaccharides containing mainly β-1,6 (gentiobiose, gentiotriose) and β-1,4 (cellobiose, cellotriose) glycosidic linkages. Transgalactosylation of lactose catalysed by β-galactosidase (EC 3.2.1.23) also results in the synthesis of β-galactooligosaccharides. The reaction yield depends on the enzyme-producing microbial source and on the lactose concentration (Mozaffar *et al.*, 1984; Prakash *et al.*, 1987).

β-Xylooligosaccharides are produced by enzymatic hydrolysis of plant xylans (Morgan *et al.*, 1992). They can also be found naturally occurring in bamboo shoots, which are eaten in Asia (Imaizumi *et al.*, 1991). The efficiency of action of endoxylanases (EC 3.2.1.8) is influenced by the presence of arabinofuranosyl side chains in the xylan polymer (Kormelink *et al.*, 1992). The interest in the use of xylanases and other enzymes by the pulp, paper and feed industries is increasing the availability of this type of industrial enzyme preparation.

EFFECTS OF OLIGOSACCHARIDES AS FEED ADDITIVES

The addition of a limited amount of oligosaccharides to animal feeds (below 1%) can result in a significant improvement in weight gain, consumption index and health status of the animal. However, such effects are highly variable according to the type of oligosaccharide employed, the class of animal (age and species) and, in particular, the conditions of husbandry.

Fructooligosaccharides (FOS) developed in Japan by Meiji Seika are the most extensively documented products as feed additives. These products are also marketed under the trade name Profeed® in the United States by Coors Biotech and in Europe by Beghin Meiji Industries. In Europe, they compete with the fructooligosaccharides (Raftilose®) produced by the controlled enzymatic hydrolysis of inulin.

When fed to 50 weaned piglets for 30 days at 0.25% and 0.5%, addition of FOS to the diet resulted in higher weight gains of 7.2 and 9.2 kg respectively, compared to the control group at 5.3 kg (Fukuyasu and Oshida, 1988). In addition, diarrhea problems were reduced. It is important to note that for similar experiments in well-controlled environments, such as those found in research facilities, the difference between test and control groups was reduced (see also Chapter 10). The use of 0.3% FOS in piglets feed resulted in an increased weight gain of 13% in field trials and only 4% in well-controlled conditions (Nakamura, 1988).

In Europe, the best results have been obtained with FOS with piglets and rabbits. In a trial with 1,500 rabbits, for example, average weight gain was increased of 6.4%, the consumption index decreased by 7.8%, and mortality rate decreased by 32% (Bastien, 1990).

Table 1 presents the results obtained in 1992 in field trials with calves when using 0.15% α-1,2-linked GOS in the feed. This field trial was organized by I.N.R.A. (Rennes, France) in collaboration with SOFIVO (Condé/Vire, France) and BioEurope. It can be seen that a very substantial effect is observed on the health of the calves. Veterinary costs, taken as an objective criterion, were reduced by 20% for the animals fed with GOS in comparison with the control group.

The effect of FOS feeding to broiler chickens on the susceptibility to *Salmonella* colonization of the intestine has been investigated (Bailey *et al.*, 1991). When FOS was fed at 0.375% of diet, little effect was observed. However, at 0.75% inclusion, 12% fewer FOS-fed birds were colonized with *Salmonella* compared with control birds. FOS (0.75%) given to chicks in combination with competitive exclusion culture (prepared from aseptically removed caeca

Table 1. Effect of feed supplemented with α-glucooligosaccharides (GOS) on the breeding of calves in Britanny, France.

	Control group (supplemented with placebo)	Trial group (supplemented with 0.15% GOS)
Starting number of calves	1345	1312
% Females	14.9	5.7
Average starting weight (kg)	49.2 ± 2.7	47.7 ± 2.8
Mortality rate (%)	1.04	1.37
Final number of calves	1331	1294
Average carcass weight (kg)	120.6 ± 11.1	121.7 ± 11.1
Average final live weight (kg)	204.4 ± 18.8	206.3 ± 18.8
Fattening period (days)	134.1 ± 2.8	134.8 ± 2.2
Average daily gain (g day^{-1})	1157	1177
Average consumption per animal (kg)	257.9 ± 9.0	263.1 ± 11.3
Consumption index	1.67	1.65
Veterinary costs per animal (FF)	74.4 ± 12.8	59.4 ± 14.4

sample from a *Salmonella*-free chicken) appeared more effective. Only four of 21 chickens (19%) challenged with 10^9 *Salmonella* sp. on day seven became colonized compared with 14 of 23 chickens (61%) given the competitive exclusion culture alone. When chickens were stressed by feed and water deprivation on day 13, and challenged with 10^9 *Salmonella* on day 14, 33 of 36 chickens (92%) fed a control diet were colonized, compared with only 9 of 36 chickens (25 %) fed a 0.75 % FOS diet. Moreover, chickens treated with FOS had a four-fold reduction in the level of *Salmonella* present in the caecum.

α-Galactooligosaccharides at a dietary level of 0.1% failed to protect weaned rabbits against an experimental challenge with *E. coli* (Maertens and Peeters, 1992), although mortality was reduced and some reduction in diarrhea score was observed.In the case of ruminants, no significant effect on body weight, milk yield or milk composition was observed when feeding dairy cows with FOS (Kobayashi and Eida, 1990). This lack of effect was attributed to the rapid hydrolysis of FOS by rumen microorganisms.

MECHANISM OF ACTION OF OLIGOSACCHARIDES

As indicated previously, a common feature of feed oligosaccharides is that they are partially or totally resistant to attack by host digestive enzymes. For this reason, they are not absorbed or metabolised in the upper digestive tract and thus are able to reach the colon, where they can interact with the microbial flora and with the intestinal membrane cells.

Glucooligosaccharides linked α-1,2, for example, were highly resistant to attack by rat jejunum enzymes during a 24 h incubation (Quirasco *et al.*, 1994). When germ-free rats were fed glucooligosaccharides (2% and 4% of diets) composed of a mixture of di- to heptasaccharides, the extent of digestion was only about 20% and the major component, (pentasaccharide) was fully resistant to the action of the endogenous enzymes (Valette *et al.*, 1993). In the case of ^{14}C-labelled FOS no $^{14}CO_2$ was released in the first 8 h by germ-free rats, while more than 50% of the FOS was expired as CO_2 under similar conditions by their conventional counterparts (Tokunaga *et al.*, 1989).

Cereal fructans are very slowly hydrolyzed by human gastric juice and by homogenates of the intestinal rat mucosa and no, or a very limited, disappearance was observed in the small intestine of rats (Nilsson *et al.*, 1988). In the case of inulin, the extent of digestion and absorption, determined using male Wistar rats in which the intestinal microflora was suppressed by an antibiotic (Nebacitin) appeared to be 18 to 26% (Nilsson and Björck, 1988). Isomaltooligosaccharides are only partly hydrolysed by the enzymes of the intestinal mucosa, and can reach the lower intestine (Kaneko *et al.*, 1992).

Specific carbon sources

Several oligosaccharides are used specifically as substrates by potentially beneficial intestinal bacteria, particularly bifidobacteria, but not by pathogenic or potentially detrimental microorganisms. This property introduces the concept of specific substrate feeding; instead of feeding humans or animals with live microorganisms it could be wiser to promote the growth of beneficial bacteria already present in the digestive system. This avoids any problems associated with the introduction of microorganisms to the gut whose properties may not be fully understood. Even if less specific, the effect of feed oligosaccharides is very close to the effect of bifidogenic factors such as N-acetylglucosamine and lactulose, which are found in human milk and processed milk-products and are specific growth factors for bifidobacteria (Modler *et al.*, 1990). This property has been well characterized in the case of fructooligosaccharides, particularly from the point of view of their interaction with bifidobacteria (Hidaka *et al.*, 1986; Hidaka *et al.*, 1990; Modler *et al.*, 1990; Hidaka and Hirayama, 1991). The addition of FOS to the human diet has been shown to increase the size of the bifidobacteria populations in the large bowel (Modler *et al.*, 1990).

Glucooligosaccharides (GOS) are metabolized by bifidobacteria, lactobacilli and *Bacteroides* spp. (Kohmoto *et al.*, 1991), while they are poorly used as substrate by clostridia, eubacteria, enterobacteria and coliforms (Table 2). Oligosaccharides are fermented mainly by the intestinal flora to short-chain fatty acids which are, in turn, at least partly absorbed and metabolised (Modler *et al.*, 1990; Hidaka and Hirayama, 1991). GOS are completely fermented by the intestinal flora, and, in heteroxenic rats inoculated with a complex human flora, the short-chain fatty acids profile in the caecum is changed, with a decrease in butyric, isobutyric and isovaleric acid proportions ($p < 0.01$) and an increase in the proportion of caproic acid ($p < 0.05$) (Valette *et al.* 1993). The consequence of the modifications in short-chain fatty acids profile is not clearly understood.

Inclusion of FOS in the diet also alters microbial metabolism in the gut in other ways. For example, when feeding rats a diet containing tyrosine and tryptophan, their "putrefactive" degradation products (phenol, *p*-cresol and indole) were absent in the faeces and urine of FOS-fed animals but present in control animals (Hidaka *et al.*, 1986).

Table 2. *In vitro* assimilation of α-1,2 glucooligosaccharides (GOS) by intestinal bacteria.

Carbon source	Glucose (control)	GOS
Bifidobacterium adolescentis	+++	++
Bifidobacterium animalis	+	+++
Bifidobacterium breve	+++	+++
Bifidobacterium longum	+++	+++
Lactobacillus acidophilus	++	++
Lactobacillus casei	+++	++
Lactobacillus fermentum	++	-
Lactobacillus gasseri	++	±
Bacteroides bivius	++	+
Bacteroides fragilis	+	+
Bacteroides intermedius	++	++
Bacteroides ovatus	+	+
Bacteroides thetaiotaomicron	+	+
Bacteroides uniformis	+	+
Clostridium butyricum	++	+
Clostridium cadaveris	+	-
Clostridium clostridioforme	+	-
Clostridium difficile	±	-
Clostridium innocuum	++	-
Clostridium paraputrificum	++	-
Clostridium perfringens	+	-
Clostridium ramosum	+++	-
Eubacterium aerofaciens	++	-
Eubacterium limosum	++	-
Eubacterium nitritogenes	+	-
Fusobacterium mortiferum	±	-
Fusobacterium necrophorum	±	-
Fusobacterium varium	±	-
Megamonas hypermegas	++	-
Mitsuokella multiacidus	+++	-
Enterobacter aerogenes	+	-
Enterobacter cloacae	+	-
Escherichia coli	+	-
Klebsiella pneumoniae	+	-
Enterococcus faecalis	+++	±
Enterococcus faecium	+++	-

Oligosaccharides may also act as inducers of enzyme production by the intestinal bacterial flora, particularly of glycolytic enzymes, thus resulting in an increased hydrolysis of insoluble carbohydrate polymers (fibres). This aspect has not been documented but could explain, to some extent, the important increase in weight gain of animals, which clearly cannot be attributed directly to the low amount of added oligosaccharides. The use of oligosaccharides as specific substrates by beneficial bacteria of the intestine explains their increase in number, which results in a more effective colonization of the intestinal system, thus preventing the establishment of pathogens or potential pathogens such as *Salmonella* spp.

Specific biological interactions

Protein-carbohydrate interactions are involved in most of the specific biological recognition processes (Sharon and Lis, 1993). For this reason, oligosaccharides are able to interact with protein receptors found on the surface of microbial cells and intestine brush border cells.

Pathogenicity of microorganisms involves, as an initial step, the attachment of the microbial cell to mucosal surfaces. This mechanism is based on the specific interaction between surface proteins (adhesins or lectins) of bacteria and carbohydrate moieties from glycolipids or glycoproteins of the mucosal surface (Morgan *et al.*, 1992; Chesson, 1993). α-D-mannose units of the gut surface, for example, are specifically recognized by *E. coli* fimbrial lectins, which allows cell adhesion and pathogenicity in the case of enterotoxigenic *E. coli* (Ofek and Sharon, 1990). Oligosaccharides are able to interfere with this recognition process provided they can interact specifically with microbial cell fimbrial lectins, and thus prevent cell adhesion and pathogenicity. It has been shown, for example, that the complex oligosaccharides of human milk are able, in addition to providing a bifidogenic factor, to inhibit adhesion of various bacterial pathogens to epithelial cells (Andersson *et al.*, 1986; Aniansson *et al.*, 1990).

Another possibility is the specific interaction of oligosaccharides with protein receptors present at the surface of immunocompetent cells of the intestinal brush border. The important immunomodulatory role of the intestinal membrane has been little studied (Chesson, 1993) and remains to be understood completely. It has been shown, for example, that a cell-free filtrate of *Lactobacillus acidophilus* culture fed to weaned piglets caused a small, but significant increase in the concentration of serum IgG (Lessard and Brisson, 1987). But nothing has appeared in the scientific literature on secretory IgA production in the digestive system in relation to oligosaccharide consumption.

Oral administration of a number of lactic acid bacteria results in a systemic augmentation of the immune response (Chesson, 1993). This necessarily involves a signal system, which may be located at the level of the memory cells of the lamina propia and Peyer's patches. Oligosaccharides may also interfere with this system and activate the immune response. This could explain the very significant effect of limited amounts of orally-fed oligosaccharides. It is also probable that some oligosaccharide molecules are able to cross the intestinal barrier and thus stimulate the blood immune system.

An additional aspect which has not been studied in connection with animal health is the influence of oligosaccharides on bacterial translocation. It is known that the gut may lose its barrier function under certain circumstances and serve as a reservoir for systemic microbial infections. This translocation phenomenon, related to the intestinal microecology (Wells, 1990), is dependent on the bacterial species involved (Wells *et al.*, 1991) and is promoted both by bacterial endotoxins (Deitch *et al.*, 1989) and antibiotics (George *et al.*, 1990). Bacterial translocation from the gut is a very important phenomenon to consider, as it has been proven to impair systemic immunity in mice (Deitch *et al.*, 1991). A fibre-free diet has been shown to promote bacterial translocation from the gut (Spaeth *et al.*, 1990). It is possible to speculate that oligosaccharides, acting as soluble fibre, may decrease bacterial translocation and thus promote the preservation of systemic immunity.

CONCLUSIONS

A wide variety of oligosaccharides (fructo-, gluco-, and galacto-oligosaccharides) is commercially available as feed additives. When added in limited amounts to animal feeds, they can result in a significant improvement in weight gain, efficiency of feed conversion and health status of the animal.

These oligosaccharides present several key advantages

- most are natural products, made of very simple sugars, without any antigenic capacity
- they do not present side effects or accumulate in animal tissues
- they are resistant to high temperatures and to the acidic pH of stomach, which avoids formulation and application problems
- they have no viability constraints like microorganisms (probiotics)
- their production cost is low and compatible with dose effect in animal feed
- they can promote directly the growth of beneficial bacteria already present in the intestine.

Unfortunately, the mechanism of action of these oligosaccharides is not fully understood and cannot be considered as resulting only from metabolism by the intestinal flora. The involvement of oligosaccharides in specific biological interactions occurring in the digestive tract needs to be more thoroughly studied. To date, the use of oligosaccharides has been limited by to the difficulty in obtaining clearly reproducible results. Efficacy appears greater in field trials than in trials under well-controlled conditions. This means that when it is not easy to demonstrate the effect of oligosaccharides when feeding animals in a hygienic environment with optimal feed, economic results still may be obtained under field conditions.

A further difficulty, at least in Europe, is the lack of regulatory status for oligosaccharides. While antibiotics and probiotics are clearly recognised by regulatory bodies, there is not a clear definition for this type of product. Maybe the recently introduced concept of Ecological Health Control Products (EHCP) will help in that direction.

In the future, elucidation of the mechanism(s) of action of oligosaccharides will allow more accurate structure/function relationships to be established leading to the design of specific carbohydrate structures with improved efficacy.

REFERENCES

Ajisaka, K., Nishida, H. and Fujimoto, H. 1987. The synthesis of oligosaccharides by reversed hydrolysis reaction of β-glucosidase at high substrate concentration and at high temperature. *Biotechnol. Lett.* **9**, 243-248.

Amarakone, S.P., Ishigami, H. and Kainuma, K. 1984. Conversion of oligosaccharides formed during starch hydrolysis by a dual enzyme system. *Denpun Kagaku* **31**, 1-7.

Andersson, B., Porras, O., Hanson, L.Å., Lagergård, T. and Svanborg-Edén, C. 1986. Inhibition of attachment of *Streptococcus-pneumoniae* and *Haemophilus-influenzae* by human milk and receptor oligosaccharides. *J. Infect. Dis.* **153**, 232-237.

Aniansson, G., Andersson, B., Lindstedt, R. and Svanbrog, C. 1990. Anti-adhesive activity of human casein against *Streptococcus-pneumoniae* and *Haemophilus-influenzae*. *Microb. Pathog.* **8**, 315-324.

Bailey, J.S., Blackenship, L.C. and Cox, N.A. 1991. Effect of fructooligosaccharide on *Salmonella* colonization of the chicken intestine. *Poultry Sci.* **70**, 2433-2438.

Bastien, R. 1990. Nouveaux régulateurs de flore. *Rech. Alim. Anim.* **434**, 56-57.

Chesson, A. 1993. Probiotics and other intestinal mediators. In *Principles of Pig Science* (D.J.A. Cole, J. Wiseman, and M.A. Varley, eds) pp. 197-214. Nottingham University Press, Loughborough, UK.

Deitch, E.A., Ma, L., Ma, W.J., Grisham, M.B., Granger, D.N., Specian, R.D. and Berg, R.D. 1989. Inhibition of endotoxin-induced bacterial translocation in mice. *J. Clin. Invest.* **84**, 36-42.

Deitch, E.A., Xu, D., Qi, L. and Berg, R.D. 1991. Bacterial translocation from the gut impairs systemic immunity. *Surgery* **109**, 269-276.

Fishbein, L., Kaplan, M. and Cough, M. 1988. Fructooligosaccharides: a review. *Vet. Hum. Toxicol.* **30**, 104-107.

Fujii, S. and Komoto, M. 1991. Novel carbohydrate sweetners in Japan. *Zuckerindustrie* **116**, 197-200.

Fukuyasu, T. and Oshida, T. 1988. Use of Neosugar® in piglets. In *Proceedings of the 3rd Neosugar® Conference*, p. 1, Tokyo, Japan, 1986.

George, S.E., Kohan, M.J., Whitehouse, D.A., Creason, J.P. and Claxton, L.D. 1990. Influence of antibiotics on intestinal tract survival and translocation of environmental *Pseudomonas* species. *Appl. Environ. Microbiol.* **56**, 1559-1564.

Heinz, F. and Vogel, M. 1991. Process for preparing a low glucose, fructose and saccharose inulooligosaccharide product. European Patent 0440074 A1.

Hidaka, H. and Hirayama, M. 1991. Useful characteristics and commercial applications of fructo-oligosaccharides. *Biochem. Soc. Trans.* **19**, 561-565.

Hidaka, H., Eida, T., Takizawa, T., Tokunaga, T. and Tashiro, Y. 1986. Effects of fructooligosaccharides on intestinal flora and human health. *Bifidobacteria Microflora* **5**, 37-50.

Hidaka, H., Hirayama, M. and Sumi, N. 1988. A fructooligosaccharide-producing enzyme from *Aspergillus niger* ATCC 20611. *Agric. Biol. Chem.* **52**, 1181-1187.

Hidaka, H., Hirayama, M., Tokunaga, T. and Eida, T. 1990. The effects of undigestible fructooligosaccharides on intestinal microflora and various physiological functions on human health. In *New Developments in Dietary Fiber* (I. Furda, and C.J. Brine, eds) pp. 105-117. Plenum Press, New York, US.

Imaizumi, K., Nakatsu, Y., Sato, M., Sedarnawati, Y. and Sugano, M. 1991. Effects of xylooligosaccharides on blood glucose, serum and liver lipids and caecum short-chain fatty acids in diabetic rats. *Agric. Biol. Chem.* **55**, 199-205.

Jeanes, A.R., Haynes, W.C., Wilham, C.A., Rankin, J.C., Melvin, E.H., Austin, M.J., Cluskey, J.E., Fisher, B.E., Tsuchiya, H.M. and Rist, C.E. 1954. Characterization and classification of dextrans from ninety-six strains of bacteria. *J. Amer. Chem. Soc.* **76**, 5041-5052.

Kaneko, T., Kohmoto, T. Kikuchi, H., Fukui, F., Shiota, M., Yatake, T., Takaky, H. and Ino, H. 1992. *Nippon Nogeikagaku Kaishi* **66**, 1211-1220.

Kobayashi, S. and Eida, T. 1990. Effects of fructo-oligosaccharides on milk-yield and milk-components of dairy cows. *J. Anim. Sci.* **3**, 21-25.

Koepsell, H.J., Tsuchiya, H.M., Hellman, N.N., Kazenko, A., Hoffman, C.A., Sharpe, E.S. and Jackson, R.W. 1953. Enzymatic synthesis of dextran. *J. Biol. Chem.* **200**, 793-801.

Kohmoto, T., Fukui, F., Takaku, A. and Mitsuoka, T. 1991. Dose-response test of isomaltooligosaccharides for increasing faecal bifidobacteria. *Agric. Biol. Chem.* **55**, 2157-2159.

Kormelink, F.J.M., Gruppen, H., Wood, T.M. and Beldman, G. 1992. Mode of action of the xylan-degrading enzymes from *Aspergillus awamori*. In *Xylans and Xylanases* (J. Visser, G. Beldman, M.A. Kusters-Van Someren and A.G.J. Voragen, eds) pp. 141-147. Elsevier, London, UK.

Kuriki, T., Yanase, M., Takata, H., Takesada, Y., Imanaka, T. and Okada, S. 1993. A new way of producing isomalto-oligosaccharide syrup by using the transglycosylation reaction of neopullulanase. *Appl. Environ. Microbiol.* **59**, 953-959.

Lessard, M. and Brisson, G.J. 1987. Effect of a *Lactobacillus* fermentation product on growth, immune response and fecal enzyme activity in weaned pigs. *Can. J. Anim. Sci.* **67**, 509-516.

Maertens, L. and Peeters, J.E. 1992. Influence of galactooligosaccharides on performances, hindgut fermentation and experimantal colibacillosis in weanling rabbits. *Med. Fac. Landbouww. Univ. Gent.* **57**, 1935-1943.

Minami, Y., Yazawa, K., Tamura, Z., Tanaka, T. and Yamamoto, T. 1983. Selectivity of utilization of galactosyl oligosaccharides by bifidobacteria. *Chem. Pharm. Bull.* **31**, 1688-1691.

Modler, H.W., McKellar, R.C. and Yaguchi, M. 1990. Bifidobacteria and bifidogenic factors. *Can. Inst. Food Sci. Technol. J.* **23**, 29-41.

Morgan, A.J., Mul, A.J., Beldman, G. and Voragen, A.G.J. 1992. Dietary oligosaccharides. New insights. *Agro Food Ind. Hi-tech.* **11/12**, 35-38.

Mozaffar, S., Nakanishi, K., Matsuno, R. and Kanukubo, T. 1984. Purification and properties of β-galactosidases from *Bacillus circulans*. *Agric. Biol. Chem.* **48**, 3053-3061.

Nakamura, K. 1988. Application of Neosugar® to piglets and sows. In *Proceedings of the 3rd Neosugar® Conference*, p. 71, Tokyo, Japan, 1986.

Nilsson, U. and Björck, I. 1988. Availability of cereal fructans and inulin in the rat intestinal tract. *J. Nutr.* **118**, 1482-1485.

Nilsson, U., Öste, R., Jägerstad, M. and Birkhed, D. 1988. Cereal fructans: *in vitro* and *in vivo* studies on availability in rats and humans. *J. Nutr.* **118**, 1325-1330.

Ofek, I. and Sharon, N. 1990. Adhesions as lectins specificity and role in infection. (K. Jann and B. Jann, eds) *Curr. Top. Microbiol. Immunol.* **151**, 91-114.

Paul, F., Lopez-Munguia, A., Remaud, M., Pelenc, V. and Monsan, P. 1992. Method for the production of α-1,2 oligodextrans using *Leuconostoc mesenteroides* B-1299. US Patent 5,141,858.

Paul, F., Oriol, E., Auriol, D. and Monsan, P. 1986. Acceptor reaction of a highly purified dextransucrase with maltose and oligosaccharides. Application to the synthesis of controlled-molecular weight dextrans. *Carbohydr. Res.* **149**, 433-441.

Prakash, S., Suyama, K., Itoh, T. and Adachi, S. 1987. Oligosaccharide formation by *Trichoderma harzianum* in lactose-containing medium. *Biotechnol. Lett.* **9**, 249-252.

Quirasco, M., Lopez-Munguia, A., Pelenc, V., Remaud, M., Paul, F. and Monsan, P. 1994. Enzymatic production of rare glucooligosaccharides containing α-1,2 glycosidic bonds. Potential applications in human and animal nutrition. *Ann. NY Acad. Sci.*, (*in press*).

Remaud-Simeon, M., Lopez-Munguia, A., Pelenc, V., Paul, F. and Monsan, P. 1994. Production and use of glucosyltransferases from *Leuconostoc mesenteroides* NRRL B-1299 for the synthesis of oligosaccharides containing α-1,2 linkages. *Appl. Biochem. Biotechnol.* **44**, 101-117.

Robyt, J.F. and Ecklund, S.H. 1983. Relative, quantitative effect of acceptors in the reaction of *Leuconostoc mesenteroides* dextransucrase. *Carbohydr. Res.* **121**, 279-286.

Roper, H. von and Koch, H. 1988. New carbohydrate-derivatives for biotechnical and chemical processes. *Starch* **40**, 453-459.

Sharon, N. and Lis, H. 1993. Carbohydrates in cell recognition. *Scient. Amer.* **1**, 74-81.

Shiomi, N. 1978. Isolation and identification of 1-kestose and neokestose from onion bulbs. *J. Fac. Agric. Hokkaido Univ.* **58**, 548-556.

Shiomi, N., Yamada, J. and Izawa, M. 1976. Isolation and identification of fructo-oligosaccharides in roots and asparagus. *Agr. Biol. Chem.* **40**, 567-575.

Spaeth, G., Berg, R.D., Specian, R.D. and Deitch, E.A. 1990. Food without fiber promotes bacterial translocation from the gut. *Surgery* **108**, 240-247.

Tokunaga, T., Oku, T. and Hosoya, N. 1989. Utilization and excretion of a new sweetener, fructooligosaccharide (Neosugar®) in rats. *J. Nutr.* **119**, 553-559.

Valette, P., Pelenc, V., Djouzi, Z., Andrieux, C., Paul, F., Monsan, P. and Szylit, O. 1993. Bioavailability of new synthesized glucooligosaccharides in the intestinal tract of gnotobiotic rats. *J. Sci. Food Agric.* **62**, 121-127.

Wells, C.L. 1990. Relationship between intestinal microecology and the translocation of intestinal bacteria. *Ant. van Leeuw.* **58**, 87-93.

Wells, C.L., Jechorek, R.P., Gillingham, K.J. 1991. Relative contributions of host and microbial factors in bacterial translocation. *Arch. Surg.* **126**, 247-252.

Yoneyama, M., Shibuya, T. and Miyake, T. 1992. Saccharides sous forme de poudre, préparation et utilisations. French Patent 2,677,359.

12 Microbial feed additives for pre-ruminants

Kyle E. Newman and Kate A. Jacques

Alltech Biotechnology Center, 3031 Catnip Hill Pike, Nicholasville, Kentucky 40356, US

INTRODUCTION

Using live microorganisms to supplement feeds for neonatal livestock is a practice that stems from investigations in humans. Metchnikoff discovered a "Bulgarian Bacillus" which was thought to be responsible for the advanced age observed in Rumanian and Bulgarian farmers (Metchnikoff, 1908). The author felt that the inclusion of milk cultured with *Lactobacillus acidophilus* and *L. delbreukii* subsp. *bulgaricus* counteracted the production of toxins which he felt led to arteriosclerosis and senility. In animals, Belonowsky (1907) infused sterile grain with *L. delbreukii* subsp. *bulgaricus* and noted a decrease in putrefaction and virulence of the feces. In 1956, Edmund Raffle noted that when antibiotics were given orally to infants with gastroenteritis the normal gut microflora was disrupted. This alteration could cause an increase in opportunistic pathogens leading to a secondary infection. However, feeding yogurt containing live cultures of lactic acid bacteria led to clinical improvement and more rapid weight gain compared to infants not receiving yogurt (Raffle, 1956).

The primary microorganisms currently used in animal feeding include bacteria such as *Lactobacillus, Enterococcus, Streptococcus, Bifidobacterium, Bacillus* spp. and the yeast, *Saccharomyces cerevisiae*. Uses of microbial supplements (microbials) in young ruminants differ somewhat depending on whether they are directed toward the neonate before or after the point in development when solid feed is consumed consistently. Applications of microbial preparations for newborn animals include dosing or drenching the animal soon after birth and inclusion of direct-fed microbial products (DFM) in either milk or milk replacer. The goals of microbial supplementation of the neonatal ruminant are similar to those for non-ruminants - rapid adaptation to solid feed by accelerating the development of a normal adult intestinal microflora and avoiding the establishment of enteropathogens. Various preparations of lactic acid-producing bacteria are available commercially and these have been used by both producers and researchers. Promoting the rapid establishment of a functional rumen microbial population prior to weaning is a second goal of microbial supplementation. In this application, viable yeast culture products added to starter feeds are in commercial use, stemming from knowledge that yeast stimulated certain rumen microorganisms in adult ruminants. Inoculants of rumen microbes given in drench form to pre-ruminants have also been of interest.

Research into manipulation of the gut microflora has followed several directions in recent years. It has involved both basic studies of gut microbial ecology and work centered on the effects of commercially available microbial preparations. The research has been driven by the growing emphasis on disease prevention as a means of reducing the use of antibiotics and also public concern about enteropathogens as a food safety issue. This chapter will focus on applications for microbial additives in the neonate through weaning, responses to the additives and their mode of action, and future development.

APPLICATIONS FOR MICROBIALS IN THE NEONATAL RUMINANT

Lactic acid-producing bacteria

Lactic acid-producing bacteria are administered to calves by drenching soon after birth and/or in milk or milk replacer. The primary goal of inoculating neonates with lactic acid bacteria is to establish a beneficial population of bacteria in the GI tract capable of competing successfully with pathogens. The known progression of intestinal microbial development and the role that lactobacilli play in the normal population explain the reasoning behind supplementing with lactobacilli.

Gut microbial ecology in the neonate

Ruminants, like all mammals, are born devoid of indigenous microorganisms. During transport through the vagina some bacteria are acquired by the neonate. This route may provide the initial inoculation of the newborn gastrointestinal tract, since predominant bacteria in the vagina include lactic acid bacteria such as enterococci, streptococci and lactobacilli. After passage through the birth canal, the neonate may become contaminated and subsequently inoculated by fecal organisms such as *Escherichia coli*. These events may help to explain the initial microflora of the neonate described by Smith (1965). In his work, *E. coli, Clostridium welchii* (now called *C. perfringens*) and streptococci are described as the first organisms to be found in the neonate followed closely by lactobacilli. Lactobacilli are slower to grow than the other organisms mentioned. Because of this, it is not surprising that the development of a noticeable *Lactobacillus* population is slow and detection of these organisms corresponds to a drop in stomach pH.

One threat to neonatal ruminant health stems from the fact that the gastrointestinal tract pH is near neutrality. Since the microbial population is in transition and extremely sensitive during this time, a monoculture can establish. If that organism is pathogenic, it can cause disease. There have been no trials that actually prove a decreased time-frame involved in the development of the gut microflora when of the neonate is supplemented with lactic acid bacteria. However, there are several studies which describe lactobacilli as a primary indicator of dietary stress. When the animal is stressed, the *Lactobacillus* population decreases (reviewed by Tannock, 1983). There is also evidence of more rapid rumen development with the addition of certain DFM.

Effects of direct fed microbials on gut ecology

Though the importance of the lactic acid bacteria in gastrointestinal ecology is accepted, the role of these bacteria is not fully understood. Other DFM may not be as universally recognized as important to the intestinal ecosystem, but there is evidence to support their use. A number of studies have demonstrated that these organisms are beneficial to the newborn by a variety of mechanisms. These mechanisms, summarized in Table 1, will be discussed in detail.

Production of lactic acid. Acetic and lactic acid are two of the most commonly used chemical preservatives. Foods such as yogurt, pickles, and sauerkraut enjoy a long shelf life

Table 1. Proposed mechanisms by which microbial additives exert beneficial responses in the neonate.

Mechanism	Effect
Lactic acid production	Detrimental to the growth of most enteric pathogens
Gut colonization	Exclusion of pathogens from binding to the gut epithelium
Inhibitory metabolites	Direct bacteriocidal activity on specific organisms
Non-specific immune response	Antigenic components of the microbial cell stimulate the immune system
Adsorption of bacteria	Adsorption of bacteria to a yeast derivative prevents colonization

because of the inhibitory activity of these acids. The antimicrobial activity of these organic acids is due to their depression of gut pH below the growth range of many bacteria and also by metabolic inhibition by the undissociated form of the acid. Inhibition of microorganisms by low pH is due to destruction of enzymes and enzyme functions in the cell and/or interference with intracellular transport. In the presence of acid, most microorganisms must either prevent H^+ ions from entering the cell or have a mechanism to export the H^+ ions as rapidly as they enter. When the H^+ ion concentration is too great for the cell to overcome then cell death occurs. Lactic acid bacteria are more resistant to lower pH than other bacteria and can thus withstand higher concentrations of lactic acid.

Production of inhibitory metabolites. Lactic acid production is only one of the mechanisms that inhibit growth of other microorganisms. In addition to organic acids, lactic acid bacteria produce a variety of secondary metabolites (hydrogen peroxide, diacetyl, ammonia and fatty acids) and antimicrobial proteins (bacteriocins). These cell products, along with maintenance of a low pH, are inhibitory to pathogens. The ability of certain lactic acid bacteria isolated from commercial products to inhibit the growth of enteric pathogens has been demonstrated *in vitro* (Newman *et al.*, 1990). In this study, pH and/or hydrogen peroxide-associated inhibition of *E. coli, Salmonella typhimurium, C. perfringens, Staphylococcus aureus,* and *Listeria monocytogenes* was noted with certain strains of *Lactobacillus*. In addition, a strain of *Enterococcus faecium* in a commercial microbial feed additive was found to produce an extracellular metabolite which inhibited *L. monocytogenes, Streptococcus agalactiae* and a number of taxonomically-related organisms (Table 2).

The effects that metabolites produced by lactic acid bacteria have on enteric pathogens have also been investigated. Mitchell and Kenworthy (1976) discovered a cell-free preparation from *L. delbreukii* subsp. *bulgaricus* that neutralized the enterotoxin from *E. coli*. Preparations containing either *L. delbreukii* or a cell-free extract indicated beneficial responses in piglets. In calves, a commercial *L. bulgaricus* fermentation product was found to improve weight gain and feed consumption while not affecting fecal lactobacilli or coliforms (Schwab *et al.*, 1980).

Table 2. Antagonistic activity of *Enterococcus faecium* strain AT1, and high molecular weight (HMW) (>10,000 Da) and low molecular weight (LMW) (<10,000 Da) cell-free extracts of *E. faecium* against indicator bacteria.

Indicator organism	Inhibitory zone width[a]		
	Viable *E. faecium*	LMW fraction	HMW fraction
Enterococcus faecium 19434[b]	10.5	0	10
Enterococcus faecalis 8043	10.5	0	9
Clostridium perfringens 3624	8	0	0
Escherichia coli 15R NAL	8	0	0
Lactobacillus acidophilus 4356	10	0	8
Lactobacillus bulgaricus 9224	0	0	0
Lactobacillus fermentum 14933	0	0	0
Listeria monocytogenes 7644	16	0	12
Pediococcus cerevisiae 8081	11.5	0	6
Sarcina lutea 383	13.5	0	0
Staphylococcus aureus 12600	8	0	0
Streptococcus agalactiae 624	0	0	9
Streptococcus agalactiae 13813	0	0	9
Streptococcus bovis 9809	0	0	0

[a] Values represent the mean diameter of the zone of inhibition (mm) using a direct antagonism test. The size of the colony of *E. faecium* was 6.5 mm.
[b] Numbers represent ATCC identification except in the case of *E. coli* which is a nalidixic acid-resistant strain.
Adapted from Newman (1990).

Colonization of the intestinal epithelium and competitive exclusion. The ability of lactic acid bacteria to compete successfully with pathogens for nutrients and colonization sites on the intestinal epithelium is often proposed to be a mechanism by which intestinal inoculants benefit animal health; however, inhibition of pathogens by lactic acid bacteria *in vivo* is difficult to detect. A number of investigators have noted decreases in certain bacterial populations associated with lactic acid bacteria supplementation. In baby pigs, alterations in fecal and intestinal coliforms were associated with a live microbial feed supplement (Table 3; Newman, 1990).

Several studies have examined the ability of microorganisms to colonize the GI tract (Savage and Dubos, 1967; Savage *et al.*, 1968; Davis and Savage, 1972). The ability of lactobacilli to colonize the GI tract appears to be linked to a certain extent to the host species (Morishita *et al.*, 1971; Savage, 1972; Fuller and Brooker, 1974). In chickens, it was shown that only *Lactobacillus* strains of avian origin were able to colonize crop epithelial cells (Fuller and Brooker, 1974). Later studies identified acidic mucopolysaccharides that aid in adhesion in

Table 3. Effects of a direct fed microbial (DFM) containing lactic acid bacteria on selected bacterial groups in the intestinal tract of growing pigs.

Bacterial Group	Control	DFM
Coliforms (log CFU g^{-1})	4.18	3.76[a]
Lactobacilli (log CFU g^{-1})	7.85	7.93
Ratio[b]	1.91	2.33[a]

[a] Significant difference (P<0.05).
[b] Ratio of the log of lactobacilli concentration and log of coliform concentration.
From Newman (1990).

the chicken crop (Brooker and Fuller, 1975). In the human gut, adhesion of lactobacilli appears to be mediated by an extracellular proteinaceous compound produced by the adhering bacteria, which provides a bridge that links the bacterium to the intestinal cell (Coconnier *et al.*, 1992). The ability to adhere to the intestinal wall certainly plays a role in intestinal colonization. At the present time, efforts to determine the genetic and physiological mechanisms involved in adhesion are under investigation. Knowledge of these mechanisms will certainly be useful in the future for development of microbial additives for neonates.

It should be noted that the extent to which microbial additives in commercial use today colonize the gut epithelium is virtually unknown; nor is it known for certain whether colonization is required for beneficial effect. In most instances the same lactic acid bacteria are indicated for use across species. This would likely preclude colonization in all but the species of origin if species specificity is a prerequisite to attachment. Little information about the source of a bacterial strain is provided with products, nor are details of strain or origin frequently included in research reports. Improvement in health and/or performance in cross-species applications suggests that something other than colonization/competitive exclusion - possibly transient acid or metabolite production - is important.

Non-specific immune response. It has been suggested that certain organisms can elicit an immune response in the host. Cellular components of inactivated microorganisms have been used for many years as vaccines (e.g. capsular material from *Haemophilus influenzae* and inactivated *Bordetella pertussis* for the control of whooping cough). Stimulation of non-specific immunity may be responsible at least in part for benefits noted with the use of *Bacillus* species as feed additives. Inclusion of *Bacillus subtilis* containing products in milk replacer for Holstein calves had no significant effects on performance parameters (Jenny *et al.*, 1991) but immunity was not examined. Pollman *et al.* (1984) demonstrated an increase in the survival rate of baby pigs supplemented with *B. subtilis*. In poultry, a reduction in mortality and the incidence of pasted vents was noted with *Bacillus* spp. supplementation (Saylor *et al.*, 1993). In these examples, the response may be due to the *Bacillus* spore rather than the actual vegetative cell. Because *Bacillus* spp. sporulate, they are more resistant to environmental extremes such as those present during feed processing. As such, *Bacillus* spp. at first glance seem ideal as feed-borne microbials. However, sporulation is essentially a survival response to harsh conditions, and the GI tract is not likely to provide a hospitable environment for growth and activity of these organisms. *B. subtilis* is an aerobic organism which can grow anaerobically to a very limited extent in the presence of high glucose concentrations (Sneath, 1986). As glucose concentrations in the GI tract are limited, it would not therefore be likely that *B. subtilis* would germinate or grow to any extent in the animal. If in some cases viable cells are not necessary to elicit a response, the cellular components may be responsible for immune modulation.

Health and performance effects of microbials in neonates

The primary purpose of adding lactic bacteria to very young ruminants is to influence gut microecology in an attempt to avoid pathogenic colonization and disease. The anatomy of the digestive tract and the complexity of the microbial ecosystem make direct evaluation of this objective difficult. Several studies have reported decreased shedding of fecal coliforms in response to *Lactobacillus* supplements, however others have stated that fecal populations do not meaningfully reflect intestinal microbial change (Ellinger *et al.*, 1978; Gilliland *et al.*, 1980; Newman, 1990). Reductions in scouring by calves have been reported for both *Lactobacillus* and *Streptococcus (Enterococcus)* supplements (Bechman *et al.*, 1977; Fox, 1988; Maeng *et al.*, 1987). Many other studies reflect only broad performance parameters which may or may not indicate important responses during the first three weeks of life when enteric disease is most prevalent. Reduction in the incidence or severity of scouring problems, though difficult to measure for statistical analysis, may have a bigger impact on labor and production costs (i.e. treatment time and expense) than on liveweight gain. Experimental reports that include detailed information about both the microbial supplement and culture data from scouring experimental animals are needed to move forward in learning about the usefulness of microbial supplements in neonatal calves.

APPLICATIONS FOR MICROBIALS PRE-AND POST-WEANING

Stimulation of rumen development

Rapid adaptation to solid feed by baby calves, the central focus of replacement calf management, depends on the development of the rumen epithelium and rumen capacity. This is dependent on access to a fibrous diet and stimulation by volatile fatty acids (VFA), the production of which requires both bacteria and substrate (Van Soest, 1982). Natural inoculation of the developing rumen with the anaerobic bacterial species that eventually form the adult rumen population probably occurs both via the feed and inter-animal contact. During rumen development, easily degraded concentrates entering the rumen are metabolized by microbial fermentation to acids and ammonia. The consumption of roughage combined with an increase in saliva production cause a buffering effect in the rumen. The results of the saliva and forage are a gradual increase in pH and a decrease in ammonia (Godfrey, 1961). This phenomenon enhances cellulolytic bacteria and the development of the adult microflora, since the vast majority of microbes found in the adult animal prefer pH values near neutrality.

Because of the interactive role played by bacteria and substrates in rumen development, the potential impact of microbial supplements has been of interest. The primary microorganisms used in starter feeds (pre-weaning) are bacteria such as *Lactobacillus, Enterococcus, Bifidobacterium, Bacillus* spp. and the yeast *S. cerevisiae*. Microbial-derived supplements such as extracts from *Aspergillus oryzae* are also added to starter feeds.

Lactic acid bacteria. Lactic acid bacteria added to starter diets have been suggested to affect rumen function in the young animal. Holstein calves supplemented with yogurt containing *L. acidophilus* tended to ruminate more at 30 days than untreated calves indicating that the supplementation may promote rumination. There were no performance benefits associated with the treated calves in this trial and any possible microbial changes were not determined (Nakanishi *et al.*, 1993).

Viable yeast culture in starter formulas. A number of investigators have reported performance and intake responses to yeast culture in both calf and lamb starter diets; however no effects of the supplement on rumen metabolism were measured (Fallon and Harte, 1987; Hughes, 1988; Jordan and Johnston, 1990). Later experiments examining the effects of viable yeast culture on rumen fermentation helped to explain the performance response. Nisbet and Martin (1991) found that the addition of yeast culture stimulated growth of the lactate-utilizing rumen bacterium, *Selenomonas ruminantium*, *in vitro*, while Williams *et al.* (1991) reported an increased rumen pH in adult cattle associated with decreased concentrations of ruminal L(+)-lactate. Hyperacidity associated with high concentrate calf starter feeds inhibits voluntary intake in young calves. Experiments in which ruminal pH was monitored continuously in young calves have shown that pH fluctuates widely over a range from below 5.0 to 5.8 (Williams *et al.*, 1985; Anderson *et al.*, 1987). Quigley *et al.* (1992) suggested that positive responses in pre-ruminants to yeast culture might be related to increasing or stabilizing pH in a manner similar to that in the adult animal. This group found that the typical increases in L(+) and D(-) ruminal lactate concentrations at 4 h post-feeding were reduced by 42 and 25%, respectively, in Jersey calves given yeast culture at 0.2% of the diet; however, no effect on liveweight gain was noted.

Fermentation extracts. Extracts from fungi such as *A. oryzae* have been marketed for several years for diets fed to both neonatal and adult ruminants. The content of these products is poorly described, but it is assumed that the extracts, although they do not contain viable organisms, do contain a certain amount of enzyme activity and, to a lesser extent, vitamins. Responses to supplementation in one trial included earlier weaning and improved ruminal microbial activity compared to calves not receiving supplement (Beharka *et al.*, 1991).

Transition to high concentrate diets: rumen inoculants

Inoculation to alter or affect rumen populations has been of occasional interest in the literature for many years (Van Soest, 1982). Suggested applications have included hastening rumen development, re-supplying microbial populations following therapeutic antibiotic use, and hastening the transition to a diet rich in rapidly fermentable carbohydrates by dosing unadapted animals with populations adapted to high starch diets. The effectiveness of inoculation in altering rumen microbial populations has been demonstrated on a practical basis by researchers working with ruminally-cannulated animals and by veterinarians with convalescent animals. Ziolecka *et al.* (1984) found that a stabilized non-viable extract of rumen contents stimulated rumen development in calves approaching weaning. Unlike the *Lactobacillus, Bacillus, Streptococcus (Enterococcus)* and yeast species currently used in microbial supplements, the complex anaerobic population of the mature ruminant is not easily adapted to industrial fermentation. A stabilized product containing adult chicken microflora has been developed and is being used in the poultry industry; however, no product has been designed for the young calf.

NUTRITIONAL PROBIOSIS: SELECTING NUTRIENT SOURCES BASED ON GUT MICROBIAL ECOLOGY

Manipulating gut microbial ecology through nutrition is not new (e.g. acidification of milk replacer), however developments in this area over recent years, such as the use of selected sugars, may signal a change in how we think about neonatal diet formulation. The scope of this chapter precludes a thorough treatment of nutritional probiosis, but the objectives for their use are closely allied to those for microbial supplements and deserve mention in this context.

Acidification of milk replacer

It is well established that most microorganisms grow best at pH values near neutrality. Few organisms are able to initiate growth below pH 4.0, some exceptions to this being yeasts, molds and lactobacilli. Fortunately, pathogenic bacteria tend to be among the most fastidious of bacteria in terms of pH requirements for growth. Actual pH minima and maxima for microorganisms depend upon several external factors including the type of acid used. Both direct acidification and addition of lactic acid-producing bacteria have been employed in order to bring intestinal pH into a range unfavorable for coliform growth. Low molecular weight organic acids (e.g. formic, acetic, lactic and propionic acids) are more effective at higher pH than high molecular weight organic and inorganic acids (e.g. citric, hydrochloric acids). Although there is a growing number of pathogens which have demonstrated adaptation to acidic environments (Leyer and Johnson, 1992; Goodson and Rowbury, 1989), low molecular weight organic acids remain a feasible method of inhibiting the growth of numerous pathogens. Acid (not specified) added to calf milk replacer caused a decrease in fecal coliform concentration during the initial four weeks of treatment (Simm et al., 1980; Table 4).

Table 4. Fecal coliform concentrations in calves receiving a milk replacer with and without acidification.

		Fecal coliforms ($\log_{10}$ g^{-1})		
Age...	2 days	2 weeks	4 weeks	7 weeks
Acidified milk replacer	9.23	8.25	7.67	7.79
Control	9.12	9.01	8.88	7.44

Adapted from Simm et al. (1980).

Dietary carbohydrate sources

Research has shown that sugars and/or complex carbohydrates affect gut microbes differentially and may benefit animal health. Fructooligosaccharides have been found to stimulate the growth of beneficial bacteria such as *Bifidobacterium* spp. (Mitsuoka et al., 1987). The use of mannose and mannan-oligosaccharides has developed from knowledge of the role that carbohydrates play in the attachment of bacteria to the gut epithelium. Mannose-specific lectins on the surface of the bacterial cell attach to epithelial cells in the animal that contain mannose derivatives. Not all bacteria have mannose-specific lectins, but strains of *Salmonella, E. coli*, and *Klebsiella* have all been isolated that bind preferentially to mannose and mannose-like derivatives (Mirelman et al., 1980). The importance of attachment lies in the role it plays in colonization and disease. If attachment and colonization are not accomplished, the invading organisms are expelled from the host by physiological mechanisms such as peristalsis and mucous secretion. The introduction of a mannose-rich material may interfere with the binding of the bacteria to the mucosal surface which would, in turn, allow the bacteria to be expelled from the animal.

The mannan-oligosaccharide (MOS) derived from yeast cell wall material has been shown to stimulate a non-specific immune response in various species of fish, rats (Onarheim, 1992), and calves (Newman *et al.*, 1993). Neonatal calves receiving 2 g of MOS per head per day added to a commercial milk replacer had an improved liveweight at weaning (Table 5) and a reduced incidence of respiratory illness (Table 6). The exact mechanism involved in these results is not clear but an interrelationship between certain carbohydrates and immune function has been implicated (Sharon and Lis, 1993).

Table 5. Effect of mannan-oligosaccharide and acidification on performance of Holstein calves.

Weight gain characteristics	Dietary modification		
	Control	Acidification[1]	Oligosaccharide[2]
Initial weight (kg)	48.15	47.99	48.03
3 wk weight (kg)	50.94	52.05	52.05
3 wk gain (kg)	2.79[a]	4.05[b]	4.02[b]
Daily gain (kg)	0.127	0.186	0.182
5 wk weight (kg)	59.97	60.95	62.02
Total gain (kg)	11.82[a]	12.95[ab]	13.98[b]
Average daily gain (kg)	0.336	0.368	0.400

[a,b] Values in the same row with different superscripts differ (P<0.05).

[1] Citric acid, electrolytes, enzymes and lactic acid bacteria.

[2] Mannan-based oligosaccharide.

Adapted from Newman *et al.* (1993).

CONCLUSIONS

The use of microbial supplements for both neonates and in starter diets fed pre-weaning has been based on an admittedly limited knowledge of gut microbial development and the roles

Table 6. Incidence of respiratory disease in calves (3 to 6 weeks) fed diets with or without mannan-oligosaccharide.

	Incidence of respiratory disease	
	Control	Mannan-oligosaccharide
Trial 1	10/15[a]	3/14
Trial 2	10/14	2/14

[a] Values represent the number of treated calves per total calves in the treatment.

Adapted from Newman et al. (1993).

played by various species in the adult, normal animal. Lactic acid-producing bacteria are the most common microbial supplement used during the first few weeks of life, when emphasis is placed on establishing beneficial species and excluding coliforms. As the goal of supplementation becomes stimulation of rumen microbial development instead of the intestinal population, viable yeast culture is an effective addition to starter feeds. Effects of viable yeast culture on rumen lactic acid-utilizing and cellulolytic species may explain the performance response seen.

Development of inoculants containing rumen microbial species is hampered by the O_2 sensitivity of anaerobes; however manipulation of gut microbial ecology by nutritional means may allow us to expand the range and effectiveness of currently-used microbial supplements.

REFERENCES

Anderson, K.L., Nagaraja, T.G. and Morrill, J.L. 1987. Ruminal metabolic development in calves weaned conventionally or early. *J. Dairy Sci.* **70**, 1000-1005.

Bechman, T.J., Chambers, J.V. and Cunningham, M.D. 1977. Influence of *Lactobacillus acidophilus* on performance of young dairy calves. *J. Dairy Sci.* **60**(Suppl. 1) 74. (Abstract).

Beharka, A.A., Nagaraja, T.G. and Morrill, J.L. 1991. Ruminal microbial and metabolic development of young calves fed calf starter supplemented with *Aspergillus oryzae* fermentation extract. *J. Dairy Sci.* **74**, 4326-4336.

Belonowsky, J. 1907. Influence du ferment lactique sur la flore des excrements des souris. *Ann. Inst. Pasteur.* **21**, 991.

Brooker, B.F. and Fuller, R. 1975. Adhesion of lactobacilli to the chicken crop epithelium. *J. Ultrastruct. Res.* **52**, 21-31.

Coconnier, M.H., Klaenhammer, T.R., Kerneis, S., Bernet, M. and Servin, A.L. 1992. Protein-mediated adhesion of *Lactobacillus acidophilus* BG2FO4 on human enterocyte and mucus-secreting cell lines in culture. *Appl. Environ. Microbiol.* **58**, 2034-2039.

Davis, C.P. and Savage, D.C. 1972. Colonization of the large bowel of suckling mice by indigenous spiral-shaped microbes. Abstr. Ann. Meet. Am. Soc. Microbiol. p. 118.

Ellinger D.K., Muller, L.D. and Glantz, P.J. 1978. Influence of feeding fermented colostrum and *Lactobacillus acidophilus* on faecal flora and selected blood parameters of young dairy calves. *J. Dairy Sci.* **61**(Suppl. 1), 126. (Abstract).

Fallon R.J. and Harte, F.J. 1987. The effect of yeast culture inclusion in the concentrate diet on calf performance. *J. Dairy Sci.* **70**(Suppl.1), 119. (Abstract).

Fox, S.M. 1988. Probiotics - intestinal inoculants for production animals. *Vet. Med.* **83**, 806-830.

Fuller, R. and Brooker, B.E. 1974. Lactobacilli which attach to the crop epithelium of the fowl. *Am. J. Clin. Nutr.* **67**, 1305-1312.

Gilliland, S.E., Bruce, B.B., Bush, L.J. and Staley, T.E. 1980. Comparison of two strains of *Lactobacillus acidophilus* as dietary adjuncts for young calves. *J. Dairy Sci.* **63**, 964-972.

Godfrey, N.W. 1961. The functional development of the calf. *J. Agr. Sci.* **57**, 173-183.

Goodson, M. and Rowbury, R.J. 1989. Habituation to normally lethal acidity by prior growth of *Escherichia coli* at a sub-lethal acid pH value. *Lett. Appl. Microbiol.* **8**, 77-79.

Hughes, J. 1988. The effect of a high strength yeast culture in the diet of early weaned calves. *Anim. Prod.* **46**, 526.

Jenny, B.F., Vandijk, H.J. and Collins, J.A. 1991. Performance and fecal flora of calves fed a *Bacillus subtilis* concentrate. *J. Dairy Sci.* **74**, 1968-1973.

Jordan R.M. and Johnston, L. 1990. Yeast culture supplemented lamb diets. *J. Anim. Sci.* **68**(Suppl. 1), 493. (Abstract).

Leyer, G.J. and Johnson, E.A. 1992. Acid adaptation promotes survival of *Salmonella* spp. in cheese. *Appl. Environ. Microbiol.* **58**, 2075-2080.

Maeng, W.J., Kim. C.W. and Shin, H.T. 1987. Effect of a lactic acid bacteria concentrate (*Streptococcus faecium* Cernelle 68) on growth rate and scouring prevention in dairy calves. *Korean J. Dairy Sci.* **9**, 204-210.

Metchnikoff, E. 1908. *The Prolongation of Life.* 1st ed. G.P. Putnam and Sons, Paris, France.

Mirelman, D., Altman, G. and Eshdat, Y. 1980. Screening of bacterial isolates for mannose-specific lectin activity by agglutination of yeasts. *J. Clin. Microbiol.* **11**, 328-331.

Mitchell, I.G. and Kenworthy, R. 1976. Investigations on a metabolite from *Lactobacillus bulgaricus* which neutralizes the effect of enterotoxin from *Escherichia coli* pathogenic for pigs. *J. Appl. Bacteriol.* **41**, 163-174.

Mitsuoka, T., Hidaka, H. and Eida, T. 1987. Effect of fructo-oligosaccharides on intestinal microflora. *Hahrung.* **31**, 427-436.

Morishita, Y., Mitsuoka, T., Kaneuchi, C., Yamamoto, S. and Ogata, M. 1971. Specific establishment of lactobacilli in the digestive tract of germ-free chickens. *Jap. J. Microbiol.* **15**, 531.

Nakanishi, Y., Arave, C.W. and Stewart, P.H. 1993. Effects of feeding *Lactobacillus acidophilus* yogurt on performance and behavior of dairy calves. *J. Dairy Sci.* **76**(Suppl. 1), 244. (Abstract).

Newman, K.E. 1990. *Antagonistic activities of lactic acid bacteria on selected gastrointestinal and pathogenic bacteria.* Ph.D. Dissertation, University of Kentucky, US.

Newman, K.E., Dawson, K.A. and Morehead, M.C. 1990. Antagonistic activities of bacterial isolates from probiotic feed supplements upon pathogenic and rumen bacteria. *J. Anim. Sci.* **68**(Suppl. 1), 505. (Abstract).

Newman, K.E., Jacques, K. and Buede, R.P. 1993. Effect of mannan oligosaccharide supplementation of milk replacer on gain, performance and fecal bacteria of Holstein calves. *J. Anim. Sci.* **71**(suppl. 1), 271. (Abstract).

Nisbet, D.J. and Martin, S.A. 1991. Effect of a *Saccharomyces cerevisiae* culture on lactate utilization by the ruminal bacterium *Selenomonas ruminantium*. *J. Anim. Sci.* **69**, 4628-4633.

Onarheim, A.M. 1992. The glucan way to fish health. *Fish Farming International* **19**, 32-33.

Pollman, D.S., Johnston, M.E., Allee, G.L. and Hines, R.H. 1984. Effect of *Bacillus subtilis* addition to carbadox medicated starter pig diets. *J. Anim. Sci.* **59** (Suppl. 1), 275. (Abstract).

Raffle, E. 1956. Yogurt in gastro-enteritis of infancy. *Lancet* **2**, 1106-1107.

Quigley, J.D., Wallis, L.B., Dowlen, H.H. and Heitman, R.N. 1992. Sodium bicarbonate and yeast culture effects on ruminal fermentation, growth, and intake in dairy calves. *J. Dairy Sci.* **75**, 3531-3538.

Savage, D.C. 1972. Associations and physiological interactions of indigenous microorganisms and gastrointestinal epithelia. *Am. J. Clin. Nutr.* **25**, 1372-1379.

Savage, D.C. and Dubos, R.J. 1967. Localization of indigenous yeast in the murine stomach. *J. Bacteriol.* **94**, 1811-1816.

Savage, D.C., Dubos, R. and Schaedler, R.W. 1968. The gastrointestinal epithelium and its autochthonous bacterial flora. *J. Exp. Med.* **127**, 67-75.

Saylor, W.W., Korver, D.R., Mullins, T.M. and Malone, G.W. 1993. Response of broiler chickens to a direct-fed microbial (*Bacillus* sp.) in the presence of anticoccidial drugs and coccidial infection. *Poult. Sci.* **72**(Suppl. 1), 58. (Abstract).

Schwab, C.G., Moore, J.J., Hoyt, P.M. and Prentice, J.L. 1980. Performance and fecal flora of calves fed a nonviable *Lactobacillus bulgaricus* fermentation product. *J. Dairy Sci.* **63**, 1412-1423.

Sharon, N. and Lis, H. 1993. Carbohydrates in cell recognition. *Sci. Amer.* **268**, 74-81.

Simm, G., Chamberlain, A.G. and Davies, A.B. 1980. The effect of acid milk replacer on faecal coliform populations in preweaned calves. *Vet. Rec.* **107**, 64.

Smith, H.W. 1965. The development of the flora of the alimentary tract in young animals. *J. Path. Bact.* **90**, 495-513.

Sneath, P.H.A. 1986. Endospore-forming Gram-positive rods and cocci. In *Bergey's Manual of Systematic Bacteriology,* vol 2, pp. 1104-1207. Williams and Wilkins, Baltimore, US.

Tannock, G.W. 1983. Effect of dietary and environmental stress on the gastrointestinal microbiota. In: *Human Intestinal Microflora in Health and Disease* (D. Hentges, ed.) pp 517-539. Academic Press, London, UK.

Van Soest, P.J. 1982. *Nutritional Ecology of the Ruminant.* Cornell University Press, Ithaca, New York, US.

Williams, P.E.V., Innes, G.M., Brewer, A. and Magadi, J.P. 1985. The effects on growth, food intake and rumen volume of including untreated or ammonia-treated barley straw in a complete diet for weaning calves. *Anim. Prod.* **41**, 63-68.

Williams P.E.V., Tait, C.A.G., Innes, G.M. and Newbold, C.J. 1991. Effects of the inclusion of yeast culture (*Saccharomyces cerevisiae* plus growth medium) in the diet of dairy cows on milk yield and forage degradation and fermentation patterns in the rumen of sheep and steers. *J. Anim. Sci.* **69**, 3016-3026.

Ziolecka A., Osinska, Z. and Ziolecki, A. 1984. The effect of stabilized rumen extract on growth and development of calves. 1. Liveweight gain and efficiency of feed utilization. *Z. Tierphysiol. Tierrernahrg. u. Futtermittelkde.* **51**, 13-20.

13 Microbial feed additives for ruminants

C. James Newbold

Rowett Research Institute, Bucksburn, Aberdeen AB2 9SB, UK

INTRODUCTION

The use of yeast and other fungi in ruminant diets does not immediately identify itself as being a product of modern biotechnology. In 1924, Eckles *et al.* published a report on the use of yeast in the diet of calves, pre-dating the elucidation of the structure of DNA by over 25 years. However, it is only in the last decade that a considerable literature concerning the use of microbial additives to improve the health and productivity of ruminant livestock has appeared. The renewed interest in microbial feed additives has occurred at least partly as a result of increasing consumer concern about the use of hormonal and antibiotic growth promoters, but has also been promoted as a result of commercial interests. Wallace and Newbold (1992) suggested that the potential market for microbial feed additives in ruminant diets, in the USA alone, was likely to exceed $200 million per annum.

A wide range of microbial feed additives for ruminants has been described, including bacterial cultures from both ruminal and non-ruminal sources (Jahn *et al.*, 1973; Ware *et al.*, 1988; Greening *et al.*, 1991; Robinson *et al.*, 1993) and mixtures of bacteria and fungi (Windschitl, 1992; St-Pierre *et al.*, 1993). However, by far the most commonly used products are those based on *Aspergillus oryzae* and/or *Saccharomyces cerevisiae*. Inclusion rates in the diet are typically in the range of 4 to 100 g per day, well below the levels fed when *S. cerevisiae* is included in the ration as a protein source (Bruning and Yokoyama, 1988).

The aims of the current article are to review the use of *A. oryzae* and *S. cerevisiae* in the diet of adult ruminants, to identify the extent and variability of the production responses that have been observed, to outline a possible model for explaining the action of fungal probiotics in ruminants and to use the model to identify the dietary and management situations in which fungal probiotics might be beneficial.

PRODUCTION RESPONSES

Milk and meat production

Responses to *A. oryzae* and *S. cerevisiae* have been recorded in lactating and growing cattle (Wiedmeier, 1989; Edwards, 1991; Gomez-Alarcon *et al.*, 1991; Williams *et al.*, 1991), buffalo, sheep and goats (Teh *et al.*, 1987; Judkins and Stobart, 1988; Jordan and Johnston, 1990; Kumar *et al.*, 1992) as well as in a variety of non-ruminant species (Terrell *et al.*, 1984; Glade, 1991; McDaniel, 1991).

Williams and Newbold (1990) summarised fifteen studies in which *A. oryzae* or *S. cerevisiae* had been added to the diet of lactating dairy cows. Responses varied from a 9% reduction to an almost 17% increase in milk yield. Overall milk yield increased on average by 5% in response to the addition of the fungi. More recently, Wallace and Newbold (1993) summarised the response to *S. cerevisiae* in growing and lactating cattle and reported that the average response to the additive was an increase in productivity of around 7.5%. While any attempt to derive an average production response to dietary additives will doubtless be influenced by a reluctance of authors to report negative results, it is clear that economic responses to *S. cerevisiae* and *A. oryzae* occur. Nevertheless, as can been seen in Figs 1 and 2, production responses to fungal cultures are highly variable and a clearer understanding of the factors controlling this variability is required before any recommendation on the usage of these additives can be made.

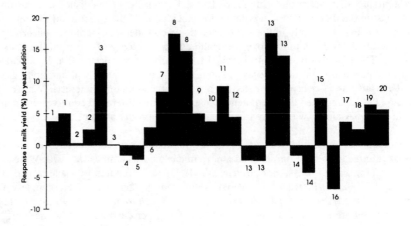

Figure 1. The response in milk yield to the addition of *Saccharomyces cerevisiae* to the diet of dairy cows.

All values based on fat corrected milk yield. 1) Harris and Lobo, 1988. 2) Quinonez *et al.*, 1988. 3) Bax, 1988. 4) Erdman and Sharma, 1989. 5) Arambel and Kent, 1990. 6) Huber *et al.*, 1989. 7) Dobos *et al.*, 1990. 8) Gunther, 1990. 9) Harris and Webb, 1990. 10) Weiss, 1991. 11) Rodriguez-Salazar *et al.*, 1991. 12) Wohlt *et al.*, 1991. 13) Williams *et al.*, 1991. 14) Alikhani *et al.*, 1992. 15) Bernard, 1992. 16) Kim *et al.*, 1992a. 17) Harris and Smith, 1992. 18) Harris *et al.*, 1992. 19) Erasmus *et al.*, 1992. 20) Piva *et al.*, 1993.

Variations in production response

Within the trials reported in the literature there are indications that the effectiveness of *S. cerevisiae* and *A. oryzae* seems to be effected by the diet and nutritional demands of the host. Harris and Lobo (1988) and Gunther (1990) with *S. cerevisiae,* and Wallentine *et al.* (1986), Kellems *et al.* (1987) and Denigan *et al.* (1992) with *A. oryzae,* found that the response to the inclusion of the additives was greater in early as opposed to mid or late lactation. Huber *et al.* (1985) observed larger responses in milk yield in response to *A. oryzae* addition as the ratio of concentrate to forage in the ration increased. Williams *et al.*

(1991) observed similar effects with *S. cerevisiae*. Spedding (1991) reported that *S. cerevisiae* stimulated weight gain in bulls fed a diet of barley by almost 19% while the response in bulls fed an *ad lib* grass silage plus 2 kg per day concentrates was 6.7%. However, Sievert and Shaver (1993) found that the response to *A. oryzae* was greater on a diet containing 35% non-fibre carbohydrates (starch, sugars, pectins and β-glucans) than on a diet containing 42% non-fibre carbohydrates, while Edwards (1991) found a greater response to *S. cerevisiae* in steers fed an *ad lib* silage plus 3 kg per day barley/soyabean meal concentrate diet than in bulls fed a fibrous by-products diet containing a high proportion of barley. Thus, while in many studies the response to fungal cultures has been greater on high concentrate diets, this is not universally true and other factors may also govern the response to the additives.

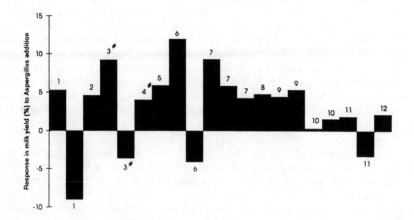

Figure 2. The response in milk yield to the addition of *Aspergillus oryzae* to the diet of dairy cows.

All values based on fat corrected milk yield except references 3[#] and 4[#]. 1) Harris *et al.*, 1983. 2) Van Horn *et al.*, 1984. 3) Huber *et al.*, 1985. 4) Huber *et al.*, 1986. 5) Marcus *et al.*, 1986. 6) Wallentine *et al.*, 1986. 7) Kellems *et al.*, 1987. 8) Kellems *et al.*, 1990. 9) Gomez-Alarcon *et al.*, 1991. 10) Sievert and Shaver, 1993. 11) Denigan *et al.*, 1992. 12) Higginbotham *et al.*, 1993.

Summarising responses to *S. cerevisiae* in beef animals, Wallace and Newbold (1993) noted that responses in cattle fed corn silage diets (Kimenai, 1990; Jacques, 1990; Hudyma *et al.* 1990; Gippert, 1992) tended to be higher than responses recorded in trials using diets based on grass silage (Drennan, 1990, Edwards, 1991, Spedding, 1991). Response to fungal cultures may also be modified by more subtle variations in the diet. Harris *et al.* (1983) recorded a 5% increase in fat corrected milk yield in response to *A. oryzae* when the diet contained sugar cane and corn silage but a 9% depression in yield when the silage was replaced by cotton seed hulls. Williams *et al.* (1991) recorded a 17.5% increase in milk yield, in response to *S. cerevisiae* addition to the diet, in cows fed a diet of 60% concentrates: 40% straw but this response fell to 14% when the straw was replaced by hay.

Quinonez *et al.* (1988) found that *S. cerevisiae* stimulated milk yield in cows fed a diet of alfalfa hay plus wheat but not when the wheat was replaced by corn.

Our understanding of the interaction between diet composition and the response of ruminants to fungal probiotics is incomplete. A better understanding of the mechanism by which fungal probiotics are believed to drive production responses should allow the prediction of dietary situations in which production benefits might be expected.

MODE OF ACTION OF MICROBIAL FEED ADDITIVES

Possible post-ruminal effects

Previous models for the action of fungal probiotics have been based on their ability to stimulate microbial activity in the rumen (Williams and Newbold, 1990; Wallace and Newbold, 1992). That model is outlined (Fig. 3) and expanded below, however it is important to note that not all of the production benefits observed with fungal probiotics can be explained based exclusively on their action in the rumen. Post-ruminal effects cannot be ruled out, as viable *S. cerevisiae* were recovered from the duodenum and ileum of sheep fed yeast culture (Newbold *et al.*, 1990). Likewise, the reduction in rectal temperature in heat-stressed animals fed both *A. oryzae* and *S. cerevisiae* may represent a direct effect on the physiology of the animal rather than a consequence of an altered rumen fermentation (Huber *et al.*, 1986; Huber *et al.*, 1989).

Increases in the numbers of total culturable bacteria that can be recovered from the rumen would appear to be one of the most consistently reported responses to both *S. cerevisiae* and *A. oryzae*. A 60% increase in the bacterial population was found in the rumen of lactating dairy cows supplemented with *S. cerevisiae* (Harrison *et al.*., 1988). Dawson (1987) reported a 51-461% increase in the bacterial population in a rumen-simulating fermentor supplemented with *S. cerevisiae,* and Wiedmeier *et al.* (1987) reported a 30% increase in the total bacterial population in the rumen of cattle supplemented with *S. cerevisiae* while *A. oryzae* increased the count by 12%. The bacterial population increased by 80% in a rumen simulator supplemented with *A. oryzae* (Frumholtz *et al.,* 1989). Varel and Kreikemeier (1993) observed increases in rumen bacterial numbers of between 50 and 100% in cattle supplemented with *A. oryzae.* While the increases in culturable bacteria in the above studies might not always reach statistical significance, studies in which fungal probiotics fail to stimulate bacterial numbers are rare (Dawson *et al.*, 1990). What is not known is to what extent the increase in culturable bacteria recovered from the rumen reflects an actual increase in bacterial biomass and to what extent it represents an increase in the viability of bacterial cells within the rumen. We failed to detect any increase in the microscopic count of bacterial cells from rumen fluid withdrawn from sheep fed *S. cerevisiae* but did note a 12% increase in acid-precipitable protein, suggesting an increase in microbial protein concentration (Newbold and McKain, unpublished observation). Increases in the flow of nitrogen from the rumen of animals fed *S. cerevisiae* and *A. oryzae* have been reported (Wanderley *et al.*, 1987; Williams *et al.*, 1990). Gomez-Alarcon *et al.* (1990), with *A. oryzae*, and Carro *et al.* (1992a), with *S. cerevisiae,* reported increases in the efficiency of synthesis of microbial protein in response to fungal addition. In some studies this has been associated with an increased flow of microbial protein leaving the rumen and an enhanced supply of amino

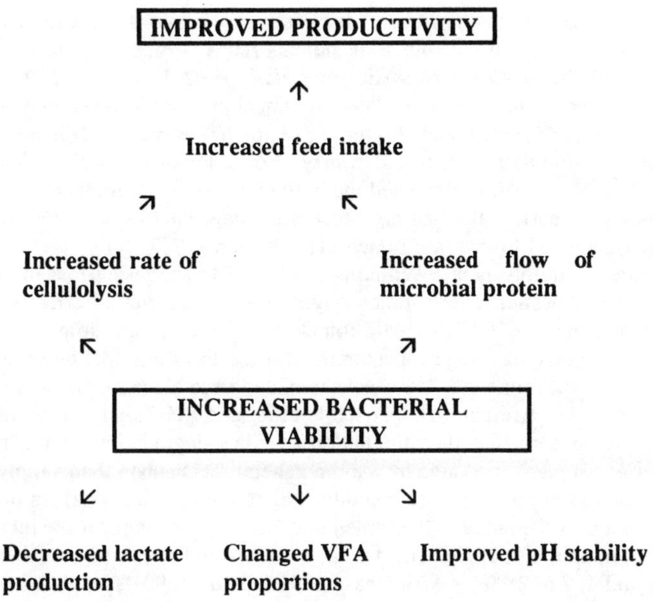

IMPROVED PRODUCTIVITY

↑

Increased feed intake

↗ ↖

**Increased rate of
cellulolysis**   **Increased flow of
microbial protein**

↖ ↗

| INCREASED BACTERIAL
VIABILITY |
|:---:|

↙ ↓ ↘

**Decreased lactate   Changed VFA   Improved pH stability
production   proportions**

Figure 3. A model for the action of fungal probiotics in ruminants.

acids entering the small intestine (Erasmus *et al.*, 1992; Caton *et al.*, 1993). However, Huhtanen (1991) and Carro *et al.* (1992b), both studying the effects of *S. cerevisiae* in cattle fed grass silage based diets, failed to find any increase in the flow of microbial protein entering the duodenum. El Hassan (unpublished but data given in Wallace and Newbold, 1993) found that *S. cerevisiae* stimulated viable bacterial numbers in a rumen simulator by 22% when the diet was frozen grass, but by only 6% when the grass was replaced by grass silage. An increase in microbial protein leaving the rumen may help explain the production benefits observed when fungal cultures are added to the diet. Increases in microbial protein supply might be expected to boost production in situations, such as dairy cows in early lactation, where duodenal protein supply is likely to limit productivity. However, it is evident that, like the production responses themselves, increases in microbial protein synthesis in response to fungal cultures are dependent on the diet fed.

Influence on fibre breakdown

In addition to increases in total viable bacteria, several authors have noted increases in the cellulolytic bacterial population in response to *A. oryzae* (Wiedmeier *et al.*, 1987; Frumholtz *et al.*, 1989; Newbold *et al.*, 1992a) and *S. cerevisiae* (Harrison *et al.*, 1988; Dawson *et al.*, 1990; Kim *et al.*, 1992b). It has been suggested that an increase in the population of cellulolytic bacteria in the rumen could account for the increases in total tract digestibility of dry matter and acid detergent fibre which have been reported in animals fed *A. oryzae* or *S. cerevisiae* (Van Horn *et al.*, 1984; Wiedmeier *et al.*, 1987). Gomez-Alarcon *et al.* (1990) noted that *A. oryzae* caused a shift in the site of dry matter digestion with significantly more dry matter being degraded in the rumen. Increases in the rate but not the extent of fibre digestion have been noted in the rumen of animals fed *A. oryzae* (Fondevila *et al.*, 1990; Newbold *et al.*, 1991) and *S. cerevisiae* (Erasmus *et al.*, 1992; Kim *et al.*, 1992c). However, as with many of the ruminal effects mediated by fungal probiotics, other studies have found no effect of *A. oryzae* (Sievert and Shaver, 1993) or *S. cerevisiae* (Mir and Mir, 1992), suggesting that the stimulation in digestion may also be modified by diet. Williams *et al.* (1991) found that *S. cerevisiae* stimulated the initial rate of hay degradation in the rumen of animals fed hay plus barley, but had no effect when concentrates were removed from the diet. The yeast appeared to increase rumen pH. Stewart (1977) found that low pH values depressed ruminal cellulolysis and Williams *et al.* (1991) suggested that the effects of *S. cerevisiae* on fibre digestion in the rumen might be mediated via an effect on rumen pH. However, Chademana and Offer (1990) found that *S. cerevisiae* stimulated dry matter degradation over a range of forage:concentrate ratios, with little effect on rumen pH, while Fondevila *et al.* (1990) found that *A. oryzae* stimulated fibre digestion in the rumen of sheep fed a diet of straw when rumen pH was stable at around pH 7 and was unaffected by *A. oryzae*. Thus it appears that the stimulation of fibre degradation in the rumen by *S. cerevisiae* and *A. oryzae* is mediated by a more general mechanism than simply an increase in rumen pH, such as an increase in the numbers of cellulolytic bacteria. An increase in the rate at which forage is degraded in the rumen may partially account for the increase in food intake observed in animals supplemented with *A. oryzae* and *S. cerevisiae* (Van Horn *et al.*, 1984; Harris and Lobo, 1988). Williams and Newbold (1990) speculated that in many studies the increase in production observed when fungal probiotics were added to the diet could be explained largely by an increase in dry matter intake.

Effects on rumen protozoa and fungi

The above discussion on the effects of fungal cultures on microbial numbers in the rumen has concentrated on bacteris. Oellermann *et al.* (1990) and Newbold *et al.* (1992b) found no effect of *A. oryzae* on the numbers of fungi or protozoa in the rumen. However, Welch and Calza (1993) found that *A. oryzae* stimulated the growth of the rumen anaerobic fungus, *Neocallimastix frontalis, in vitro*. More work is required to clarify the effects of *A. oryzae* and *S. cerevisiae* on protozoal and fungal activities in the rumen.

Mechanism of stimulation of rumen bacteria

In addition to a general increase in bacterial numbers, leading to an increase in protein synthesis and fibre digestion, it is possible that fungal probiotics stimulate specific groups of rumen bacteria (Oellermann *et al.*, 1990; Dawson, 1993, Beharka and Nagaraja, 1991; Varel and Kreikemeier, 1993) causing more subtle effects such as changes in volatile fatty acid and lactic acid concentrations in the rumen (Fig. 3). What remains unclear is how small levels of fungal inclusion in the diet stimulate microbial numbers in the rumen. A number of mechanisms by which *S. cerevisiae* and *A. oryzae* might stimulate bacterial numbers in the rumen have been proposed (Rose, 1987; Wallace and Newbold, 1992), some of which are discussed below.

As noted above, *S. cerevisiae* increased rumen pH in animals fed high concentrate diets (Williams *et al.*, 1991), while Frumholtz *et al.* (1989) reported similar results with *A.*

oryzae. Increasing rumen pH will increase the efficiency of the rumen fermentation as low rumen pH values decreased the growth of many rumen bacteria (Russell *et al.*, 1979; Russell and Dombrowski, 1980). Williams *et al.* (1991) suggested that the increase in rumen pH resulted from a decrease in lactic acid concentrations observed when the products were fed. However, the concentrations of lactic acid in the rumen of animals fed balanced diets are low (<5 mM) and unlikely to cause large changes in rumen pH (Wallace and Newbold, 1992). Only on high concentrate diets in conditions approaching acidosis (Slyter, 1976) or in animals consuming large quantities of acidic silage (Tutt, 1972) is lactic acid likely to cause large depressions in rumen pH. Rose (1987) and Williams (1989) speculated on the buffering capacity of the yeast cell wall; however, Ryan (1990) could find no effect of *S. cerevisiae* on the buffering capacity of rumen fluid. Supplementation of the diet with *S. cerevisiae* decreased soluble sugar concentrations in the rumen of steers fed a hay plus barley diet (Williams *et al.*, 1991). Rapid bacterial growth in the rumen occurs in the presence of high soluble sugar concentrations (Hungate, 1966) and removal of sugars may have slowed growth, decreasing the production of acidic fermentation products. Based on the ability of *S. cerevisiae* to utilise a wide range of sugars (Panchal *et al.*, 1984), Williams (1988) suggested that yeast might accumulate sugars directly from rumen fluid. Removal of oligosaccharides by *S. cerevisiae* would also benefit the cellulolytic bacteria by removing sugars that might otherwise depress cellulolysis (Mould *et al.,* 1983); however, the possibility of yeast accumulating sugars from rumen fluid does not appear to have been tested experimentally.

Low numbers of yeasts (but not *S. cerevisiae*) and moulds occur naturally in the rumen (Lund, 1974). However, it seems unlikely that either *S. cerevisiae* (Newbold *et al.*, 1990) or *A. oryzae* (Fondevila *et al.*, 1990) grow in the rumen. A lack of growth should not be confused with a lack of metabolic activity; Ingledew and Jones (1982) found that *S. cerevisiae* was metabolically active in rumen fluid for up to 6 h, and El Hassan *et al.* (1993) isolated viable *S. cerevisiae* cells from the rumen up 72 h after the last meal containing a commercial yeast culture. Wallace *et al.* (1993) found that *S. cerevisiae* accumulated intracellular malic acid when incubated in autoclaved rumen fluid. Malate stimulated the growth of the prominent Gram-negative rumen bacterium *S. ruminantium* in medium containing lactic acid (Nisbet and Martin 1990). No growth occurred on malate and it was shown that malate stimulated the uptake of lactic acid from the medium. Based on the concentration of dicarboxylic acids in both *A. oryzae* and *S. cerevisiae,* Nisbet and Martin (1990, 1991, 1993) suggested that a stimulation in the numbers of *S. ruminantium* by malate present in fungal probiotics might occur *in vivo.* Edwards (1991) and Girard *et al.* (1993) found that *S. cerevisiae* increased the number of lactate-utilizing bacteria recovered from rumen fluid and lower rumen lactate concentrations have been noted in animals supplemented with both *S. cerevisiae* and *A. oryzae* (Williams *et al.*, 1991; Newbold *et al.*, 1992a). Wallace *et al.* (1993) found no effect of adding malate to the rumen on the numbers of lactate-utilizing bacteria, however malate did appear to stimulate the cellulolytic bacterial population and fibre digestion. Kung *et al.* (1982) found that malate, at levels over 100 times higher than that likely to be supplied by *S. cerevisiae* or *A. oryzae*, stimulated ruminal fermentation and the persistency of milk yield in dairy cattle. More work is required to elucidate fully the extent to which malate and other dicarboxylic acids can explain the action of fungal cultures *in vivo.*

Oxygen scavenging by yeast

Rose (1987) initially suggested that yeast might scavenge oxygen thus stimulating the growth of anaerobic bacteria in the rumen. The rumen is widely considered to be anaerobic; nevertheless, the rumen gas, even in non-fistulated animals, contains between 0.5 and 1.0% oxygen (McArthur and Multimore, 1962). Hillman *et al.* (1985) found detectable levels of dissolved oxygen *in situ* shortly after feeding. The oxygen concentration then declined below the levels of detection between 10 and 30 min after feeding. Czerkawski (1969) calculated that oxygen transfer from saliva, food and diffusion from the blood of the host animal might account for 38 l of oxygen entering the rumen of a sheep per day. Newbold *et al.* (1993) reported rates of oxygen uptake by rumen fluid, in the absence of yeast, of 100 nmol ml^{-1} min^{-1}. Assuming a rumen volume in sheep to be 6 l, this equates to an oxygen flux of 16 l per day. Oxygen is toxic to anaerobic bacteria, inhibiting the growth of rumen bacteria in pure culture (Marounek and Wallace, 1984) and the adhesion of cellulolytic rumen bacteria to cellulose (Roger *et al.*, 1990). Newbold *et al.* (1993) compared the ability of different strains of *S. cerevisiae* to stimulate bacterial numbers in a rumen simulating fermentor and the ability of the yeast to stimulate oxygen uptake by rumen fluid. The ability of different strains of *S. cerevisiae* to stimulate oxygen uptake by rumen fluid appeared to be related to their capacity to stimulate the bacterial viable count (Newbold *et al.*, 1993; Fig. 4).

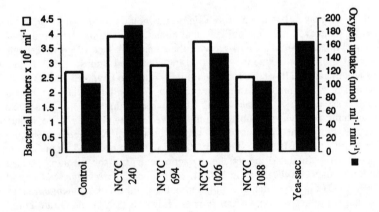

Figure 4. The effect of *Saccharomyces cerevisiae* NCYC 240, NCYC 694, NCYC 1088, NCYC 1026 and the commercial yeast culture, Yea-sacc®, on oxygen uptake by rumen fluid *in vitro* and bacterial numbers in Rusitec.

Respiration-deficient mutants of *S. cerevisiae* enriched by repeated subculturing in the presence of ethidium bromide failed to stimulate bacterial numbers under conditions in which the parent strains were found to be beneficial (Newbold *et al.*, 1993, Table 1). Furthermore the stimulatory activity of *S. cerevisiae* could be mimicked by taking extra care to exclude oxygen from the rumen simulating fermentor, Rusitec, and the stimulatory activity of the yeast was less pronounced under decreased oxygen conditions (Newbold *et al.*, 1993). Thus the suggestion made by Rose (1987) that the probiotic activity of yeast is at least partially derived from its ability to remove potentially harmful oxygen from the rumen would appear to have been confirmed by the experimental evidence. Interestingly, *A. oryzae* had no effect on oxygen uptake by rumen fluid.

Table 1. Effect of *Saccharomyces cerevisiae* NCYC 240 and a respiration deficient mutant of *S. cerevisiae* NCYC 240 rho° on microbial numbers in the rumen simulating fermentor, Rusitec.

	Control	*S. cerevisiae* NCYC 240	*S. cerevisiae* NCYC 240 rho°
Total viable bacteria (x 10^8 ml^{-1})	2.8	5.1	2.7
Cellulolytic bacteria (x 10^6 ml^{-1})	3.5	37.3	5.3

Mode of action of *A. oryzae*

Autoclaved *A. oryzae* failed to stimulate bacterial numbers in mixed fermentations, while *A. oryzae* that had been sterilised by gamma-irradiation rather than autoclaving retained most of its stimulatory activity (Newbold *et al.*, 1991). Either a heat-sensitive nutrient is destroyed by autoclaving or *A. oryzae* has a metabolic activity that is destroyed by heat but not irradiation. The wide range of polysaccharidase enzymes produced by *Aspergillus* spp. (Fogarty and Kelly, 1979) and in particular *A. oryzae* (Walsh and Stewart, 1969) had led to the suggestion that enzymic attack of plant fibres by *Aspergillus* might be an important factor in the stimulation of forage degradation in the rumen when *A. oryzae* was fed (Wiedmeier *et al.*, 1987; Fondevila *et al.*, 1990). When the release of reducing sugars from a variety of carbohydrates by aqueous extracts prepared from rumen organisms and *A. oryzae* was measured (Newbold, 1992), rates of sugar release were similar with extracts from both *A. oryzae* and rumen organisms (Newbold, 1992; Fig. 5). In view of low inclusion rate of *A. oryzae* in the diet, it might appear unlikely that activities from *A. oryzae* will contribute significantly to the hydrolysis of polysaccharides *in vivo*.

However, the activities of *A. oryzae* and rumen organisms did appear to differ when plant material was used as substrate. Rates of reducing sugar release from hay and straw were similar with both *A. oryzae* and rumen organisms, but the release of total sugars from forage incubated with *A. oryzae* extract was over twice that released by rumen microbes (Table 2). The ratio of reducing to total sugars recovered from incubations with rumen organisms was around 1, suggesting that single sugar residues were the major end products of these incubations. With *A. oryzae*, the ratio of reducing to total sugars recovered was above 2, consistent with larger oligomers being the major end product of the incubations. When extract prepared from rumen organisms and *A. oryzae* were mixed in a 95:5 ratio, the release of reducing and total sugars from hay was higher than would have been predicted from the arithmetic addition of the activities in the two extracts. No similar synergy was observed

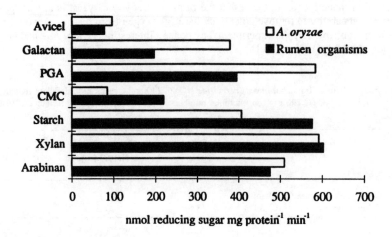

Figure 5. Hydrolysis of polysaccharides by extracts prepared from mixed rumen organisms or *Aspergillus oryzae*.

with straw as substrate. Thus the activities in the rumen microbes and *A. oryzae* were apparently complementary, but again the effect may be diet-dependent. Based on the rates of degradation of esterified p-coumaric and ferulic acids by rumen fluid plus *A. oryzae in vitro*, Varel *et al.* (1993) speculated that esterase enzymes in *A. oryzae* may be important in stimulating fibre digestion when the fungi are added to ruminant diets. Ether, ester bridges formed by ferulic acid form bonds between polysaccharide and lignin in Graminaceous plant cell walls (Ralph and Helm, 1993) and may limit cell wall degradation (Hartley and Ford, 1989). Varel *et al.* (1991) suggested that microbes capable of degrading such bonds may act as catalysts to fibre degradation in the rumen. Thus the finding by Varel *et al.* (1993) that *A. oryzae* contained measurable amounts of feruloyl esterase is consistent with the apparent synergism between enzyme extracts prepared from rumen microbes and *A. oryzae* (Newbold, 1992; Table 2).

Model for mode of action of *S. cerevisiae* and *A oryzae*

From the above it is clear that the model of Wallace and Newbold (1992) should now be modified to include the removal of oxygen and the provision of exogenous fibre-degrading enzymes among the mechanisms by which fungal probiotics stimulate bacterial numbers in the rumen. However, it would be premature to attribute the effects of either *S. cerevisiae* or *A. oryzae* in the rumen to a single mechanism. It is also clear that, although superficially similar in their action in the rumen, the current generation of fungal probiotics based on *S. cerevisiae* and *Aspergillus* differ in the mechanism by which they stimulate bacterial numbers. In addition, with *S. cerevisiae* it has been noted that not all strains of the yeast are

Table 2. Release of sugars from hay and straw by extracts prepared from rumen organisms, *Aspergillus oryzae* fermentation extract or by a 95:5 mixture of rumen organisms and *A. oryzae* fermentation extract.

	Mixed rumen organisms	*A. oryzae*	Rumen organisms plus *A. oryzae*	
			Measured	Predicted
Hay				
Reducing sugars released (nmol mg protein^{-1} min^{-1})	300	332	387	302
Total sugars released (nmol mg protein^{-1} min^{-1})	316	816	431	341
Straw				
Reducing sugars released (nmol mg protein^{-1} min^{-1})	78	150	94	82
Total sugars released (nmol mg protein^{-1} min^{-1})	115	356	114	127

capable of stimulating digestion in the rumen (Jouany *et al.*, 1991; Newbold and Wallace, 1992). It is also likely that the method of growing the culture will effect the final probiotic activity. Care should therefore be taken in selecting fungal probiotics to ensure not only that the parent culture is capable of stimulating the rumen fermentation but also that the preparation retains this activity in large scale production (e.g. the effect of high temperatures during the pelleting of concentrate feeds).

Relating the mode of action of fungal probiotics to their action *in vivo*.

Any proposal for a mechanism by which fungal probiotics stimulate bacterial numbers in the rumen must also try to explain responses to the products observed *in vivo*. As noted earlier, production responses to the addition of fungal probiotics appear to be modified by the composition of the diet. Clearly responses to *S. cerevisiae* and *A. oryzae* are only likely to occur in dietary and management situations where animals are likely to respond to increases in protein synthesis or fibre degradation. However, even at a ruminal level the responses to fungal probiotics appear to be diet-dependent. A complex microbial ecosystem such as the rumen has many potential limiting factors; removal of one potential constraint (e.g. toxic concentrations of oxygen) will not stimulate growth if another is still limiting (e.g. substrate supply). Thus Carro *et al.* (1992a) found that *S. cerevisiae* caused a greater stimulation in bacterial protein synthesis on a high concentrate diet (high substrate availability) than on high forage diet (low substrate supply). Similarly, *S. cerevisiae* stimulated lactic utilising bacteria in bulls fed a high concentrate diet, when lactate fluxes in the rumen were high, but not in sheep fed a forage /concentrate diet when lactate fluxes were low (Newbold, unpublished observations).

Responses to *S. cerevisiae* appeared to be greater in beef cattle fed corn (Kimenai, 1990; Jacques, 1990; Hudyma *et al.*, 1990; Gippert, 1992) as opposed to grass silage (Drennan, 1990; Edwards, 1991; Spedding, 1991). El Hassan (unpublished, but data given in Wallace and Newbold, 1993) found that *S. cerevisiae* stimulated bacterial numbers in Rusitec when the diet was fresh frozen grass but not when silage prepared from the same forage was fed. It is known that diets containing a high proportion of grass silage support a low rate of microbial protein synthesis in the rumen (ARC, 1984). The reason for the low efficiency of synthesis is not entirely resolved, but in great part it must reflect the poor ATP yield obtained in the rumen from silage fermentation products (Thomas and Thomas, 1985). Under such circumstances, where it is the energy supply that is the primary limitation, it is unlikely that a decrease in dissolved oxygen due to the presence of *S. cerevisiae* will boost microbial growth.

The effects of diet on the action of *Aspergillus* in the rumen are harder to predict without more details on the interactions between the enzymes from the fungi and those of the rumen. Newbold (1992; Table 2) noted difference in the interactions between extracts from *A. oryzae* and rumen microbes to release sugars from hay compared to straw. Similarly, *A. oryzae* stimulated the rate of degradation of bromegrass but not alfalfa in the rumen (Varel and Kreikemeier (1993). Tapia *et al.* (1989) found that the response in dry matter disappearance to the addition of *Aspergillus niger*, *A. oryzae*, *Trichoderma harzium* and *Penicillium* spp. varied with the fibrous substrate used. It may be necessary to match the source of fungal enzyme with the type of forage to maximise the response in rumen dry matter digestion.

CONCLUSIONS

Presumptive modes of action for fungal probiotic preparations containing *S. cerevisiae* and *A. oryzae* have been proposed. Based on these suggestions, it should be possible to develop a second generation of rumen probiotics with enhanced but essentially similar activities. These need not be based on either *S. cerevisiae* or *A. oryzae*. Although the proposed modes of action for *S. cerevisiae* and *A. oryzae* differ, they share a basic property in that each is based on the ability of enzymes in the preparation to function in the rumen for a short time after feeding. There has been much speculation on the benefits to ruminant nutrition that might be gained through the application of recombinant DNA technology to rumen bacteria (Teather, 1985; Forsberg *et al.*, 1986; Hespell, 1987). However it has been argued that when rumen bacteria have been modified to express a new desired activity, natural selection will militate against the successful *in vivo* establishment of these organisms (Russell and Wilson,

1988). Might not fungal probiotics, which are fed daily, be a more convenient way of introducing novel activities into the rumen ?

REFERENCES

Agricultural Research Council. 1984. *The Nutrient Requirements of Ruminant Livestock.* Supplement 1. Commonwealth Agricultural Bureaux, Slough, UK.

Alikhani, M., Hemken, R.W. and Xin, Z. 1992. Effects of yeast supplementation of alfalfa silage or alfalfa hay fed to lactating dairy cows. *J. Anim. Sci.* **69** (Suppl. 1), 499. (Abstract).

Arambel, M.J. and Kent, B.A. 1990. Effect of yeast culture on nutrient digestibility and milk yield response in early to midlactation dairy cows. *J. Dairy Sci.*, **73**, 1560-1563.

Bax, J.A. 1988. An investigation into the response of dairy cows to supplementation with yeast culture. pp. 223-224. In: 2nd International Symposium on New Techniques in Agriculture (C.J.C. Phillips, ed.) Univ. College of North Wales, UK.

Beharka, A.A. and Nagaraja, T.G. 1991. Effects of *Aspergillus oryzae* extract (Amaferm) on ruminal fibrolytic bacteria and *in vitro* fiber degradation. In *21st Biennial Conference on Rumen Function*, p. 32, Chicago, Illinois. (Abstract).

Bernard, J.K. 1992. Influence of supplemental yeast on the performance of Holstein cows during early lactation. *J. Dairy Sci.* **75** (Suppl 1), 312. (Abstract).

Bruning, C.L. and Yokoyama, M.T. 1988. Characteristics of live and killed brewers yeast slurries and intoxication by intraruminal administration to cattle. *J. Anim. Sci.* **66**, 585-591.

Carro, M.D., Lebzien, P. and Rohr, K. 1992a. Influence of yeast culture on the *in vitro* fermentation (Rusitec) of diets containing variable portions of concentrates. *Anim. Feed Sci. Technol.* **37**,-209-220.

Carro, M.D., Lebzien, P. and Rohr, K. 1992b. Effects of yeast culture on rumen fermentation, digestibility and duodenal flow in dairy cows fed a silage based diet. *Livestock Prod. Sci.* **32**, 219-229.

Caton, J.S., Erickson, D.O., Carey, D.A. and Ulmer, D.L. 1993. Influence of *Aspergillus oryzae* fermentation extract on forage intake, site of digestion, in situ degradability, and duodenal amino acid flow in steers grazing cool-season pasture. *J. Anim. Sci.* **71**, 779-787.

Chademana, I. and Offer, N.W. 1990. The effect of dietary inclusion of yeast culture on digestion in the sheep. *Anim. Prod.* **50**, 483-489.

Czerkawski, J.W . 1969. Methane production in ruminants and its significance. *World Rev. Nutr. Diet.* **11**, 240-282.

Dawson, K.A. 1987. Mode of action of the yeast culture, Yea-sacc®, in the rumen: a natural fermentation modifier. In *Biotechnology in the Feed Industry* (T.P. Lyons, ed.) pp. 119- 125. Alltech Technical Publications, Nicholasville, Kentucky, US.

Dawson, K.A. 1993. Current and future role of yeast culture in animal production: a review of research over the last six years. In *Biotechnology in the Feed Industry* (T.P. Lyons, ed.) pp. 269-291. Alltech Technical Publications, Nicholasville, Kentucky, US.

Dawson, K.A., Newman, K.E. and Boling, J.A. 1990. Effects of microbial supplements containing yeast and lactobacilli on roughage-fed ruminal microbial activities. *J. Anim. Sci.* **68**, 3392-3398.

Denigan, M.E., Huber, J.T., Aldhadrami, G. and Al-Dehneh, A. 1992. Influence of feeding varying levels of Amaferm on performance of lactating dairy cows. *J. Dairy Sci.* **75**, 1616-1621.

Dobos, R.C., Dickens, A.J. and Norris, T.L. 1990. Yea-sacc®[1026] for dairy cattle in low concentrate input systems: effects on milk yield and composition in an Australian experiment. In *Biotechnology in the Feed Industry* (T.P. Lyons, ed.) pp. 518-519. Alltech Technical Publications, Nicholasville, Kentucky, US.

Drennan, M. 1990. Effect of yeast culture on feed intake and performance of finishing bulls. In *Biotechnology in the Feed Industry* (T.P. Lyons, ed.) p. 495. Alltech Technical Publications, Nicholasville, Kentucky, US.

Eckles, C.H., Williams, V.M., Wilbur, J.W., Palmer, L.S. and Harshaw, H.M. 1924. Yeast as a supplementary feed for calves. *J. Dairy Sci.* **7**, 421-439.

Edwards, I.E. 1991. Practical uses of yeast culture in beef production: insight into its mode of action. In *Biotechnology in the Feed Industry* (T.P. Lyons, ed.) pp. 51-65, Alltech Technical Publications, Nicholasville, Kentucky, US.

El Hassan, S.M., Newbold, C.J. and Wallace, R.J. 1993. The effect of yeast in the rumen and the requirement for viable yeast cells. *Anim. Prod.* **54**, 504. (Abstract).

Erasmus, L.J., Botha, P.M. and Kistner, A. 1992. Effect of yeast culture supplementation on production, rumen fermentation, and duodenal nitrogen flow in dairy cows. *J. Dairy Sci.* **75**,- 3056-3065.

Erdman, R.A. and Sharma, B.K. 1989. Effect of yeast culture and sodium bicarbonate on milk yield and composition in dairy cows. *J. Dairy Sci.* **72**, 1929-1932.

Fogarty, W.M. and Kelly, C.T. 1979. Developments in microbial extracellular enzymes. In *Topics in Enzyme and Fermentation Biotechnology* (A. Wiseman, ed.) pp. 45-102. John Wiley, Chichester, UK.

Fondevila, M., Newbold, C.J., Hotten, P.M. and Ørskov, E.R. 1990. A note on the effect of *Aspergillus oryzae* fermentation extract on the rumen fermentation of sheep fed straw. *Anim. Prod.* **51**, 422-425.

Forsberg, C.W., Crosby, B. and Thomas, D.Y. 1986. Potential for manipulation of the rumen fermentation through the use of recombinant DNA techniques. *J. Anim. Sci.* **63**, 310-325.

Frumholtz, P.P., Newbold, C.J. and Wallace, R.J. 1989. Influence of *Aspergillus oryzae* fermentation extract on the fermentation of a basal ration in the rumen simulation technique (Rusitec). *J. Agric. Sci., Camb.* **113**, 169-172.

Gippert, T. 1992. Effect of Yea-sacc®[1026] on performance of growing calves. In *Biotechnology in the Feed Industry* (T.P. Lyons, ed.) p. x8. Alltech Technical Publications, Nicholasville, Kentucky, US.

Girard, D., Jones, C.R. and Dawson, K.A. 1993. Lactic acid utilization in rumen-simulating cultures receiving a yeast culture supplement. *J. Anim. Sci.* **71** (Suppl. 1), 288. (Abstract).

Glade, M. 1991. Dietary yeast culture supplementation of mares during late gestation and early lactation. In *Biotechnology in the Feed Industry* (T.P. Lyons, ed.) pp. 351-354. Alltech Technical Publications, Nicholasville, Kentucky, US.

Gomez-Alarcon, R.A., Dudas, C. and Huber, J.T. 1990. Influence of cultures of *Aspergillus oryzae* on rumen and total tract digestibility of dietary components. *J. Dairy Sci.* **73**, 703-710.

Gomez-Alarcon, R.A., Huber, J.T., Higginbotham, G.E., Wiersma, F., Ammon, D. and Taylor, B. 1991. Influence of feeding *Aspergillus oryzae* fermentation extract on the milk yields, eating patterns, and body temperatures of lactating cows. *J. Anim. Sci.* **69**, 1733-1740.

Greening, R.C., Smolenski, W.J., Bell, R.L., Barsuhna, K., Johnson, M.M. and Robinson, J.A. 1991. Effects of ruminal inoculation of *Megasphaera elsdenii* strain 407A (UC-12497) on ruminal pH and organic acids in beef cattle. *J. Anim. Sci.* **69** (Suppl. 1), 518. (Abstract).

Gunther, K.D. 1990. Yeast culture : success under German dairy conditions. *The Feed Compounder.* January, pp. 17-20.

Harris, B. and Lobo, R. 1988. Feeding yeast culture to lactating dairy cows. *J. Dairy Sci.* **77**, (Suppl. 1), 276. (Abstract).

Harris, B. and Smith, W.A. 1992. Feeding dairy cattle in early lactation for maximum efficiency In *Biotechnology in the Feed Industry,* (T.P. Lyons, ed.), pp 99-107. Alltech Technical Publications, Nicholasville, Kentucky, US.

Harris, B. and Webb, D.W. 1990. The effect of feeding a concentrated yeast culture product to lactating dairy cows. *J. Dairy Sci.*, **73** (Suppl. 1), 26.6 (Abstract).

Harris, B., Van Horn, H.H., Manookian, K.E., Marshall, S.P., Taylor, M.J. and Wilcox, C.J. 1983. Sugar cane silage, sodium hydroxide and steam pressure treated sugar cane bagasse, corn silage, cottonseed hulls, sodium bicarbonate and *Aspergillus oryzae* product in complete rations for lactating cows. *J. Dairy Sci.* **66**, 1474-1485.

Harris, D., Dorminey, D.E. and Webb, D.W. 1992. The effect of Yea-sacc®[1026] supplementation on milk yield and composition under large herd management conditions *J. Dairy Sci.*, **75** (Suppl. 1), 313. (Abstract).

Harrison, G.A., Hemken, R.W., Dawson, K.A., Harmon, R.J. and Barker, K.B. 1988. Influence of addition of yeast culture supplement to diets of lactating cows on ruminal fermentation and microbial populations. *J. Dairy Sci.* **71**, 2967-2975.

Hartley, R.D. and Ford, C.W. 1989. Phenolic constituents of plant cell walls and wall biodegradability. In *Plant cell wall polymers: biogenesis and biodegradation* (N.G. Lewis and M.G. Paice, ed.). pp. 137-145. American Chemical Society, Washington, DC, US.

Hespell, R.B. 1987. Biotechnology and modifications of the rumen microbial ecosystem. Proc. Nutr. Soc. **46**, 407-413.

Higginbotham, G.E., Bath, D.L. and Butler, L.J. 1993. Effect of feeding an *Aspergillus oryzae* extract on milk production and related responses in a commercial dairy herd. *J. Dairy Sci.* **76**, 1484-1489.

Hillman, K., Lloyd, D. and Williams, A.G. 1985. Use of a portable quadrupole mass spectrometer for the measurement of dissolved gas concentrations in ovine rumen liquor in situ. *Curr. Microbiol.* **12**, 335-340.

Huber, J.T., Higginbotham, G.E. and Ware, D. 1985. Influence of feeding Vitaferm, containing an enzyme-producing culture from *Aspergillus oryzae*, on performance of lactating cows. *J. Dairy Sci.* **68** (Suppl. 1), 30. (Abstract).

Huber, J.T., Higginbotham, G.E. and Gomez-Alarcon, R. 1986. Influence of feeding an *A. oryzae* culture during hot weather on performance of lactating dairy cows. *J. Dairy Sci.* **69** (Suppl. 1), 290. (Abstract).

Huber, J.T., Sullivan, J., Taylor, B., Burgos, A. and Cramer, S. 1989. Effect of feeding Yea-sacc®[1026] on milk production and related responses in a commercial dairy herd in Arizona. In *Biotechnology in the Feed Industry* (T.P. Lyons, ed.), pp. 35-38. Alltech Technical Publications, Nicholasville, Kentucky, US.

Hudyma, W., Gray, D. and Stallknecht, G. 1990. Effect of Yea-sacc®[1026] Farm Pak on performance of crossbred steer calves fed corn silage. In Biotechnology in the Feed Industry (T.P. Lyons, ed.) pp. 529-530. Alltech Technical Publications, Nicholasville, Kentucky, US.

Huhtanen, P. 1991. Effects of yeast culture supplement on digestion of nutrients and rumen fermentation in cattle fed on a grass silage barley diet. *J. Agric. Sci. Finland* **64**, 443-453.

Hungate, R.E. 1966. *The Rumen and Its Microbes*. Academic Press, New York, US.

Ingledew, W.M. and Jones, G.A. 1982. The fate of live brewers yeast slurry in bovine rumen fluid. *J. Inst. Brewing*, **88**, 18-20.

Jacques, K.A. 1990. Effects of Yea-sacc®[1026] in diets to fed finishing beef cattle. In *Biotechnology in the Feed Industry* (T.P. Lyons, ed.) pp. 51-65. Alltech Technical Publications, Nicholasville, Kentucky, US.

Jahn, E., Chandler, P.T. and Miller, C.N. 1973. Lactational responses of dairy cows inoculated with live adapted rumen microorganisms. *J. Dairy Sci.* **56** (Suppl. 1), 643. (Abstract).

Jouany, J.P., Fonty, G., Lassalas, B., Dore, J., Gouet, P. and Betin, G. 1991. Effect of live yeast cultures on feed degradation in the rumen as assessed by *in vitro* measurements. *21st Biennial Conference on Rumen Function*, p. 7. Chicago, US. (Abstract).

Jordan, R.M. and Johnston, L. 1990. Yeast culture supplemented lamb diets. *J. Anim. Sci.*, **68** (Suppl. 1), 493. (Abstract).

Judkins, M.B. and Stobart, R.H. 1988. Influence of two levels of enzyme preperation on ruminal fermentation, particulate and fluid passage and cell wall digestion in wether lambs consuming a 10 or 25% grain diet. *J. Anim. Sci.* **66**, 1010-1015.

Kellems, R.O., Johnston, N.P., Wallentine, M.V., Lagerstedt, A., Andrus, D., Jones, R. and Huber, J.T. 1987. Effect of feeding *Aspergillus oryzae* on performance of cows during early lactation. *J. Dairy Sci.* **70** (Suppl. 1), 219. (Abstract).

Kellems, R.O., Lagerstedt, A. and Wallentine, M.V. 1990. Effect of feeding *Aspergillus oryzae* fermentation extract or *Aspergillus oryzae* plus yeast culture plus mineral and vitamin supplement on performance of Holstein cows during a complete lactation. *J. Dairy Sci.* **73**, 2922-2928.

Kim, D.Y., Figueroa, M.R., Dawson, D.P., Batallas, C.E., Arambel, M.J. and Walters, J.L. 1992a. Efficacy of supplemental viable yeast culture with or without *Aspergillus oryzae* on nutrient digestibility and milk production in early to midlactation dairy cows. *J. Dairy Sci.* **75** (Suppl. 1), 206. (Abstract)

Kim, D.Y., Wandersee, M.K., Batallas, C.E., Dawson, B.A., Kent, M.R., Figueroa, M.R., Arambel, M.J. and Walters, J.L. 1992b. Effect of added yeast culture with or without Aspergillus oryzae on rumen fermentation and nutrient digestibility when fed to nonlactating Holstein cows. *J. Dairy Sci.* **75** (Suppl. 1), 206. (Abstract).

Kim, D.Y., Wandersee, M.K., Batallas, C.E., Dawson, B.A., Kent, M.R., Figueroa, M.R., Arambel, M.J. and Walters, J.L. 1992c. Effect of feeding yeast culture with or without *Aspergillus oryzae* on dry matter disappearance in three different forage types. *J. Dairy Sci..* **75** (Suppl. 1), 206. (Abstract)

Kimenai, R. 1990. Yea-sacc®[1026] effects on bull beef performance and carcass characteristics in a low concentrate input program. In *Biotechnology in the Feed Industry* (T.P. Lyons, ed.), p. 496. Alltech Technical Publications, Nicholasville, Kentucky.

Kumar, U., Sareen, V.K. and Singh, S. 1992 . Effect of Yea-sacc®[1026] yeast culture on yield and composition of milk from murrah buffaloes. In *Biotechnology in the Feed Industry,* (T.P. Lyons, ed.) pp. x4-x5. Alltech Technical Publications, Nicholasville, Kentucky.

Kung, L., Huber, J.T., Krummrey, J.D., Allison, L. and Cook, R.M. 1982. Influence of adding malic acid to dairy cattle rations on milk production, rumen volatile acids, digestibility, and nitrogen utilization. *J. Dairy Sci.* **65**, 1170-1174.

Lund, A. 1974. Yeasts and moulds in the bovine rumen. *J. Gen. Microbiol.* **81**, 453-462.

Marcus, K.M., Huber, J.Y. and Cramer, S. 1986. Influence of feeding VitaFerm during hot weather on performance of lactating cows in a large dairy herd. *J. Dairy Sci.* **69** (Suppl. 1), 188. (Abstract).

Marounek, M. and Wallace, R.J. 1984. Influence of culture E$_h$ on the growth and metabolism of the rumen bacteria *Selenomonas ruminantium, Bacteroides amylophilus, Bacteroides succinogenes* and *Streptococcus bovis* in batch culture. *J. Gen. Microbiol.* **130**, 223-229.

McArthur, J.M. and Multimore, J.E. 1962. Rumen gas analysis by gas solid chromatography. *Can. J. Anim. Sci.*, **41**, 187-192.

McDaniel, G. 1991. Effect of Yea-sacc®[1026] on reproductive performance of broiler breeder males and females. In *Biotechnology in the Feed Industry* (T.P. Lyons, ed.) pp. 413-415. Alltech Technical Publications, Nicholasville, Kentucky, US.

Mir, Y.S. and Mir, Z. 1992. Effect of addition of live-yeast culture (*Saccharomyces cerevisiae*) on feed digestibility, degradability in the rumen and performance of steers. *J. Anim. Sci..* **70** (Suppl. 1), 309. (Abstract).

Mould, F.L., Ørskov, E.R. and Mann, S.O. 1983. Associative effects of mixed feeds. I. Effects of type and level of supplementation and the influence of the rumen fluid pH on cellulolysis in vivo and dry matter digestion of various roughages. *Anim. Feed Sci. Technol.* **10**, 15-30.

Newbold, C.J. 1992. Probiotics: a new generation of rumen modifiers? *Med. Fac. Landbouww. Univ. Gent.* **57/4b**, 1925-1933.

Newbold, C.J. and Wallace, R.J. 1992. The effect of yeast and distillery by-products on the fermentation in the rumen simulation technique (Rusitec). *Anim. Prod.* **54**, 504. (Abstract).

Newbold, C.J., Williams, P.E.V., McKain, N., Walker, A. and Wallace, R.J. 1990. The effects of yeast culture on yeast numbers and fermentation in the rumen of sheep. *Proc. Nutr. Soc.* **49**, 47A. (Abstract).

Newbold, C.J., Brock, R. and Wallace, R.J. 1991. Influence of autoclaved or irradiated *Aspergillus oryzae* fermentation extract on the fermentation in the rumen simulation technique (Rusitec). *J. Agric. Sci., Camb.* **116**, 159-162.

Newbold, C.J., Frumholtz, P.P. and Wallace, R.J. 1992a. Influence of *Aspergillus oryzae* fermentation extract on rumen fermentation and blood constituents in sheep given diets of grass hay and barley. *J. Agric. Sci. Camb.* **119**, 423-427.

Newbold, C.J., Brock, R. and Wallace, R.J. 1992b. The effect of *Aspergillus oryzae* fermentation extract on the growth of fungi and ciliate protozoa in the rumen. *Lett. Appl. Microbiol.* **15**, 109-112.

Newbold, C.J., Wallace, R.J. and McIntosh, F.M. 1993. The stimulation of rumen bacteria by *Saccharomyces cerevisiae* is dependent on the respiratory activity of the yeast. *J. Anim. Sci.* **71** (Suppl. 1), 280. (Abstract).

Nisbet, D.J. and Martin, S.A. 1990. Effect of dicarboxylic acids and ·*Aspergillus oryzae* fermentation extract on lactate uptake by the ruminal bacterium *Selenomonas ruminantium*. *Appl. Environ. Microbiol.* **56**, 3515-3518.

Nisbet, D.J. and Martin S.A. 1991. The effect of *Saccharomyces cerevisiae* culture on lactate utilization by the ruminal bacterium *Selenomonas ruminantium*. *J. Anim. Sci.* **69**, 4628-4633.

Nisbet, D.J. and Martin, S.A. 1993. Effects of fumarate, L-malate, and an *Aspergillus oryzae* fermentation extract on D-lactate utilization by the ruminal bacterium *Selenomonas ruminantium*. *Curr. Microbiol.* **26**, 133-136.

Oellermann, S.O., Arambel, M.J., Kent, B.A. and Walters, J.L. 1990. Effect of graded amounts of *Aspergillus oryzae* fermentation extract on ruminal characteristics and nutrient digestibility in cattle. *J. Dairy Sci.* **73**, 2412-2416.

Panchal, C.J., Russell, I., Sills, A.M. and Stewart, G.G. 1984. Genetic manipulation of brewing and related yeast strains. *Food Technol* **38**, 99-111.

Piva, G., Fusconi, G. and Belladonna, S. 1993. Effect of yeast culture on milk yield and composition in dairy cows in late lactation. *J. Anim. Sci.* **71** (Suppl. 1), 288. (Abstract).

Quinonez, J.A., Bush, L.A., Nalsen. T. and Adams. G.D. 1988. Effect of yeast culture on intake and production of dairy cows fed high wheat rations. *J. Dairy Sci.* **71** (Suppl. 1), 275 (Abstract).

Ralph, J. and Helm, R.F. 1993. Lignin/hydroxycinnamic acid/polysaccharide complexes: synthetic models for regiochemical characterization. In *Forage Cell Wall Structure and Digestibility*. (H.G. Jung, D.R. Buxton, R.D. Hatfield, J. Ralph, eds.) pp. 201-246. ASA-CSSA-SSSA, Madison, US.

Robinson, J.A., Greening, R.C., Smolenski, W.J., Bell, R.L., Ogilvie, M.L. and Barsuhn, K. 1993. Effects of inoculum size of *Megasphaera elsdenii* 407A on ruminal pH, lactate and VFA in a bovine model of acute acidosis. *J. Anim. Sci.* **71** (Suppl 1), 269. (Abstract).

Rodriguez-Salazar, O., Herrera-Saldana, R., Gonzalez-Munoz, S. and Miranda-Romero, L.A. 1991. The effect of Yea-sacc® (*Saccharomyces cerevisiae*) on dry matter degradability and milk production. *J. Anim. Sci.* **74** (Suppl. 1), 105. (Abstract).

Roger, V., Fonty, G., Komisarczuk-Bony, S. and Gouet, P. 1990. Effects of physicochemical factors on the adhesion to cellulose (Avicel) of the ruminal bacteria *Ruminococcus flavefaciens* and *Fibrobacter succinogenes* subsp. *succinogenes*. *Appl. Environ. Microbiol.* **56**, 3081-3087.

Rose, A.H. 1987. Yeast culture, a microorganism for all species: a theoretical look at its mode of action. In *Biotechnology in the Feed Industry* (T.P. Lyons, ed.) pp. 113-118. Alltech Technical Publications, Nicholasville, Kentucky, US.

Russell, J.B. and Dombrowski, D.B. 1980. Effect of pH on the efficiency of growth by pure cultures of rumen bacteria in continuous culture. *Appl. Environ. Microbiol.* **39**, 604-610.

Russell, J.B. and Wilson, D.B. 1988. Potential opportunities and problems for genetically altered rumen microorganisms. J. Nutr. **118**, 271-279.

Russell, J.B., Sharp, W.M. and Baldwin, R.L. 1979. The effect of pH on maximum bacterial growth rate and its possible role as a determinant of bacterial competition in the rumen. *J. Anim. Sci.* **48**, 251-255.

Ryan, J.P. 1990. The suggestion that the yeast cell *Saccharomyces cerevisiae* may absorb sufficient hydrogen ions to increase ruminal pH is untenable. *Biochem. Soc. Trans.* **18**, 350-351.

Sievert, S.J. and Shaver, R.D. 1993. Effects of nonfiber carbohydrate level and *Aspergillus oryzae* fermentation extract on intake, digestion and milk production in lactating dairy cows. *J. Anim. Sci.* **71**, 1032-1040.

Slyter, L.L. 1976. Influence of acidosis on rumen function. *J. Anim. Sci.*, **43**, 910-929.

Spedding, A. 1991. Effects of Yea-sacc®[1026] on performance of beef bulls fed cereal or silage beef diets containing monensin. In *Biotechnology in the Feed Industry*, (T.P. Lyons, ed.) pp. 333-336. Alltech Technical Publications, Nicholasville, Kentucky, US.

St-Pierre, N.R., Easton, M.D. and Wolfe, B. 1993. Effect of feeding a combination of yeast culture, *A. oryzae* extracts and probiotics on lactating dairy cows. *J. Dairy Sci.* **76** (Suppl. 1), 281. (Abstract)

Stewart, C.S. 1977. Factors affecting the cellulolytic activity of rumen contents. *Appl.Environ. Microbiol.* **33**, 497-502.

Tapia, M.N., Herrera-Saldana, R., Mex, S., Russos, S., Viniegra, G and Gutierrez, M. 1989. The effect of four fungal compounds as probiotics on *in vitro* dry matter disappearance of different feedstuffs. *J. Anim. Sci.*, **67** (Suppl. 1), 521. (Abstract).

Teather, R.M. 1985. Application of gene manipulation to rumen microflors. *Can. J. Anim. Sci.* **65**, 563-574.

Teh, T.H., Sahlu, T., Escobar, E.N. and Cushaw, J.L. 1987. Effect of live yeast culture and sodium bicarbonate on lactating goats. *J. Dairy Sci.* **70** (Suppl. 1), 200. (Abstract).

Terrel, S.S., Vaughn, J.B., Bertrand, W.E., Knowles, R.P. and Bassham, H.H. 1984. On trial: an enzyme-producing food supplement for dogs. *Vet. Med. Small Anim. Pract.* **79**, 1733 - 1745.

Thomas, C. and Thomas, P.C. 1985. Factors affecting the nutritive value of grass silages. In Recent Advances In Animal Nutrition. (W. Haresign and D.J.S. Cole, eds.) pp. 223-256. Butterworths, London, UK.

Tutt, J.B. 1972. Acid silage as a probable cause of enteritis in a dairy herd. *Vet. Rec.* **90**, 91-92.

Van Horn, H.H., Harris, B., Taylor, M.J., Bachman, K.C. and Wilcox, C.J. 1984. By-product feeds for lactating dairy cows: effects of cottonseed hulls, sunflower hulls, corrugated paper, peanut hulls, sugercane bagasse and whole cottonseed with additives of fat, sodium bicarbonate and *Aspergillus oryzae* product on milk production. *J. Dairy Sci.* **67**, 2922-2938.

Varel, V.H. and Kreikemeier, K.K. 1993. Influence of feeding *Aspergillus oryzae* fermentation extract (Amaferm) on in situ fiber degradation, ruminal parameters and bacteria in non-lactating cows fed alfalfa or bromegrass hay. *J. Anim. Sci.* **71** (Suppl. 1), 287. (Abstract).

Varel, V.H., Jung, H.G. and Krumholtz, L.R. 1991. Degradation of cellulose and forage fiber fractions by ruminal cellulolytic bacteria alone and in coculture with phenolic monomer-degrading bacteria. *J. Anim. Sci.* **69**, 4993-5000.

Varel, V.H., Kreikemeier, K.K., Jung, H.G. and Hatfield, R.D. 1993. *In vitro* stimulation of forage fiber degradation by ruminal microorganisms with *Aspergillus oryzae* fermentation extract. *Appl. Environ. Microbiol.*, **59**, 3171-3176.

Wallace, R.J. and Newbold, C.J. 1992. Probiotics for ruminants. In *Probiotics: the Scientific Basis*. (R. Fuller, ed.) pp. 317-353. Chapman and Hall, London, UK.

Wallace, R.J. and Newbold, C.J. 1993. Rumen fermentation and its manipulation: the development of yeast cultures as feed additives. In *Biotechnology in the Feed Industry* (T.P. Lyons, ed.) pp. 173-192. Alltech Technical Publications, Nicholasville, Kentucky.

Wallace, R.J., Newbold, C.J. and McIntosh, F.M. 1993. Influence of *Saccharomyces cerevisiae* NCYC 240 and malic acid on bacterial numbers and fibre degradation in the sheep rumen. *J. Anim. Sci.*, **71** (Suppl.. 1), 287. (Abstract).

Wallentine, M.V., Johnston, N.P., Andrus, D., Jones, R., Huber, J.T. and Higginbotham, G. 1986. The effect of feeding an *Aspergillus oryzae* culture-vitamin mix on the performance of lactating dairy cows during periods of heat stresS. *J. Dairy Sci.* **69**, (Suppl. 1), 294. (Abstract).

Walsh, J.H. and Stewart, C.S. 1969. A simple method of the assay of cellulolytic activity of fungi. *International Biodeterioration Bulletin* **5**, 15-20.

Wanderley, R.C., Al-Dehneh, A., Theurer, C.B., DeYoung, D.W. and Huner, J.T. 1987. Fiber disappearance and nitrogen flow from the rumen of cows fed differing amounts of grain with or without fungal addition. *J. Dairy Sci.* **70** (Suppl. 1), 180. (Abstract).

Ware, D.R., Read, P.L. and Manfredi, E.T. 1988. Lactation performance of two large dairy herds fed *Lactobacillus acidophilus* strain BT 1386 in a switchback experiment. *J. Dairy Sci.* **71** (Suppl. 1), 219. (Abstract).

Weiss, D. 1991. Effect of Yea-sacc®[1026] on milk yield and composition at a German dairy. In *Biotechnology in the Feed Industry*. (T.P. Lyons, ed.) pp. 305-306. Alltech Technical Publications, Nicholasville, Kentucky, US.

Welch, R.O. and Calza, R.E. 1993. Amaferm stimulates the growth of the rumen fungus *Neocallimastix frontalis* ED188. *J. Anim. Sci.* **71** (Suppl..1), 280. (Abstract).

Wiedmeier, R.D. 1989. Optimizing the utilization of low-quality forages through supplementation and chemical treatment. In *9th Annual Utah Beef Cattle Field Day*, pp. 17-21. Brigham Young University, Provo, Utah, US.

Wiedmeier, R.D., Arambel, M.J., and Walters, J.L. 1987. Effect of yeast culture and Aspergillus oryzae fermentation extract on ruminal characteristics and nutrient digestibility. *J. Dairy Sci.* **70**, 2063-2068.

Williams, P.E.V. 1988. Understanding the biochemical mode of action of yeast culture. In *Biotechnology in the Feed Industry* (T.P. Lyons, ed.) pp. 79-100. Alltech Technical Publications, Nicholasville, Kentucky, US.

Williams, P.E.V. 1989. The mode of action of yeast culture in ruminant diets: a review of the effect on rumen fermentation patterns. In *Biotechnology in the Feed Industry,* (T.P Lyons, ed.), pp. 64-84. Alltech Technical Publications, Nicholasville, Kentucky.

Williams, P.E.V. and Newbold, C.J. 1990. Rumen probiosis: the effects of novel microorganisms on rumen fermentation and ruminant productivity. In *Recent Advances in Animal Nutrition* (W. Haresign and D.J.A. Cole, eds) pp. 211-227. Butterworths, London, UK.

Williams, P.E.V., Walker, A., and MacRae, J.C. 1990. Rumen probiosis: the effects of addition of yeast culture (viable yeast (*Saccharomyces cerevisiae*) plus growth medium) on duodenal protein flow in wether sheep. *Proc. Nutr. Soc.* **49**, 128A. (Abstract).

Williams, P.E.V., Tait, C.A.G., Innes, G.M. and Newbold, C.J. 1991. Effects of the inclusion of yeast culture (*Saccharomyces cerevisiae* plus growth medium) in the diet of dairy cows on milk yield and forage degradation and fermentation patterns in the rumen of sheep and steers. *J. Anim. Sci.*. **69**, 3016-3026.

Windschitl, P.M. 1992. Effects of probiotic supplementation of hull-less barley and corn based diets on bacterial fermentation in continous culture of ruminal contents. *Can. J. Anim. Sci.* **72**, 265-272.

Wohlt, J.E., Finkelstein, A.D. and Chung, C.H. 1991. Yeast culture to improve intake, nutrient digestibility and performance by dairy cattle during early lactation. *J. Dairy Sci.* **74**, 1395-1400.

14 Transgenic plants with improved energy characteristics

Claire Halpin, Geoffrey A. Foxon and P. Anthony Fentem

Plant Biotechnology Section, Zeneca Seeds, Jealott's Hill Research Station, Bracknell, Berks RG12 6EY, UK

INTRODUCTION

In writing this review the authors are conscious that it may well be out of date by the time of its publication. There are many projects engineering transgenic plants that are in progress but where results are not yet available. In addition, transformation of important crop plants such as maize, wheat and barley only has become possible in recent years (Fromm *et al.*, 1990; Gordon-Kamm *et al.*, 1990; Vasil *et al.*, 1992). As a consequence it is anticipated that there will be a rapid increase in the number of reports of "improved" transgenic crop plants in the near future.

This review is restricted to alterations in energy-limiting characteristics of major economic importance such as cell wall digestibility and starch and oil content. All the progress in improving these characteristics in crop plants has so far been achieved by conventional plant breeding. The use of mutants, both induced and naturally occurring, has also played an important role in these breeding programmes. Attempts to augment these programmes by transgenic techniques are as yet in their infancy. This review will therefore try to present a balanced view of transgenic approaches in the context of the other methodologies available to the plant breeder.

Strategies for trait manipulation in transgenic plants

A number of strategies exist for manipulating the activity of biochemical pathways, and hence phenotypic quality traits, by genetic engineering. By introducing extra copies of an endogenous gene, plants can be induced to over-express the protein encoded by that gene (e.g. Shah *et al.*, 1986). If the protein is a rate-limiting enzyme for the synthesis of an important energy product such as starch, this may result in an increased accumulation of that product. Activities of endogenous enzymes may also be extended in duration, or introduced into other plant organs by reinsertion of the gene linked to alternative promoter sequences. In addition the activities of enzymes can be down-regulated by introducing antisense RNA (Smith *et al.*, 1988; Van der Kroll *et al.*, 1989) which is complementary to and binds to the endogenous messenger RNA for the target enzyme, preventing its translation (Murray and Crockett, 1992). A similar effect can be provided by a different method, by the introduction of partial length sense genes (Smith *et al.*, 1990). At its most sophisticated, the transgenic approach facilitates the introduction into crop plants of novel enzymic activities and, indeed, entire novel biochemical pathways, enabling the synthesis of new high-energy products.

Advantages and disadvantages of the transgenic approach

Plants with improved energy content can of course be obtained using classical breeding approaches linked to biochemical measurements of the components of interest. Near infra red analysis (NIR), for example, is increasingly being used to screen maize genotypes for improved cell wall digestibility (Russell *et al.*, 1989). The screen and breed approach is well established and proven. This is not yet the case for molecular approaches. A prerequisite for any transgenic experiment is knowledge of the biochemistry of the pathway which is to be manipulated, including the determination of rate-limiting or control points. Genes encoding the enzymes involved in these reactions then have to be cloned from either cDNA or genomic DNA libraries. Promoter sequences which will control expression in the correct plant tissue at the desired developmental time have either to be selected or isolated as have sequences encoding targeting information which will direct the activity to the appropriate subcellular compartment. Finally, efficient methods have to be developed for transforming and regenerating the crop species and variety of interest. Although enormous potential exists for the use of transgenic methodologies in improving crop varieties, for many applications these prerequisites have not yet been met. This uncertainty of success has been a deterrent to industrial companies when considering investment in research to generate an improved plant by genetic engineering. In addition, tight regulatory controls have to be complied with in the release of transgenic material which inevitably delays the progress of a new plant variety to commercial exploitation.

Despite these problems, genetic engineering has many advantages over conventional breeding for the production of novel crop varieties and may indeed be the only way to improve certain traits. Many useful genetic mutations are recessive, making it difficult and time-consuming to breed them into high-yielding varieties especially in polyploid crops. This problem can be overcome using antisense or truncated sense technologies since these types of introduced genes act as dominant suppressors regardless of the ploidy level or the copy number of the target gene. In addition, antisense experiments typically produce plants with a range of phenotype, from near total suppression of the activity of interest to marginal effects. This enables an analysis of how much inhibition of activity is necessary to produce the desired phenotype and facilitates the selection of plants for further breeding or commercialisation. This level of control is not possible using conventional mutation techniques where there may be a total or an inappropriate level of loss of gene expression. Even in situations where conventional breeding of an improved character is comparatively simple, the transgenic approach may offer the potential for directly modifying high-yielding disease-resistant varieties, considerably reducing development times.

IMPROVING CELL WALL DIGESTIBILITY

Lignin and plant digestibility

While the cell contents of forage plants are completely digestible, the nutritional value of the cell wall varies considerably between species and even between tissues. The wall is composed of structural carbohydrates in grasses (predominantly cellulose and glucuronoarabinoxylan), protein and lignin. It has been known for a long time that as a plant tissue ages and becomes progressively more lignified there is a reduction in cell wall digestibility of that tissue. This relationship has been exemplified in many forage plants including maize (Phipps and Weller, 1979; Reeves, 1987), alfalfa (Reeves, 1987; Buxton and Russell, 1988) and several grass species (Jung and Vogel, 1986; Buxton and Russell, 1988). In maize, an increase of 2.8% to 5.0% in lignin resulted in a decreased degradability from 65% to 18% (Cone and Engles, 1990). However, the composition and distribution of lignin in different cell types is probably as important as the absolute amount present. In particular the syringyl component of lignin (derived from sinapyl alcohol) has been shown to account for a greater proportion of the variability in digestibility between grasses than is accounted for by the total lignin concentration (Reeves, 1985). In addition, the observation that in grass species, treatment of wall material with alkali increases its digestibility has focused attention on the role of alkali-extractable phenolic acids such as ferulic and *p*-coumaric acid in limiting digestibility (Hartley, 1972; Burritt *et al.*, 1984). These phenolics have been implicated in potential cross-linking between cell wall polymers. In particular, ferulic acid and its dimers may be responsible for cross-linking polysaccharides and lignin (Scalbert *et al.*, 1985; Lam *et al.*, 1992a,b). The reason why phenolic compounds decrease cell wall digestibility is not understood but may be related to a reduction of pore size in the cell wall caused by these lignin-carbohydrate cross-links. Pore size has been correlated with limitation of degradative enzyme diffusion in primary cell walls (McCann *et al.*, 1990). In addition, phenolic acids have been shown to be mildly toxic to the rumen microflora (Akin *et al.*, 1988). Clearly, manipulating the content and composition of lignin in plant cell walls is a valid target for increasing plant digestibility.

Target enzymes for manipulating lignin biosynthesis

Lignin biosynthesis might be altered by decreasing the activity of lignin biosynthetic enzymes with antisense RNA technology. This could provide a means of decreasing the total amount of lignin deposited or of altering its composition to improve forage digestibility. Genes for a number of enzymes on the lignin pathway have been isolated, but not all of these offer suitable targets for down-regulation. Lignin is a product of the phenylpropanoid pathway (Fig. 1) which also supplies phenolic precursors for other important compounds such as anthocyanins (providing protection from UV light), phytoalexins (important in disease resistance), flavonoids and tannins (Hahlbrock and Scheel, 1989). The enzyme phenylalanine ammonia-lyase (PAL) controls the entry to the phenylpropanoid pathway and is highly regulated during plant development. It is likely that interfering with PAL levels would affect many biological functions and might be seriously deleterious to the plant. This was confirmed by Elkind *et al.* (1990) who introduced a heterologous bean PAL gene into tobacco under the control of the constitutively expressed cauliflower mosaic virus (CaMV) 35S promoter. Paradoxically many of the transgenic plants produced had lower than normal PAL activity and a corresponding reduced lignin deposition in stem xylem. However the plants also exhibited a number of unusual and aberrant phenotypes including stunted growth, altered leaf shape and texture, reduced pollen viability and altered flower morphology and pigmentation. Clearly alteration of PAL activity has too many diverse effects to be useful and the same is probably true for the other early enzyme on the lignin pathway, cinnamate 4-hydroxylase (C4H).

After PAL and C4H there follows a series of hydroxylation and methylation reactions (catalysed by the enzymes cinnamate 3-hydroxylase (C3H), ferulate 5-hydroxylase (F5H) and an O-methyltransferase (OMT)) that produce ferulic and sinapic acid from *p*-coumaric acid. These three acid derivatives undergo a series of reductions giving rise to the three cinnamyl alcohols or monolignols, coumaryl, coniferyl and sinapyl alcohols, which are the basic building blocks for lignin. The monolignols are thought to be exported to the cell wall where they undergo peroxidase- or laccase-catalysed polymerisation. Again, few of the enzymes concerned in these reactions are thought to be dedicated solely to lignin (and lignan) biosynthesis and therefore make poor targets for specific trait manipulation. Only the enzymes cinnamoyl-CoA reductase (CCR) and cinnamyl alcohol dehydrogenase (CAD)

Figure 1. Lignin biosynthetic pathway in higher plants. PAL, phenylalanine ammonia-lyase; C4H, cinnamate 4-hydroxylase; C3H, cinnamate 3-hydroxylase; OMT, O-methyltransferase; F5H, ferulate 5-hydroxylase; CCR, cinnamoyl-CoA reductase; CAD, cinnamyl alcohol dehydrogenase.

function after all possible branch points in the pathway. In addition, while a number of different O-methyltransferases exist in plant tissues, one bispecific isozyme is thought to be responsible for the two methylation reactions in lignin precursor biosynthesis (Bugos *et al.*, 1991; Gowri *et al.*, 1991). Blocking one of these steps might be expected to produce a plant potentially deficient in lignin, or having lignin with an altered monomer composition. Manipulation of the polymerisation of precursors into lignin is also a possibility provided that lignin-specific peroxidases and laccases could be identified. Finally, specific transferases may be involved in attaching *p*-coumaric and ferulic acid to grass cell wall polymers (Kohler and Kauss, 1992), although there has been little research in this area to date.

Mutant plants with improved digestibility

The feasibility of improving forage digestibility through manipulation of lignin biosynthesis is supported by studies on low-lignin or brown midrib mutants (*bmr*) which have been found or induced in a number of forage species including maize (4 independent lines: bm_1, bm_2, bm_3 and bm_4) sorghum (3 lines: bmr_6, bmr_{12} and bmr_{18}) and pearl millet (1 line). The data concerning these mutants has been comprehensively reviewed by Cherney *et al.* (1991). The brown midrib mutants are characterised by a red-brown colour in lignified tissues such as leaf midribs and stem sclerenchyma. This unusual phenotype is associated with reduced quantities of lignin (Muller *et al.*, 1971) and a corresponding increase in digestibility (Barnes *et al.*,

1971) whether measured *in vivo* or *in vitro*. In addition, feeding trials have shown that intake of brown midrib silage is increased compared to normal silage (Muller *et al.*, 1972). Despite these substantial benefits, brown-midrib plants have not been extensively used in conventional breeding programmes since the *bmr* trait appears to be adversely linked to yield, *bmr* plants giving lower grain and stover yields than their normal counterparts.

Biochemical evidence suggests that *bmr* plants are deficient in lignin biosynthetic enzymes, most likely due to mutation in one of the genes encoding these enzymes. The best studied case is that of maize bm_3 which has been shown to be severely deficient in catechol O-methyl transferase with only 10% of the activity found in normal plants (Grand *et al.*, 1985). Both OMT and CAD activities are apparently lower in sorghum bmr_6 (Bucholtz *et al.*, 1980; Pillonel *et al.*, 1991). Work in this laboratory has shown that OMT activity is also lower in sorghum bmr_{12} and bmr_{18}, and that CAD activity is lower in maize bm_1. The maize CAD cDNA has been cloned and the position of the CAD gene within the maize genome can now be mapped. The identification of the maize CAD cDNA and also a maize OMT clone (Collazo *et al.*, 1992) may enable genetic engineering to be used as a rapid alternative to conventional breeding for introducing low-lignin improved digestibility traits into elite crops. Expression of antisense RNA can be used specifically to decrease the expression of these enzymes, allowing potentially a range of new *bmr* effects. This approach may have the benefits of separating the improved digestibility of *bmr* from the reduction in yield if these two traits are not causally related.

Transgenic plants with altered lignin

Transformation of crops such as maize has only very recently been achieved and is still not routine. In consequence many investigators have concentrated on trait manipulation in more accessible material such as tobacco, which is easy to transform (Horsch *et al.*, 1985). "Proof of concept" can more rapidly be achieved in such material to underpin the more difficult and lengthy progress towards commercial crop improvement. Work in this laboratory has concentrated on analysing the effects of decreased CAD activity in tobacco plants expressing CAD antisense RNA. Lignin from these plants has been shown to be modified both in composition and structure although the total amount of lignin is not obviously altered (Halpin *et al.*, 1993). Interestingly, plants with very low CAD activity (15% of normal or less) show a strong red-brown pigmentation in the xylem ring, similar to the phenotype of brown midrib mutants. Increased quantities of cinnamyl aldehydes, especially sinapyl aldehyde have been detected in the transgenic plant lignin. Incorporation of aldehydes into lignin has previously been shown to occur in the low CAD/low OMT brown midrib mutant sorghum bmr_6 (Pillonel *et al.*, 1991). These similarities with the *bmr* phenotype suggest that reduction of CAD activity by genetic manipulation in elite forages may lead to improved digestibility.

In experiments similar to those described above, other groups have attempted to genetically manipulate OMT activity in tobacco which, if the brown-midrib model holds true, should also lead to digestibility improvements. Dwivedi *et al.* (1993) showed that both the monomer composition and the quantity of lignin is reduced in tobacco plants expressing antisense RNA for OMT. Plants reduced in OMT activity by 15-35% apparently had, on average, 9% less total lignin than control plants with a reduction of 15% in syringyl monomers (from sinapyl alcohol). Whether or not these plants are improved in digestibility has not been determined.

Several reports describe the effects of altering peroxidase gene expression in transgenic plants.

Lagrimini *et al.* (1990) overproduced the major anionic peroxidase of tobacco by introducing a chimeric peroxidase gene under the control of the constitutively expressed CaMV 35S promoter. The resulting plants had ten-fold increased peroxidase activity and higher than usual levels of lignin in normal and wounded pith tissue (Lagrimini, 1991). No examination of lignin levels in other tissues was reported. Transformed plants also had the unique phenotype of chronic severe wilting, through loss of turgor in leaves, which was initiated at time of flowering. Sherf *et al.* (1993) tried to decrease the activity of a peroxidase thought to be important in suberin formation by expressing an antisense gene in tomato. Although all detectable activity of the specific peroxidase was eliminated, no change in suberin composition or deposition was found. These studies highlight the difficulty in determining and manipulating the specific role of enzymes for which related isozymes of similar or identical function exist. In fact one recent report (Beffa *et al.*, 1993) demonstrated that, in situations like this, plants can compensate for a deficiency in enzyme activity induced by antisense technology by producing a functionally equivalent replacement protein. This strongly suggests that only single or low copy number genes may be appropriate targets for efficient antisense down-regulation.

IMPROVING NON-STRUCTURAL CARBOHYDRATES

Storage carbohydrates in animal feeds

Non-structural carbohydrates are important determinants of the energy value of crops used in animal feeds. The major carbohydrate stored in the endosperm of feed grains such as maize, sorghum, and barley is, of course, starch. While plant breeding has produced varieties or hybrids in which starch constitutes up to 80% of seed weight, there is potential to increase this still further, by a combination of plant breeding and biotechnology. In vegetative tissues of crops harvested for forage the amounts of starch and water-soluble carbohydrates (WSC) present strongly influence energy content. The actual carbohydrates stored vary according to the plant species and the tissue concerned. Thus starch and WSC (primarily sucrose) are quantitatively equally important as storage carbohydrates in the leaves of maize, as well as a number of temperate grasses studied (Chatterton *et al.*, 1989). WSC in maize stalks are, however, almost entirely composed of sucrose and glucose (Setter and Flannigan, 1986). Leaves and stems of a number of grass species additionally store high concentrations of oligomers of fructose collectively referred to as fructans or levans (β-2,6-linked polymers of D-fructofuranose units).

It is important to understand the mechanisms which control the synthesis and metabolism of stored non-structural carbohydrates in both grain and vegetative tissues in order to increase their concentrations by biotechnological means. The cloning of a number of genes for enzymes involved in carbohydrate biochemistry has now been achieved and it is possible to generate transgenic plants in which the activities of these enzymes are either enhanced or in different tissues. By this method the mechanisms limiting carbohydrates composition can be elucidated, opening the way to the creation of genetically engineered crops with enhanced content of these storage compounds.

Target enzymes for manipulating starch biosynthesis

The rate and duration of starch synthesis in grain crops are determined by activities of the enzymes of the starch synthesis pathway in the developing endosperm. Starch synthesis from hexose phosphates takes place in specialised plastids known as amyloplasts. The amyloplast enzymes which are exclusively involved in synthesising starch are ADP glucose (ADPG) pyrophosphorylase, soluble and granule-bound forms of starch synthase, and branching enzyme isoforms. These enzymes are considered to regulate the amount of starch synthesised and much attention has been paid to their biochemical and molecular characterisation.

ADPG pyrophosphorylase has been proposed to control the rate of starch synthesis in green tissues. The enzyme is subject to allosteric inhibition by phosphate and activation by 3-phosphoglycerate. These properties are important in regulating the flux to starch in response to short term changes in light intensity (Preiss, 1982). Short term regulation of flux to starch is not so important in non-photosynthetic tissues such as maize endosperm, where starch synthesis is cumulative, building up over several days, followed by a period where the rate steadily declines toward grain maturity. In such tissues, regulation of the synthesis of starch enzymes is proposed to play a major role in governing flux, rather than short term regulation of enzyme activity. Nonetheless, when care is taken to prevent proteolytic degradation during its isolation, ADPG pyrophosphorylase from maize endosperm has been demonstrated to be regulated by phosphate and 3-phosphoglycerate (Plaxton and Preiss, 1987), and has been proposed to play a role in regulating starch synthesis in this tissue. This tetrameric enzyme is composed of two different subunits. Genes encoding these subunits have been cloned from many sources including maize (Smith-White and Preiss, 1992), wheat (Olive *et al.*, 1989) and potato (Mueller-Roeber *et al.*, 1990).

Starch synthases are also proposed to play a role in regulating the flux of starch precursors. These enzymes occur in both a soluble form and a form which is bound to the starch granule. The relationships between these two forms of the enzyme have recently received attention (Smith, 1990). The individual roles of soluble starch synthase isoforms and granule bound starch synthase in building up the starch granule are now being elucidated (Maddelein *et al.*, 1993). The soluble forms of starch synthase are unusually temperature labile and have been suggested to limit starch synthesis particularly at high temperatures (Jenner *et al.*, 1993). The "waxy" gene, considered to encode granule bound starch synthase (but see Smith, 1990) has been cloned for some years (Shure *et al.*, 1983). Soluble starch synthase isoforms have been purified from peas (Denyer and Smith, 1992) and maize (Ma *et al.*, 1992) and the corresponding genes will shortly be cloned.

Branching enzymes both determine the branching structure of starch and influence the amount of starch synthesised by determining the number of starch chains available for elongation by starch synthases. The branching enzyme isoforms found in maize have been purified, their individual roles in starch branching determined (Guan and Preiss, 1993a) and the genes for these polypeptides cloned (Guan and Preiss, 1993b). Genes for branching enzyme isoforms have also been cloned from pea (Bhattacharya *et al.*, 1990) and potato (Kossman *et al.*, 1991).

Attempts to manipulate the of these enzymes, by over-expression of the genes, by insertion of "similar" genes from other organisms, or by down-regulation of the genes by RNA antisense techniques, should reveal the "flux control coefficients" of the starch pathway enzymes. This should, in turn, identify the best means of increasing the amount of starch laid down in starchy tissues. Attempts so far have been restricted to the manipulation of ADPG pyrophosphorylase.

Transgenic plants with altered starch content

In transgenic potato plants containing an antisense gene to ADPG pyrophosphorylase under the control of a constitutive promoter, the activity of the enzyme in tubers was reduced to 2-5% of wild type (Mueller-Roeber *et al.*, 1992). The tuber starch content correspondingly declined to 2-5% of wild type and this decrease was accompanied by a large increase in the soluble sugar content of the tuber. Interestingly there was a massive reduction in the expression of storage protein genes suggesting that the control of protein synthesis and starch synthesis is in some way linked.

While demonstrating the importance of ADPG pyrophosphorylase in synthesising starch in storage tissues, these results do not indicate the "control strength" of the enzyme. This would require studies of a number of plants with the enzyme down-regulated to different extents. An alternative, more useful, approach is to increase the enzyme expressed in plant tissues. This has been achieved in potato (Stark *et al.*, 1992) where expression has been obtained of a mutated *E. coli* ADPG pyrophosphorylase gene (which differs in its allosteric control from the plant enzyme) fused to a plastid-targeted transit peptide under the control of a tuber specific promoter. This resulted in tubers with starch content increased by 35-60%, without any effects on the growth and development of the rest of the plant. While demonstrating the importance of the allosteric regulation of ADPG pyrophosphorylase in determining starch synthesis rate in potato tubers, these results cannot yet be extrapolated to other starchy tissues, such as maize and barley endosperm. Similar experiments with ADPG pyrophosphorylase in transgenic corn will shortly be performed and the isolation of starch synthase and branching enzyme genes means that similar experiments with these enzymes will be made in the near future.

Target enzymes for manipulating sucrose accumulation

Levels of sucrose and glucose accumulated in different plant tissues are regulated by the activities of the enzymes catalysing sucrose synthesis, membrane proteins controlling the transport and sequestration of sucrose within the tissues and the rates of sucrose catabolism. The key enzyme regulating the rate of sucrose synthesis is sucrose phosphate synthase. The gene for this enzyme has been cloned from maize (Worrel *et al.*, 1991) and spinach (Klein *et al.*, 1993). Sucrose synthase plays a role in determining the rate of sucrose metabolism in sink tissues and in regulating unloading of sucrose from the phloem. Genes for this enzyme have been cloned from a number of sources including maize (Werr *et al.*, 1985) and potato (Salanoubat and Balliard, 1987). Invertase activity is involved in the catabolism of sucrose to hexoses in sink tissues, and the gene has been cloned from plant sources such as tomato (Klann *et al.*, 1993). Rates of sucrose import by cells of storage tissues and sucrose sequestration into the vacuoles of these cells are regulated by membrane bound sucrose carrier proteins. A sucrose-proton symport protein has been cloned from spinach leaves (Riesmeier *et al.*, 1992) and it is to be expected that transporters from other sources will be cloned in the near future.

Transgenic plants with altered sugar content

In recent experiments transgenic plants have been created with altered activities of enzymes involved in sucrose synthesis and the effects on carbohydrate partitioning measured. The maize leaf sucrose phosphate synthase gene has been cloned into transgenic tomato plants

(Micallef *et al.*, 1993). The increased enzyme activity in the leaves resulted in an increased partitioning of carbohydrate into the fruit. Tomato plants have also been created that express an invertase antisense gene in the fruit (Klann *et al.*, 1993). The low invertase activity resulted in high sucrose, low hexose fruit, and field trials are being conducted to see whether total sugar content is enhanced. Transgenic tobacco plants have been created expressing a yeast invertase gene either in the cytosol, vacuole or apoplast (Sonnewald *et al.*, 1993). In all cases expression in leaves caused an increase in the content of both starch and sugars. Sucrose export from the leaves, however, was impaired and resulted in a depression in photosynthesis.

While these experiments are preliminary, and have not involved plants used for animal feeds, genetic engineering aimed at increasing partitioning into storage carbohydrates in tissues of forage crops is likely in the near future.

Target enzymes for manipulating fructan biosynthesis

Fructans are major storage carbohydrates in the leaves and stems of many temperate grass species. They occur in high molecular weight forms in some grasses (*Dactylus* and *Phleum* spp.) and lower molecular weight forms in others (*Lolium* and *Festuca* spp.). Synthesis of fructans from sucrose requires two distinct fructosyl transferase enzymes (Pollock and Cairns, 1991). The first, sucrose-sucrose fructosyl transferase (SST), transfers fructose residues from sucrose to the terminal fructose residues of an acceptor, initially sucrose and then the growing fructan chain, leading to an increased number of β-2,6 fructose-fructose bonds. The second enzyme, fructan-fructan fructosyl transferase (FFT), catalyses transfructosylation between fructans leading to chain elongation, but not to a net synthesis of fructan. Identification and isolation of SST has so far proved difficult due to contaminating β-fructofuranosidase activities. FFT has recently been extracted and assayed from wheat (Pollock and Housely, 1993). It will be a little time however before fructan synthetic enzymes are purified and the genes cloned, allowing manipulation of the amounts of these compounds in transgenic plants.

INCREASING SEED OIL CONTENT

Increasing the oil content of oilseeds is undoubtedly a means of increasing their potential energy value. However, oil crops such as soya, sunflower and rapeseed commonly find their way into animal feeds as processed products, usually seed meal, rather than as whole seed. The relationship between enhanced seed oil content and the energy value of the crop is therefore not a simple one. This relationship is more direct in a crop such as maize, where the oil-containing seed is fed directly to livestock.

Contribution of conventional breeding

Increasing the proportion of oil in maize grain has for many years been proposed as a means of increasing the energy value for animal feed. Traditional plant breeding and selection methods (Alexander, 1988) have developed "Illinois High Oil" lines from Burrs White, Alexho Synthetic, Stiff Stalk and Reid Yellow Dent lines with kernel oil content raised from 4% to 21%. In hybrids produced using these lines seed oil content can be raised up to 8% without adversely affecting yield. Raising the oil content higher than 8% has been found to decrease yield. However, it is not known whether this yield depression is a physiological consequence of the high oil content, or merely because high oil content was selected without adequate attention to other parameters affecting yield and stress resistance.

High oil corns have been found to increase gain:feed ratios in broiler chicks and egg number:feed ratios in laying hens (Han *et al.*, 1987). Significant increases in gain:feed ratios were also recorded in young pigs and growing-finishing swine (Adams and Jensen, 1987).

In the high oil corns so far derived, oil content has been raised primarily by increasing the size of the germ (embryo and scutellum) with respect to the endosperm. This trait is associated with slower loss of water during grain maturation and consequent high water content at harvest. As well as being a problem during grain storage, this causes disease problems. In addition, handling and transport of the seed is difficult due to the potential for damage to the large embryos. These problems could be reduced if high oil corn lines could be produced with "normal" size embryos containing a higher concentration of oil. In producing such lines, traditional plant breeding could be augmented considerably by genetic engineering.

Target enzymes for manipulating seed oil content

The oil content of the maize embryo is determined by the rate and duration of oil synthesis during grain growth. The onset of oil synthesis in developing oilseeds is accompanied by an induction of the enzymes of fatty acid synthesis, while the decline in oil synthesis late in grain filling is accompanied by a decline in fatty acid synthetic capacity. It has been proposed that the rate of oil synthesis is limited by the activities of these enzymes while the duration is determined by the period over which these enzymes remain active. Genes for a number of the component enzymes of the fatty acid synthetic pathway have recently been cloned, for example acyl carrier protein (ACP) (Safford *et al.*, 1988), ß-ketoacyl ACP reductase (Slabas *et al.*, 1992), enoyl reductase (Slabas and Fawcett, 1992) and condensing enzymes (Kinney *et al.*, 1993).

The enzyme acetyl CoA carboxylase (ACCase) is widely accepted to control the rate of fatty acid synthesis in animal tissues. Studies on metabolite concentrations in chloroplasts suggest that this enzyme also has a high "flux control coefficient" in leaves (Post-Beitenmiller *et al.*, 1992). It has been proposed that ACCase controls the rate of lipid synthesis in developing oilseeds. The coincidence of the decline of ACCase activity with the drop in lipid synthetic capacity in developing rapeseed suggests that the enzyme also regulates the duration of oil synthesis. Genes coding for ACCase have been cloned from rapeseed, wheat (Elborough *et al.*, 1994), maize and *Arabidopsis* (Yanai *et al.*, 1993). Increased oil deposition in the corn embryo may therefore result from over-expression of ACCase via insertion of extra gene copies. Promoter elements such as those from the ACP gene have been isolated to target expression of the transgenes to the developing embryo. Extending the duration of ACCase activity will be achievable by reinserting the gene under the control of a "late seed development" promoter such as those isolated from storage protein genes.

CONCLUSIONS

The biochemical pathways, for the synthesis of key plant components affecting energy characteristics (lignin, carbohydrates and oils) have been established. Strategies for increasing the energy content of plant material have been postulated based on knowledge of these pathways, and on biochemical studies of the "flux control coefficients" of individual enzymes. In many cases the genes encoding these enzymes have now been isolated and cloned. It is therefore possible to alter the activities of these enzymes in transgenic plants and examine their influence on plant composition. Such studies have so far been limited to "models", using easily transformed plants such as tobacco and potato. The rapid progress in transformation of plants used for animal feed such as maize, wheat and barley means that similar manipulations can now be undertaken in these crops and the potential for improving their energy content can be evaluated.

REFERENCES

Adams, K.L. and Jensen, A.H. 1987. High-fat maize diets for pigs and sows. *Anim. Feed Sci. Technol.* **17**, 201-212.

Akin, D.E., Rigsby, L.L., Theodorou, M.K. and Hartley, R.D. 1988. Population changes of fibrolytic rumen bacteria in the presence of phenolic acids and plant extracts. *Anim. Feed Sci. Technol.* **19**, 261-275.

Alexander, D.E. 1988. Breeding special nutritional and industrial types. In *Corn and Corn Improvement* (Sprague, G.F. and Dudley, J.W., eds.) pp. 869-880. American Society of Agronomy, Crop Science of America and Soil Science Society of America, Inc., US.

Barnes, R.F., Muller, L.D., Bauman, L.F. and Colenbrander, V.F. 1971. *In vitro* dry matter disappearance of brown midrib mutants of maize (*Zea mays* L.). *J. Anim. Sci.* **33**, 881-884.

Beffa, R.S., Neuhaus, J.-M. and Meins, F. 1993. Physiological compensation in antisense transformants: specific induction of an "ersatz" glucan endo-1,3-β-glucosidase in plants infected with necrotizing virus. *Proc. Natl. Acad. Sci., USA* **90**, 8792-8796.

Bhattacharya, M.K., Smith, A.M., Ellis, T.H.N., Hedley, C. and Martin, C. 1990. The wrinkled-seed characteristic of pea described by Mendel is caused by a transposon-like insertion in a gene encoding starch-branching enzyme. *Cell* **60**, 115-122.

Bucholtz, D.L., Cantrell, R.P., Axtell, J.D. and Lechtenberg, V.L. 1980. Lignin biochemistry of normal and brown midrib mutant sorghum. *J. Agric. Food Chem.* **28**, 1239-1241.

Bugos, R.C., Chiang, V.L.C. and Campbell, W.H. 1991. cDNA cloning, sequence analysis and seasonal expression of lignin-bispecific caffeic acid/5-hydroxyferulic acid O-methyltransferase of aspen. *Plant Mol. Biol.* **17**, 1203-1215.

Burritt, E.A., Bittner, A.S., Street, J.C. and Anderson, M.J. 1984. Correlations of phenolic acids and xylose content of cell walls with in vitro dry matter digestibility of three maturing grasses. *J. Dairy Sci.* **67**, 1209-1213.

Buxton, D.R. and Russell, J.R. 1988. Lignin constituents and cell wall digestibility of grass and legume stems. *Crop Sci.* **28**, 553-558.

Chatterton N.J., Harrison P.A., Bennet J.H. and Asay K.H. 1989. Carbohydrate partitioning in 185 accessions of Gramineae grown under warm and cool temperatures. *J. Plant Physiol.* **134**, 169-179.

Cherney, J.H., Cherney, D.J.R., Akin, D.E. and Axtell, J.D. 1991. Potential of brown-midrib, low-lignin mutants for improving forage quality. *Adv. Agron.* **46**, 157-198.

Collazo, P., Montoliu, L., Puigdomenech, P. and Rigau J. 1992. Structure and expression of the lignin O-methyltransferase gene from *Zea mays* L. *Plant Mol. Biol.* **20**, 857-867.

Cone, J.W. and Engles, F.M. 1990. Influence of growth temperature on anatomy and in vitro digestibility of maize tissues. *J. Agric. Sci., Camb.* **114**, 207-212.

Denyer, K. and Smith, A.M. 1992 The purification and characterisation of two forms of soluble starch synthase from developing pea embryos. *Planta* **186**, 609-617.

Dwivedi, U.N., Yu, J., Datla, R.S.S., Campbell, W.H., Podila, G.K. and Chiang, V.L. 1993. Expression of lignin-specific aspen O-methyltransferase antisense gene in tobacco and woody species to reduce lignin content. In *Proceedings of the 7th International Symposium on Wood and Pulping Chemistry*. Vol. 2, pp. 633-639. Beijing, P.R. China.

Elborough, K., Simon, J.W., Swinhoe, R., and Slabas, A.R. 1994. Studies on wheat acetyl CoA carboxylase and the cloning of a partial cDNA. *Plant Mol. Biol.* **24**, 21-34.

Elkind, Y., Edwards, R., Mavandad, M., Hendrick, S.A., Dixon, R.A. and Lamb, C.J. 1990. Abnormal plant development and down-regulation of phenylpropanoid biosynthesis in transgenic tobacco containing a heterologous phenylalanine ammonia-lyase gene. *Proc. Natl. Acad. Sci., USA* **87**, 9057-9061.

Fromm, M.E., Morrish, F., Armstrong, C., Williams, R., Thomas, J. and Klein, T.M. 1990. Inheritance and expression of chimeric genes in progeny of transgenic maize plants. *Bio/technology* **8**, 833-839.

Gordon-Kamm, W.J., Spencer, T.M., Mangano, M.L., Adams, T.R., Daines, R.J., Start, W.G., O'Brien, J.V., Chambers, S.A., Adams, W.R., Willetts, W.G., Rice, T.B., Mackey, C.J., Krueger, E.W., Kausch, A.P. and Lemeux, P.G. 1990. Transformation of maize cells and regeneration of fertile transgenic plants. *Plant Cell* **2**, 603-618.

Gowri, G., Bugos, R.C., Campbell, W.H., Maxwell, C.A. and Dixon, R.A. 1991. Stress responses in Alfalfa (*Medicago sativa* L.). X. Molecular cloning and expression of S-adenosyl-L-methionine:caffeic acid 3-O-methyltransferase, a key enzyme of lignin biosynthesis. *Plant Physiol.* **97**, 7-14.

Grand, C.P., Pamentier, P., Boudet, A.. and Boudet. A.M. 1985. Comparisons of lignins and of enzymes involved in lignification in normal and brown midrib (bm_3) mutant corn seedlings. *Physiol. Veg.* **23**, 905-911.

Guan, H.P. and Preiss, J. 1993a. Differentiation of the properties of the branching isozymes for maize (*Zea mays*). *Plant Physiol.* **102**, 1269-1273.

Guan, H.P. and Preiss, J. 1993b. Differentiation of properties of maize branching isozymes. *Plant Physiology*. **102** (Suppl.), 52. (Abstract).

Hahlbrock, K. and Scheel, D. 1989. Physiology and molecular biology of phenylpropanoid metabolism. *Annu. Rev. Plant Physiol. Plant Mol. Biol.* **40**, 347-369.

Halpin, C., Knight, M.E., Schuch, W., Campbell, M.M. and Foxon, G.A. 1993. Manipulation of lignin biosynthesis in transgenic plants expressing cinnamyl alcohol dehydrogenase antisense RNA. *J.Cell Biochem.* Suppl. **17A**, 28. (Abstract).

Han, Y., Parsons, C.M. and Alexander, D.E. 1987. Nutritive value of high oil corn for poultry. *Poultry Sci.* **66**, 103-111.

Hartley, R.D. 1972. *p*-Coumaric and ferulic acid components of cell walls of ryegrass and their relationship with lignin and digestibility. *J. Sci. Food Agric.* **23**, 1347-1354.

Horsch, R.B., Fry, J.E., Hoffmann, N.L., Eicholtz, D., Rogers, S.G. and Fraley, R.T. 1985. A simple and general method for transferring genes into plants. *Science* **227**, 1229-1231.

Jenner, C.F., Siewek, K. and Hawker, J.S. 1993. The synthesis of [^{14}C]starch from [^{14}C]sucrose in isolated wheat grains is dependent upon the activity of soluble starch synthase. *Aust. J. Plant Physiol.* **20**, 329-335.

Jung, H.G. and Vogel, K.P. 1986. Influence of lignin on digestibility of forage cell wall material. *J. Anim. Sci.* **62**, 1703-1712.

Kinney, A.J., Hitz, W.D., Yadav, N.S. and Perez-Grau, L. 1993. Genes of fatty acid biosynthesis in developing oilseeds. *Plant Physiology* **102** (Suppl.), 1. (Abstract).

Klann, E.M., Chetelat, R. and Bennet A.B. 1993. Role of acid invertase as a determinant of sugar accumulation in transgenic tomato fruit. *Plant Physiol.* **102** (Suppl.) 32. (Abstract).

Klein, R.R., Crafts-Brandner, S.J. and Salvucci, M.E. 1993. Cloning and developmental expression of the sucrose phosphate-synthase gene from spinach. *Planta* **190**, 498-510.

Kohler, A. and Kauss, H.   1992.   Biosynthesis of hydroxycinnamate esters of cell wall polysaccharides in endomembranes from parsley cells. Abstracts of the Sixth Cell Wall Meeting (Sassens, M.M.A., Derksen, J.W.M., Emons, A.M.C. and Wolter-Arts, A.M.C., eds) p. 99. University Press, Nijmegen, Netherlands.

Kossman, J., Visser, R.G.F., Mueller-Roeber, B., Willmitzer, L. and Sonnewald, U. 1991. Cloning and expression analysis of a potato cDNA that encodes branching enzyme: evidence for co-expression of starch biosynthetic genes. *Mol. Gen. Genet.* **230**, 39-44.

Lagrimini, L.M.   1991.   Wound-induced deposition of polyphenols in transgenic plants overexpressing peroxidase. *Plant Physiol.* **96**, 577-583.

Lagrimini, L.M., Bradford, S. and Rothstein, S. 1990. Peroxidase-induced wilting in transgenic tobacco plants. *The Plant Cell* **2**, 7-18.

Lam, T. B. T., Iiyama, K. and Stone, B. A. 1992a. Cinnamic acid bridges between cell wall polymers in wheat and phalaris internodes. *Phytochemistry* **31**, 1179-1183.

Lam, T. B. T., Iiyama, K and Stone, B. A. 1992b. Changes in phenolic acids from internode walls of wheat and phalaris during maturation. *Phytochemistry* **31**, 2655-2658.

Ma, S., Ramamoorthy, R., Powers, J.R., Harriman, R.W., Preiss, J. and Wasserman, B.P. 1992. Purification and characterisation of soluble starch synthase from maize. Abstr. Papers Amer. Chem. Soc. **203**, 1-3.

Maddelein, M., Liebessart, N., Delrue, B., D'Hulst, C., Van den Koornhuyse, N., Decq, A. and Ball, S.G. 1993. Amylopectin type I and II define 2 independent steps for the building of the starch granule. *Plant Physiol.* **102** (Suppl.), 27. (Abstract).

McCann, M.C., Wells, B. and Roberts, K. 1990. Direct visualization of cross-links in the primary plant cell wall. *J. Cell Sci.* **96**, 323-324.

Micallef, B.J., Roh, K.S. and Sharkey, T.D. 1993. Altering photosynthetic performance in plants by genetically manipulating sucrose biosynthesis. *Plant Physiology* **102** (Suppl.), 32. (Abstract).

Mueller-Roeber, B.T., Kossman, J., Hannah, L.C., Willmitzer, L. and Sonnewald, U. 1990. One of two different ADP-glucose pyrophosphorylase genes from potato responds strongly to elevated levels of sucrose. *Mol. Gen. Genet.* **224**, 36-146.

Mueller-Roeber, B., Sonnewald, U. and Willmitzer, L. 1992. Inhibition of the ADP-glucose pyrophosphorylase in transgenic potatoes leads to sugar-storing tubers and influences tuber formation and expression of tuber storage protein genes. *EMBO Journal* **11**, 1229-1238.

Muller, L.D., Barnes, R.F., Bauman, L.F. and Colenbrander, V.F. 1971. Variations in lignin and other structural components of brown midrib mutants of maize (*Zea mays* L.). *Crop Sci.* **11**, 413-415.

Muller, L.D., Lechtenberg, V.L., Bauman, L.F., Barnes, R.F. and Rhykerd, C.L. 1972. *In vitro* evaluation of a brown midrib mutant of *Zea mays* L. *J. Anim. Sci.* **35**, 883-889.

Murray, J.A.H. and Crockett, N. 1992. Antisense techniques: an overview. In *Antisense RNA and DNA* (James, A.H. and Murray, E.D., eds) pp. 1-49. Wiley-Liss, Modern Cell Biology Series Vol. II, New York, US.

Olive, M.R. Ellis, R.J. and Schuch, W.W. 1989. Isolation and nucleotide sequences of cDNA clones encoding ADP-glucose pyrophosphorylase polypeptides from wheat leaf and endosperm. *Plant Mol. Biol.* **12**, 525-538.

Phipps, R.H. and Weller, R.F. 1979 The development of plant components and their effects on the composition of fresh and ensiled forage maize. 1. The accumulation of dry matter, chemical composition and the nutritive value of forage maize. *J. Agric. Sci., Camb.* **92**, 471-483.

Pillonel, C., Mulder, M.M., Boon, J., Forster, B. and Binder, A. 1991. Involvement of cinnamyl-alcohol dehydrogenase in the control of lignin formation in *Sorghum bicolor* L. Moench. *Planta* **185**, 538-544.

Plaxton, W.C. and Preiss, J. 1987. Purification and properties of nonproteolytic degraded ADP glucose pyrophosphorylase from maize endosperm. *Plant Physiol.* **83**, 105-112.

Pollock, C.J., and Cairns, A..J. 1991. Fructan metabolism in grasses and cereals. *Annu. Rev. Plant Physiol. Plant Mol. Biol.* **42**, 77-102.

Pollock, C.J. and Housely, T.L. 1993. The extraction and assay of 1-ketose:sucrose fructosyl transferase from leaves of wheat. *Plant Physiol.* **102**, 537-539.

Post-Beittenmiller, D., Roughan, G. and Ohlrogge, J.B. 1992. Regulation of plant fatty acid biosynthesis. Analysis of acyl coenzyme A and acyl-acyl carrier protein substrate pools in spinach and pea chloroplasts. *Plant Physiol.* **100**, 923-930.

Preiss, J. 1982. Biosynthesis of starch and its regulation. In *Encyclopaedia of Plant Physiology* Vol. 13A (F.A. Loewus and W. Tanner, eds) pp. 397-417. Springer Verlag, Berlin, Germany.

Reeves, J.B. 1985. Lignin composition and in vitro digestibility of feeds. *J. Anim. Sci.* **60**, 316-322.

Reeves, J.B. 1987. Lignin and fiber compositional changes in forages over a growing season and their effects on in vitro digestibility. *J. Dairy Sci.* **70**, 1583-1594.

Riesmeier, J.W., Willmitzer, L. and Frommer, W.B. 1992. Isolation and characterization of a sucrose carrier cDNA from spinach by functional expression in yeast. *EMBO Journal* **11**, 4705-4713.

Russell, J.D., Murray, I. and Frazer, A.Z. 1989. Near- and mid-infrared studies of the cell wall structure of cereal straw in relation to rumen degradability. In *Physico-chemical Characterisation of Plant Residues for Industrial and Feed Use* (A. Chesson, and E.R. Ørskov, eds) pp. 13-24. Elsevier Applied Science, London, UK.

Safford, R., Windust, J.H.C., Lucas, C., De Silva, J., James, C.M., Hellyer, A., Smith, C.G., Slabas, A.R. and Hughes, S.G. 1988. Plasmid-localised seed acyl-carrier protein of *Brassica napus* is encoded by a distinct, nuclear multigene family. *Eur. J. Biochem.* **174**, 287-295.

Salanoubat, M. and Balliard, G. 1987. Molecular cloning and sequencing of sucrose synthase cDNA from potato (*Solanum tuberosum* L.) a preliminary characterisation of sucrose synthase mRNA distribution. *Gene* **60**, 47-56.

Scalbert, A., Monties, B., Lallemand, J-Y., Guittet, E. and Rolando, C. 1985. Ether linkage between phenolic acids and lignin fractions from wheat straw. *Phytochemistry* **24**, 1359-1362.

Setter, T.L. and Flannigan, B.A. 1986. Sugar and starch redistribution in maize in response to shade and ear temperature treatment. *Crop Sci.* **26**, 575-579.

Shah, D.M., Horsch, R.B., Klee, H.J., Kishore, G.M., Winter, J.A., Turner, N.E., Hironaka, C.M., Sanders, P.R. Gasser, C.S., Aykent, S., Siegel, N.R., Rogers, S.G. and Fraley, R.T. 1986. Engineering herbicide tolerance in transgenic plants. *Science* **233**, 478-481.

Sherf, B.A., Bajar, A.M. and Kolattukudy, P.E. 1993. Abolition of an inducible highly anionic peroxidase activity in transgenic tomato. *Plant Physiol.* **101**, 201-208.

Shure, M., Wessler, S. and Fedoroff, N. 1983. Molecular identification and isolation of waxy locus in maize. *Cell* **35**, 225-233.

Slabas, A.R., Chase, D., Nishada, I., Murata, N., Sidebottom, C., Safford, R., Sheldon, P.S., Kekwick, R.G.O., Hardie, D.G. and Mackintosh, R.W. 1992. Molecular cloning of higher plant 3-oxoacyl-(acyl carrier protein) reductase. *Biochem. J.* **283**, 321-326.

Slabas, A.R. and Fawcett, T. 1992. The biochemistry and molecular biology of plant lipid biosynthesis. *Plant Mol. Biol.* **19**, 169-191.

Smith, A.M. 1990. Evidence that the 'waxy' protein of pea (*Pisum sativum* L.) is not the major starch-granule-bound starch synthase. *Planta* **182**, 599-604.

Smith, C.J.S., Watson, C.F., Bird, C.R., Ray, J., Schuch, W. and Grierson., D. 1990. Expression of a truncated tomato polygalacturonase gene inhibits expression of the endogenous gene in transgenic plants. *Mol. Gen. Genet.* **224**, 477-481.

Smith, C.J.S., Watson, C.F., Ray, J., Bird, C.R., Morris, P.C., Schuch, W. and Grierson, D. 1988. Antisense RNA inhibition of polygalacturonase gene expression in transgenic tomatoes. *Nature* **334**, 724-726.

Smith-White, B.J. and Preiss, J. 1992. Comparison of proteins of ADP glucose pyrophosphorylase from diverse sources. *J. Mol. Evolution* **34**, 449-464.

Sonnewald U., Schaewen, A. and Willmitzer, L. 1993. Subcellular manipulation of sucrose metabolism in transgenic plants. *J. Exp. Bot.* **44** (Suppl.) 293-296. (Abstract).

Stark, D.M., Timmerman, K.P., Barry, G.F., Preiss, J. and Kishore, G.M. 1992. Regulation of the amount of starch in plant tissues by ADP glucose pyrophosphorylase. *Science* **258**, 287-292.

Van der Kroll, A.R., Mol, J.N.M. and Stuitje, A.E. 1989. Modulation of eukaryotic gene expression by complementary RNA or DNA sequences. *Biotechniques* **6**, 958-976.

Vasil, V., Castillo, A.M., Fromm, M.E. and Vasil, I.K. 1992. Herbicide resistant fertile transgenic wheat plants obtained by microprojectile bombardment of regenerable embryonic callus. *Bio/technology* **10**, 667-674.

Werr, W., Frommer, W-B., Maas, S. and Starlinger, P. 1985. Structure of the sucrose synthase gene on chromosome 9 of *Zea mays* L. *EMBO Journal* **4**, 1373-1380.

Worrel, A.C., Bruneau, J-M. Summerfelt, K., Beresey, M. and Voelker, T.A. 1991. Expression of a maize sucrose phosphate synthase in tomato alters leaf carbohydrate partitioning. *Plant Cell* **3**, 1121-1130.

Yanai, Y., Mitsukawa, N., Liu, Y., Whittier, R. and Shimada, H. 1993. RFLP mapping of an Arabidopsis acetyl-CoA carboxylase gene. *Plant Physiol.* **102** (Suppl.), 382. (Abstract).

15 Dietary enzymes for increasing energy availability

Hadden Graham and Derick Balnave[1]

Finnfeeds International Ltd., Marlborough, Wiltshire SN8 1AA, UK, and [1]Department of Animal Science, University of Sydney, Camden, N.S.W. 2570, Australia

INTRODUCTION

Supplementary enzymes have been widely researched and used in diets for non-ruminants over the past decade, and developments relating to improvements in energy availability from feeds will be discussed in this chapter. Applications to ruminant diets have also started to attract attention, but little information is yet available. This area will not be dealt with in detail.

The full economic and nutritional value of the cereal grains has rarely been realised in non-ruminant feeding regimens. Often, growth rate and feed conversion fail to achieve their optimum potential, and litter quality is affected adversely when individual cereals are included at high concentrations in poultry diets (Pettersson, 1988; GrootWassink *et al.*, 1989). Poor nutrient utilisation, by young animals in particular, has been blamed on the compromising of the neonatal digestive system by cereal structural carbohydrates. These non-starch polysaccharides, and especially the arabinoxylans and mixed-linked β-glucans present in the endosperm cell walls of cereal grains, have been implicated as major causative factors in this response. The mechanisms by which these compounds are thought to interfere with digestion and the potential for feed enzymes to overcome such problems are discussed below.

Microbial enzymes

Microbial enzymes have been used widely used for over forty years in the food, brewing, textile and pulp manufacturing industries. These enzymes are produced in culture fermentations from specific bacteria or fungi. Due to the selection of natural mutants and, more recently, to intra- and inter-generic gene manipulation, microbes can be made to produce excessive quantities of one particular enzyme or group of enzymes. However, in their impure form as used in the feed industry, all enzyme products contain a range of activities. As shown in Table 1, two "cellulase" preparations derived from the same microorganism, *Trichoderma longibrachiatum*, differed considerably in their enzyme activities and, therefore, relative substrate specificities. Further, inappropriate enzyme activities in impure products can exert a positive or negative effect in an animal which is unrelated to the enzyme and substrate of interest. Enzyme products ideally should be characterised as completely as possible prior to use. However, it should be noted that reported enzyme activities are dependent on the conditions of the assay and, thus, laboratory tests often give a poor indication of the effectiveness of the enzyme(s) when fed to an animal.

Although the positive effects of microbial enzymes on animal production have been recognised for a number of years, it is only in the recent past that they have been used commercially. This development has been due mainly to two factors, a reduction in cost and an improvement in heat stability. The former is the result of the increasing production of enzymes for other industries. Their improved stability, resulting from better stabilisation processes, now allows enzymes to be added to feed prior to pelleting. Thus, properly stabilised feed enzymes can now survive feed conditioning at 85°C for 15 min followed immediately by steam pelleting (Graham and Inborr, 1992).

Table 1. Enzyme activities (units per g enzyme) analysed in two "cellulase" preparations derived from *Trichoderma longibrachiatum.*

Enzyme activity	Cellulase 1	Cellulase 2
Xylanase	450	7300
β-Glucanase	3700	810
Polygalacturonase	20	10
Arabinosidase	6	88
Protease	3900	1500

Production of digestive enzymes by animals

The processes of digestion, whereby complex feed components are broken down to constituents which can be absorbed and utilised by the animal, result from the action of the endogenous enzymes found throughout the gastro-intestinal tract. While amylase may be secreted in the saliva, the major sites of enzyme production in the animal are the stomach (proventriculus in birds), where acid proteases are produced; the pancreas, where most of the lipase, amylase and proteases are secreted; and the mucosa of the small intestine, where enzymes such as disaccharidases and peptidases are found. Thus, animals produce enzymes capable of digesting all major feed components with the exception of the fibre fraction. The microbial population of the hind-gut of non-ruminants produces an array of enzymes, including those capable of degrading fibre. However, this degradation occurs too far down the tract to eliminate the negative effects some fibres have on nutrient digestion and for the end-products of fibre digestion to be absorbed and utilised efficiently by the animal. Consequently, an opportunity exists to improve energy availability through the addition of microbial fibre-degrading enzymes to animal feeds.

Another opportunity for enzyme supplementation exists in the young animal, where insufficient endogenous enzyme production sometimes can limit performance. This situation can be compromised further during periods of stress, such as post-weaning in piglets (Lindeman *et al.*, 1986), and by factors which interfere with enzyme function, such as dietary-induced high intestinal viscosity. Under these conditions, supplementation with enzymes such as proteases and amylases, in addition to the fibre-degrading enzymes discussed above, can be beneficial.

Feed chemistry

Diets fed in modern pig and poultry production systems are based on cereals, their by-products and protein concentrates of animal and plant origin. Thus, profitability is highly dependent on the relative costs and nutritive values of these dietary ingredients. In recent years, methods have been developed which allow increasingly more complete chemical analysis of feeds and, thus, a better scientific evaluation of their nutritional worth. The potential nutritive value of a feedstuff ideally should be related directly to its nutrient composition, and especially to its concentrations of starch, sugars, protein and fat (Table 2). However, the nutritive value is often limited, particularly for younger animals, by the presence of plant cell walls. Cell walls, which equate to dietary fibre, surround the nutrients within the cell preventing access to the animal's own digestive enzymes. Furthermore, a fraction of the non-starch polysaccharides (NSP) of some cell walls are water-soluble, and cause viscosity problems in the gut, with adverse effects on nutrient digestibilities. Those that are water-insoluble are considered to be biologically relatively inert.

Table 2. Typical composition (g kg^{-1} dry matter) and energy content (MJ kg^{-1}) of some common feedstuffs.

Component	Maize	Wheat	Barley	Peas	Soya meal	Canola meal
Crude fat	50	20	30	20	30	40
Crude protein	100	130	110	230	530	370
Starch + sugars	730	710	640	470	90	80
Cell walls	90	110	190	230	220	320
GE	18.8	18.5	18.5	18.4	19.7	19.8
DE - pigs	16.6	16.1	14.9	15.4	16.9	10.3
AME - poultry	15.9	14.9	13.2	11.8	12.1	7.6

GE, gross energy; DE, digestible energy; AME, apparent metabolisable energy

In feedstuffs, the important NSP include cellulose, which is found mainly in the hull and husk fractions of seeds and the vegetative parts of the plant, pectic polysaccharides found mainly in plant protein feedstuffs, and the mixed-linked β-glucans and arabinoxylans in cereal grains. The β-glucans predominate in the endosperm walls of barley and oats and arabinoxylans in the endosperm of wheat, rye and triticale.

MODE OF ACTION OF DIETARY ENZYMES

Poultry

In the 1950's Fry and co-workers (1958) reported that soaking wheat, rye and barley in water prior to feeding greatly improved poultry performance. They deduced that this could be due to the release of enzymes from the grains during soaking and germination and went on to show that a crude microbial amylase could mimic the effects of the soaking process. However, the cost of microbial enzymes, and probably their poor stability, prevented any commercial applications at that time.

During the 1960's renewed interest was shown in the use of microbial enzymes. Efforts to improve the nutritive value of cereals concentrated initially on barley and rye and it was only in the 1980's that attention was drawn to the feeding quality of wheat. The studies defining the anti-nutritive factors in these feeds, their effect on digesta viscosity and nutrient digestibility, and the development of xylanases and β-glucanases capable of their degradation have been reviewed by a number of workers (Chesson, 1987; Annison and Choct, 1991; Campbell and Bedford, 1992; Classen and Bedford, 1992). Studies with fractionated enzymes established that β-glucanase was the effective enzyme for barley and that supplementation of barley- and oat-based diets with this enzyme improved chick production and essentially eliminated litter problems (Hesselman, 1983). Subsequent studies demonstrated that supplementary arabinoxylanases (pentosanases) had similar beneficial effects when added to wheat- and rye-based diets (Pettersson, 1988; Classen and Bedford, 1992).

Furthermore, Choct and Annison (1990) observed that the arabinoxylan plus β-glucan concentration of seven different cereals was very highly correlated (r = -0.98) with apparent metabolisable energy (AME) and this correlation was slightly better than that observed between the arabinoxylan concentration and AME (r = -0.95). This suggests that advantages are to be derived from supplementing cereal diets with an enzyme product containing both arabinoxylanase and β-glucanase activities. The failure of the Sibbald rapid true ME assay to detect problem wheats with a low AME identified by the classical AME assay with broiler chickens (Mollah *et al.*, 1983) probably reflects the low food intake, and associated limited development of intestinal viscosity, associated with the former assay. In broiler chickens the anti-nutritive effects of cereals would appear to decline as the bird ages (Pettersson, 1988; Rogel *et al.*, 1987).

Where responses to xylanases and β-glucanases have been observed in chickens, they are often greater than expected, even assuming the enzymes to be capable of degrading the target polysaccharides totally. Research to define the effects of these supplementary enzymes on digestion found that they significantly improved the absorption of nutrients such as starch, protein and fat (Table 3). It was proposed that the enzymes acted by:

- Disrupting the cereal cell walls, allowing a greater digestion of encapsulated nutrients
- Reducing digesta viscosity, allowing increased movement of endogenous enzymes and (digested) nutrients.

Addition of suitable enzymes to wheat-based broiler diets can reduce digesta viscosity caused primarily by the arabinoxylans, and thus improve chick production. Recently, this phenomenon was extensively investigated in Canada (Bedford and Classen, 1991). In this study, a wheat-based diet was used as a control, and rye was included at 0, 20, 40 and 60% of the diet, partly replacing wheat. A xylanase was included at 0, 0.1, 0.2, 0.4, 0.8 and 1.6% of the diets, which were fed to broiler chicks from 0-21 days of age. Rye was used since, although arabinoxylans are the main soluble fibre in both wheat and rye, they tend to be present at higher concentrations in rye and give rise to higher viscosity than do those in wheat.

Table 3.   Effect of enzyme addition to a wheat/rye based broiler diet.

	Control	Control + enzyme[1]	Improvement (%)
Liveweight (g at 15 d)	282	373[*]	32
Feed: gain (g:g, 1-15 d)	1.46	1.28[*]	12
Sticky droppings (%,8 d)	31	11[*]	67
Intestinal length (cmkg⁻¹ body wt.)	290	220[*]	24
Ileal apparent digestibility (%)			
organic matter	71	75[*]	6
crude protein	70	76[*]	9
starch	96	99[*]	3
NSP	33	36	9

[1]Xylanase-based enzyme.
[*]Differs from control (P<0.05).
From Pettersson (1988).

Addition of rye to the wheat-based control diet significantly reduced chick growth, even at the lowest inclusion level (Fig. 1). However, this effect was eliminated by the addition of xylanase,

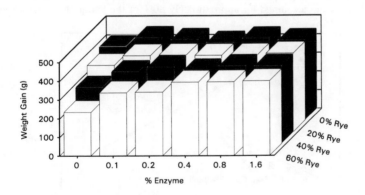

Figure 1. Weight gain to three weeks in chicks fed wheat (60-0%)- and rye (0-60%)-based diets with 0-1.6% of an arabinoxylanase added. From Bedford and Classen (1991).

with progressively more enzyme needed to restore productivity at higher rye concentrations. Measurements of foregut digesta viscosity in these chicks gave a similar picture; increasing concentrations of rye greatly increased digesta viscosity, while the addition of the xylanase to these diets reduced viscosity (Fig. 2).

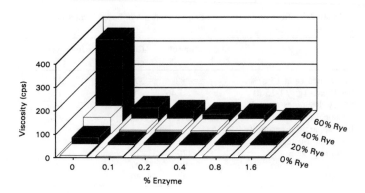

Figure 2. Foregut viscosity in chicks fed wheat (60-0%) and rye (0-60%) based diets fed with 0-1.6% of an arabinoxylanase added. From Bedford and Classen (1991).

Correlation analysis demonstrated significant (P<0.01) logarithmic relationships between digesta viscosity and both weight gain and feed efficiency (Fig. 3). The same researchers then isolated and fractionated the soluble carbohydrate from the foregut digesta. This identified a high molecular weight fraction, greater than 500 kDa which, while representing only 10% of the total polysaccharide present, accounted for approximately 80% of the variation in digesta viscosity.

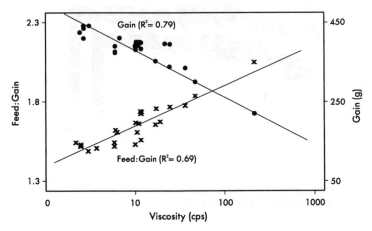

Figure 3. Relationships between foregut viscosity and weight gain and feed conversion in chicks fed wheat/rye diets. From Bedford and Classen (1991).

This high molecular weight carbohydrate proved to have a very complex structure, with a number of different components present including arabinoxylans, mixed-linked β-glucans and some associated protein. Further, the arabinoxylan, which has a β-1,4-linked xylose backbone, was very highly substituted with arabinose side-chains.

A similar relationship between digesta viscosity and chick performance has been established with barley diets (Graham *et al.*, 1993). In this case supplementation with appropriate β-glucanases reduces viscosity and generally leads to an improvement in chick performance.

A reduced rate of digestion is not the only problem encountered with increased intestinal viscosity. Despite the increase in gut motility associated with viscous intestinal environment, the rate of feed passage is also significantly reduced. The result is that feed throughput, and intake, is decreased and this limits the nutrient assimilation rates. Since feed transit is slowed, the flushing effect of the feed is reduced and intestinal bacteria are able to multiply and migrate to the upper reaches of the small intestine (Campbell and Bedford, 1992).

Intestinal microorganisms also digest and utilise the starch and proteins in the digesta, and effectively compete with the host for nutrients. This further exacerbates the problem for the host animal. Increased digesta viscosity generally has a greater effect on lipids compared to starch and protein. This is presumably due to the relatively large size of the lipid micelles, which have greater difficulty in moving through more viscous digesta. In addition, some intestinal bacteria produce bile acid-degrading enzymes which further reduce the lipid digesting capabilities of the host (Campbell *et al.*, 1983). As a consequence, birds fed diets which produce highly viscous digesta are prone to fat-soluble vitamin deficiencies (rickets is particularly common) as these vitamins are co-absorbed with the fat micelles. Since bile acids are also thought to stabilise pancreatic proteases in the intestine, protein digestion will also be compromised further. Inclusion of bile acids or antibiotics in such rations can alleviate many of the problems described above.

Pigs

The success of enzyme supplementation in poultry led to an interest in enzyme addition to pig diets. Early trials established that β-glucanases could improve performance in barley-fed pigs (Thomke *et al.*, 1980). Trials with ileal-cannulated pigs fed a wheat middlings/barley diet indicated the same mode of action as in poultry; enzymes improved the digestion in the small intestine of nutrients such as starch, lipids and protein, but had little or no effect on fibre polysaccharides (Graham *et al.*, 1988).

Pigs tend to show less response to feed enzyme supplements·than do chickens. Unlike the chick, the viscosity of the digesta in the intestines of piglets is relatively unaffected by dietary arabinoxylans or β-glucans. This appears to be related to a number of factors including a long digesta residence time in the stomach, a high digesta water content and possible fibre-degrading activity prior to the ileum (Graham *et al.*, 1988).

The potential value of enzymes in pig feeds has been demonstrated by a trial with animals fed either wheat or barley based diets from 11 to 25 kg (Bohme, 1990). Inclusion of the appropriate multi-enzyme preparation improved pig production, presumably due to better nutrient digestion (Table 4). Further, the coefficient of variation in final liveweight tended to be reduced with enzyme addition, probably reflecting a better performance by the smaller animals. These diets were fed without antibiotics, and there was also a tendency for the enzyme-fed pigs to have a lower incidence of digestive disorders. This response could be due to an enzyme-mediated improvement in digestion, reducing the substrate available for microbial proliferation, and thus overgrowth, in the posterior digestive tract. In addition oligosaccharides released by supplementary enzymes from NSP could contribute to the maintenance of a healthy gut flora.

Table 4. A comparison of piglet growth and health when fed wheat- or barley-based diets with and without added enzymes.

	Wheat	Wheat + enzymes[1]	Barley	Barley + enzymes[1]
Initial weight (kg)	11.1	10.6	11.0	11.1
Final weight (kg)	25.0	25.0	24.7	25.1
CV[2] in final weight (%)	6	3	7	2
Days on trial	34.2	32.0	35.9	32.1
Daily gain (g)	406	450	382	436
Feed:gain (g:g)	1.80	1.63*	1.91	1.62*
Antibiotic treatments (number of interventions)	24	11	17	6

From Bohme (1990).
* Differs from corresponding control (P<0.05).
[1]Xylanase / β-glucanase based multi-enzyme products.
[2]Coefficient of variation

COMMERCIAL APPLICATIONS

Barley based diets

Poultry. Feeding trials designed to develop enzymes for use in commercial barley-based broiler diets have been concentrated in areas where barley is grown as a major cereal and white-skinned broilers are accepted by the consumer. Under these conditions a barley/enzyme combination competes economically with wheat, and thus feeding trials were designed to test this application.

In a series of 29 trials carried out in 13 countries, primarily on commercial farms, broiler production on wheat-based diets was compared with diets containing, on average, 46% barley plus a commercial β-glucanase-based multi-enzyme product. On average, broilers were grown to 44 days of age and a total of more than 400,000 broilers were used. In these trials, the barley-enzyme combination replaced wheat without any significant (P>0.05) detrimental effect on broiler production (Table 5). The improvement in the productive value of the barley, in the presence of β-glucanase, can be accommodated by increasing the AME of barley by about 10%. This

Table 5. A summary of 29 trials with over 400,000 broilers comparing productivity on wheat-based control diets with enzyme-supplemented barley diets where, on average, 46% of the wheat was replaced with barley.

	Wheat-based diets	Barley + enzyme[1] diets
Liveweight at 44 days (g)	1851	1881
Feed:gain, 1-44 days (g)	2.08	1.99

[1]β-glucanase based multi-enzyme product

allows barley an AME of about 12.9 MJ kg^{-1}, which is similar to that of wheat. Thus, when barley is cheap relative to wheat, it can be included in broiler diets to a maximum of about 500 kg per tonne. In areas such as Scandinavia, the UK, Spain and Western Canada, where β-glucanase-supplemented barley diets are widely used at certain times of the year, broiler producers also report improvements in litter quality relative to standard wheat-based diets, reflecting the added value of the enzyme in reducing digesta viscosity.

Pigs. Barley is widely used in pig feeds in many countries, particularly in immediate post-weaning diets. However, inclusion is often limited to 250-300 kg tonne to avoid decreases in growth rate. The possibility of using dietary enzymes to improve the nutritional value of barley in a similar way to that observed with poultry was tested in a grower/finisher trial employing six pens each of six animals on each of three diets (Dr. P. Gill, personal communication). Pigs were fed *ad libitum* from 20 to 100 kg liveweight. The diets contained either wheat or barley (670 kg per tonne) with wheatfeed (75 kg per tonne), canola meal (75 kg per tonne) and soyabean oil (2.5 kg per tonne) as the other primary ingredients. All diets contained 0.70% available lysine, while the digestible energy values were 13.6 MJ kg^{-1} for the wheat diet and 13.0 MJ kg^{-1} for the barley diets.

The control diets gave similar liveweight gain but the lower energy barley diet gave a significantly ($P<0.01$) poorer feed conversion (Table 6). Addition of the β-glucanase-based multi-enzyme product to the barley diet improved ($P<0.05$) weight gain and feed conversion. However, the killout percentage was lower ($P<0.01$) for both the barley-based diets, which presumably reflected a greater gut-fill on these diets. Thus, the response of pigs to β-glucanase was similar to that of poultry and the digestible energy of barley for pigs was apparently increased by about 6%, to 14.1 MJ kg^{-1}.

Wheat based diets

Poultry. When formulating commercial wheat-based poultry diets, feed enzymes can be considered in two ways. Firstly, they can be provided as an addition to the normal formulation thereby giving a benefit in feed efficiency. Secondly, enzyme inclusion can allow an increment

Table 6. Pig production on diets based on wheat, or on barley fed with and without supplementary enzymes. Details of diets given in the text.

	Wheat-based	Barley-based	Barley-based + enzymes[1]
Initial weight (kg)	20.3	20.8	20.9
Final weight (kg)	99.8	100.3	101.4
Daily gain (kg)	0.76[a]	0.75[a]	0.84[b]
Feed:gain	2.69[d]	3.04[c]	2.72[d]
Killout (%)	77.3[d]	75.4[c]	75.2[c]

[1] β-glucanase based multi-enzyme product
Means within a row not sharing a superscript differ significantly
[a-b] $P<0.05$, [c-d] $P<0.01$.

in the ME value of wheat, thus allowing energy to be sourced from wheat instead of more expensive oil.

The cost-benefits of the two approaches were illustrated in a broiler trial with six pens of 115 birds each per diet (Dr C. Belyavin, personal communication). The birds were fed from one to 42 days of age, with a control diet formulated to contain about 600 kg wheat per tonne, with soyabean meal, full-fat soybeans and soya oil as the other primary ingredients. This diet was fed with or without a xylanase-based multi-enzyme product. This enzyme product was also added to another diet formulated on the assumption that the enzyme would increase the ME of wheat by 6%. In practice, this resulted in an increase in wheat levels of about 40 kg per tonne, with a decreased inclusion of soya oil. All diets had the same concentrations of lysine and methionine + cystine.

This broiler trial showed no differences in liveweight at 42 days of age (Table 7). However, adding the enzyme product to the wheat control diet significantly ($P<0.05$) improved feed conversion, by about 6%. This increased the margin over feed (price received for the processed broiler minus day-old chick and feeding costs) by more than UK £0.04 per bird. Even allowing for the 6% increase in the ME of wheat the enzyme still gave a 3% improvement in feed conversion, suggesting that for this particular wheat the 6% increase in ME was an underestimate. However, this approach gave a margin over feed which was similar to that obtained by simple addition of the enzyme product to the diet.

In practice, the preferred method of enzyme addition to wheat-based poultry diets depends very much on the desired benefits. Commercial compound feed producers, often in a competitive situation, tend to opt for the add-on benefits of a better feed conversion, while integrated companies are more likely to look for the savings in diet costs offered by using a higher ME value for wheat. As with barley, enzyme supplementation of wheat-based broiler diets substantially reduces litter problems.

Pigs. Suitable enzymes can be added to wheat-based piglet diets to give a cost-effective response, as indicated in Table 4. However, piglet diets often contain readily digestible, and

Table 7. Broiler production from diets based on wheat with or without added enzyme and formulated with or without the assumption that the enzyme improves the metabolisable energy of wheat by 6%.

	Wheat-based	Wheat-based + enzyme[1]	Wheat-based (+ 6% ME) + enzyme[1]
Liveweight (42 d, g)	2154	2222	2236
Feed:gain (1-42 d)	1.73[a]	1.62[b]	1.68[ab]
Margin over feed (UK £ per bird)	0.399	0.441	0.449

[1]Xylanase based multi-enzyme product
[a-b]Means within a row not sharing a superscript differ significantly (P<0.05).

expensive, feedstuffs such as milk powder, fishmeal and cooked cereals. Further, diet specifications are often in excess of animal requirements for maintenance and growth. As a result, adding an enzyme to improve digestion may have little or no effect.

The alternative mode of application is to use feed enzymes to allow a greater inclusion of less expensive feedstuffs, such as soyabean meal and uncooked cereals, while maintaining animal performance. One example of how this can be achieved is taken from a trial on a commercial Canadian farm. In this trial four pens of 10 pigs per diet were each fed one of two diets *ad libitum* for five weeks. The expensive control diet, costing UK £134 per tonne, contained 100 kg per tonne whey powder and 40 kg per tonne fishmeal. This diet was reformulated to the same energy and amino acid contents, replacing 60 kg per tonne whey powder and 20 kg per tonne fishmeal with soyabean meal and a feed enzyme preparation. This allowed a saving of over UK £10 per tonne feed. Over the trial period, liveweight gain and feed conversion for piglets fed the two diets were similar (P>0.1; Table 8). Consequently feed costs per kg liveweight gain were reduced by 11% with the less expensive enzyme-supplemented diet.

Other feedstuffs

Over the past few years enzymes have been included in commercial pig and poultry diets containing high concentrations of feedstuffs as divergent as maize, oats, rice, sorghum and tapioca. While many of these application may have been cost-effective, there is insufficient data to establish the effect that the enzymes had on the energy availability of any of these feedstuffs. However, it is likely that appropriate enzymes can improve the nutritive value of these feeds.

Considerable attention has been given to the effects that enzymes might have on the feeding value of plant protein feedstuffs. One approach has been to look at the possibility of replacing heat treatments with enzyme supplements. This has been tested in a chick trial, using field beans (*Vicia faba* L.) with autoclaving as the heat treatment (Castanon and Marquardt, 1989). Addition of an enzyme product containing a cellulase and a protease significantly (P<0.05) improved weight gain and feed conversion of the raw field bean diet but not the diet containing heat-treated

Table 8. Piglet performance when fed an expensive diet (100 kg whey powder and 40 kg fishmeal per tonne) or a less expensive, lower quality diet (40 kg whey powder and 20 kg fishmeal per tonne) supplemented with an enzyme product.

	Control Diet	Enzyme[1]-supplemented diet
Initial weight (kg)	6.7	6.7
Final weight (kg)	19.6	20.5
Daily gain (kg)	368	394
Feed:gain	1.55	1.49
Feed:gain	20.8	18.4

[1]Xylanase based multi-enzyme product

beans (Table 9). However, the enzyme-treated raw beans did not achieve the productivity level of the autoclaved beans.

Table 9. The effect of a dietary enzyme supplement on chickens fed diets containing raw or autoclaved field beans.

Diet	Weight gain (g, 7-21 d)	Feed:gain (g:g, 7-21 d)
Raw beans	114.7[a]	2.58[a]
Raw beans + Enzymes[1]	120.1[b]	2.44[b]
Autoclaved beans	130.7[c]	2.16[c]
Autoclaved beans + Enzymes[1]	132.2[c]	2.14[c]

From Castanon and Marquardt (1989).
[a-c]Means in a column not sharing a superscript differ significantly (P<0.05).
[1]Cellulase and protease.

Because of the widespread use of soyabean products in animal feeds, any enzyme-mediated improvement in the nutritive value of this feedstuff would have major implications for animal production. An indication of the possibilities of improving soyabeans with enzymes was obtained in a balance study with laying hens (Slominski and Campbell, 1990). In this study, the addition of a polysaccharidase enzyme preparation increased fibre polysaccharide degradation in the hens from 2% to 37% (P<0.05). However, the consequences of this improvement measured in terms of animal productivity in unknown. It should be noted that enzymatic release of free sugars such as arabinose and xylose in the intestine is of little value to animal performance, since these pentose sugars are poorly metabolised by poultry (Longstaff *et al.*, 1988; Schutte *et al.*, 1992) and pigs (Yule and Fuller, 1992). Thus, increased fibre digestion may not always give a positive response in animal growth, and exo-acting enzymes and glycosidases which give rise to free sugars should be used with caution.

Brake (1992) showed that supplementation of a maize/soyabean diet with α-galactosidase increased egg production, presumably due to a higher energy availability. Whether this effect was due to the α-galactosidase alone or to other enzyme activities present in the product used is uncertain. However, if the oligosaccharides of the raffinose series found in many legumes used as plant protein feedstuffs were to be digested, the available energy in these products would be increased and enzyme treatment would also help alleviate digestive disorders associated with these carbohydrates.

RUMINANT APPLICATIONS

Forages fed to ruminants have many of the cell wall fibres found in cereals, including cellulose, xylans and the pectic polysaccharides. In forages, however, two factors have a particular influence on digestion, namely phenolic compounds and the cuticle. The major phenolic material in forages is lignin, a randomized, 3-dimensional phenylpropanoid polymer. This polymer is thought to be linked to the arabinoxylans through ferulic acid bridging units which are, in turn, ester linked to carbohydrate and ether linked to the lignin (Lam *et al.*, 1992). Lignin is both hydrophobic and chemically relatively inert and, because of its close association with cell wall carbohydrate, limits the extent of microbial degradation of the fibre component of the diet.

The aerial parts of forages are protected by a hydrophobic cuticle, which is formed of cutin and waxes. Cutin is a polymer of fatty acids, often C_{16} and C_{18}, and various hydroxylated and epoxylated derivatives. The fatty acids are esterified and etherified with phenolic units in a complex manner (Kolattukudy *et al.*, 1981). The waxes associated with the cutin are esters of very long chain fatty acids and long chain alcohols. The hydrophobic nature of the cuticle protects the forage surface and extensive microbial colonisation is only possible on cut edges or by invasion through the stomata. As indicated previously, there has been little research into the effect of supplementing complete ruminant feeds with enzymes. However, inclusion of cutinases and polysaccharidases that can either disrupt the cuticle or open up the cell wall structure could lead to a greater initial rate of microbial colonization, but probably would take no effect on the final extent of degradation. Chesson (1991) has indicated that this has been observed with cell wall degrading enzymes, but presented no data to support this claim. However, an extract of *Aspergillus oryzae*, which could contain significant enzyme activity, has been shown to have these exact effects (Fondevila *et al.*, 1990), as has pre-treatment of roughages with polysaccharidases (Nakashima *et al.*, 1988). An increase in the rate of digestion would be expected to increase forage intake, often the limiting factor in feeding high-yielding ruminants. The greatest challenge to supplementing complete ruminant feeds will be to ensure adequate enzyme survival in the highly proteolytic conditions in the rumen.

FUTURE DEVELOPMENTS

Major developments in the understanding and application of feed enzymes are likely to occur over the next few years, due primarily to:
1. The use of high-yielding micro-organisms to produce less expensive enzymes.

2. A better understanding of the mode of action of enzymes, allowing more specific enzyme products to be formulated.

3. The development of applications to feedstuffs other than wheat and barley, and to animals other than pigs and poultry.

The present, first generation of enzyme products is designed to supplement the insufficient enzyme production of the young animal, while degrading the oligo- and polysaccharides that can hinder digestion by host-animal enzymes. The next generation of enzymes will probably be targeted at other anti-nutritive factors found in feedstuffs, including protease inhibitors, phenolics and lectins. What further generations of feed enzymes will prove to be is very much open to speculation. However, it is not unlikely that specific anti-microbial enzymes could be used to provide a "consumer friendly" control of the microbial population of the animal gastrointestinal tract (Scott, 1988).

Substantial progess has been made over the past decade in the understanding of the mode of action and commercial application of feed enzymes. However, this area of biotechnology is still very much in its infancy and considerable progress can be expected in the next few years.

REFERENCES

Annison, G. and Choct, M. 1991. Anti-nutritive activities of cereal non-starch polysaccharides in broiler diets and strategies minimizing their effects. *World's Poultry Sci.* **47**, 232-242.

Bedford, M.R. and Classen, H.L. 1991. Reduction of intestinal viscosity through manipulation of dietary rye and pentosanase concentration is effected through changes in the carbohydrate composition of the intestinal aqueous phase and results in improved growth rate and food conversion efficiency of broiler chicks. *J. Nutr.* **122**, 560-569.

Bohme, H. 1990. Experiments on the efficacy of enzyme supplements as a growth promoter for piglets. *Landbauforsch. Volkenrode* **40**, 213-217.

Brake, J. 1992. Production of broiler breeders increases when fed diets containing commercial enzyme preparations - possible method to improve performance in hot climates. In Proc. XIX World's Poultry Congress, pp. 416-419, Amsterdam, The Netherlands.

Campbell, G.L. and Bedford, M.R. 1992. Enzyme applications for monogastric feeds: a review. *Can. J. Anim. Sci.* **72**, 449-466.

Campbell, G.L., Campbell, L.D. and Classen, H.L. 1983. Utilisation of rye by chickens: effect of microbial status, diet irradiation and sodium taurocholate supplementation. *Br. Poultry Sci.* **24**, 191-203.

Castanon, J.I.R. and Marquardt, R.R. 1989. Effect of enzyme addition, autoclave treatment and fermenting on the nutritive value of field beans (*Vicia faba* L.). *Anim. Feed Sci. Tech.* **26**, 71-79.

Chesson, A. 1987. Supplementary enzymes to improve the utilisation of pig and poultry diets. In *Recent Advances in Animal Nutrition 1987* (W. Haresign and D. J. A. Cole, eds) pp. 71-89. Butterworths, London, UK.

Chesson, A. 1991. Impact of biotechnology on livestock feeds and feeding. *Med. Fac. Landbouww. Rijksuniv. Gent.* **56**, 1365-1391.

Choct, M. and Annison, G. 1990. Anti-nutritive activity of wheat pentosans in broiler diets. *Br. Poultry Sci.* **31**, 811-821.

Classen, H.L and Bedford, M.R. 1992. The use of enzymes to improve the nutritive value of poultry feeds. In *Recent Advances in Animal Nutrition 1992* (W. Haresign and D. J. A. Cole, eds) pp. 95-116. Butterworth-Heinemann Ltd., Oxford, UK.

Fondevila, M., Newbold, C.J., Hotten, P.M. and Ørskov, E.R. 1990. A note on the effect of *Aspergillus oryzae* fermentation extract on the rumen fermentation of sheep given straw. *Anim. Prod.* **51**, 422-425.

Fry, R.E., Allred, J.B., Jensen, L.S. and McGinnis, J. 1958. Influence of enzyme supplementation and water treatment on the nutritional value of different grains for poults. *Poultry Sci.* **37**, 372-375.

Graham, H. and Inborr, J. 1992. Stability of enzymes during processing. *Feed Mix* **1**, 18-23.

Graham, H. Bedford, M. and Choct, M. 1993. High gut viscosity can reduce poultry performance. *Feedstuffs* **65**, 14-15.

Graham, H., Löwgren, W., Pettersson, D. and Åman, P. 1988. Effect of enzyme supplementation on digestion of a barley/pollard based pig feed. *Nutr. Rep. Int.* **38**, 1073-1079.

GrootWassink, J.W.D., Campbell, G.L. and Classen, H.L. 1989. Fractionation of crude pentosanase (arabinoxylanase) for improvement of the nutritional value of rye diets for broiler chickens. *J. Sci. Food Agric.* **46**, 289-300.

Hesselman, K. 1983. Effects of β-glucanase supplementation to barley based diets for broiler chickens. PhD thesis. Swedish University of Agricultural Science, Uppsala, Sweden.

Kolattukudy, P.E., Espelie, K.E. and Soliday, C.L. 1981. Hydrophobic layers attached to cell walls. Gutin, suberin and associated waxes. In *Encyclopaedia of Plant Physiology*, Vol. 13B (W. Tanner and F.A. Loewus, eds) pp. 225-254. Springer, Berlin, Germany.

Lam, T.B.T., Iiyama, K. and Stone, B.A. 1992. Cinnamic acid bridges between cell wall polymers in wheat and phalaris internodes. *Phytochemistry* **31**, 1179-1183

Lindeman, M.D., Cornelius, S.G., El Kandelgy, S.M., Moser, R.L. and Pettigrew J.E. 1986. Effect of age, weaning and diet on digestive enzyme levels in the piglet. *J. Anim. Sci.* **62**, 1298-1307.

Longstaff, M.A., Knox, A. and McNab, J.M. 1988. Digestibility of pentose sugars and uronic acids and their effect on chick weight gain and caecal size. *Br. Poultry Sci.* **29**, 379-393.

Mollah, Y., Bryden, W.L., Wallis, I.R., Balnave, D. and Annison, E.F. 1983. Studies on low metabolisable energy wheats for poultry using conventional and rapid assay procedures and the effects of processing. *Br. Poultry Sci.* **24**, 81-89.

Nakashima, Y., Ørskov E.R., Hotten, P.M., Ambo, K. and Takase, Y. 1988. Rumen degradation of straw. 6. Effect of polysaccharidase enzymes on degradation characteristics of ensiled rice straw. *Anim. Prod.* **47**, 421-427.

Pettersson, D. 1988. Composition and nutritive value for broiler chickens of wheat, rye and triticale. PhD thesis. Swedish University of Agricultural Science, Uppsala, Sweden.

Rogel, A.M., Annison, E.F., Bryden, W.L. and Balnave, D. 1987. The digestion of wheat starch in broiler chickens. *Aust. J. Agric. Res.* **38**, 639-649.

Schutte, J.B., De Jong, J., Van Weerden, E.J. and Van Baak, M.J. 1992. Nutritional value of D-xylose and L-arabinose for broiler chicks. *Br. Poultry Sci.* **33**, 89-100.

Scott, D. 1988/9. Antimicrobial enzymes. *Food Biotech.* **2**, 119-132.

Slominski, B. and Campbell, L.D. 1990. Non-starch polysaccharides of canola meal: quantification, digestibility in poultry and potential benefit of dietary enzyme supplenmentation. *J. Sci. Food Agric.* **53**, 175-184

Thomke, S., Rundgren, M. and Hesselman, K. 1980. The effect of feeding high-viscosity barley to pigs. In Proceedings of the 31st Meeting of the European Association of Animal Production p. 5. Commission on Animal Production, Munich, Germany.

Yule, M.A. and Fuller, M.F. 1992. The utilisation of orally administered D-xylose, L-arabinose and D-galacturonic acid in the pig. *Int. J. Food Sci. Nutr.* **43**, 31-40.

16 Biotechnology in the treatment of animal manure

Marleen Vande Woestyne and Willy Verstraete

Centre of Environmental Studies, University of Gent, B-9000 Gent, Belgium

INTRODUCTION

In traditional agricultural practice, livestock farming and agronomy were closely integrated. Animal excrement (faeces and urine) was applied to land as source of minerals and organic compounds to improve crop growth and the plant biomass produced was, in turn, used as animal feed. Straw served as bedding material and also as an absorbent of urine in animal sheds and stables. The resulting mixture of straw and animal excreta was allowed to accumulate, ferment to a residual slow-release organic fertiliser, and spread on land in spring and autumn.

Livestock management practices have evolved considerably during the last few decades. The development of intensive confined rearing resulted in the replacement of straw bedding by slatted floors, thus producing large quantities of livestock slurries. Manure surpluses now present a considerable disposal problem in certain regions of the European community. The scope of the problem in Europe compared to the rest of the world is illustrated by Table 1 which gives livestock numbers in relation to the utilised agricultural areas.

Table 1. Relative numbers of cattle, pig and poultry found in various regions of the world in relation to utilised agricultural area compared with overall world numbers expressed as 100.

Country	Cattle	Pigs	Poultry
EC-10[1]	300	567	293
Europe	207	470	254
World	100	100	100
USSR	74	73	84
USA	88	57	160
S. America	158	49	66
Africa	84	11	49

Adapted from Lee and Coulter (1990).
[1]Belgium, Denmark, W. Germany, France, Greece, Ireland, Italy, Luxembourg, Netherlands and United Kingdom.

For pigs, the EC-10 average is five times that of the world average and for cattle and poultry there is a three-fold difference. The approximate daily volumes excreted by cattle, pigs and laying hens respectively are 33, 5 and 0.11 litres. These volumes correspond respectively to

12, 1.8 and 0.04 tonnes per year. On this basis, the estimated waste production per ha of utilised agricultural area for different European countries has been calculated (Table 2).

Table 2. Estimate of livestock waste production (tonnes ha^{-1} yr^{-1}) based on the livestock density reported in the Eurostat Regions Statistical Yearbook 1989.

Country	Cattle	Pigs	Laying hens
Belgium	25.2	7.7	1.2
Denmark	10.1	5.9	0.5
France	8.0	0.7	0.2
Germany (FGR)	14.4	3.6	0.4
Greece	2.3	0.5	0.2
Ireland	11.8	0.3	0.1
Italy	6.0	1.1	0.6
Luxembourg	19.2	34.6	0.1
Netherlands	28.8	51.8	40.0
Portugal	3.0	5.4	-
Spain	2.3	4.1	-
United Kingdom	7.9	14.2	0.8

Adapted from Fleming (1993).

In recent years the negative aspects of intensive animal husbandry have become apparent. These can be summarised as:

- difficulties in disposing of slurry on the farm itself or in its vicinity as slurry production exceeds the land area available for optimum application
- importation of feed ingredients from other countries or regions resulting in surpluses of animal manure which, in turn, may lead to saturation of soils with mineral nutrients such as phosphate and nitrate and pollution of ground and surface water
- emission of odours, especially the emission of ammonia.

Treatment is one of the possibilities available to deal with the problem of manure surpluses. This chapter provides an overview of the application of biotechnology to the processing of manure and odour abatement and includes descriptions of promising new technologies still under investigation.

UNIT OPERATIONS FOR MANURE TREATMENT

Current technology provides a wide range of unit processes to recover products from concentrated organic wastes such as manure. The primary aim of any particular treatment can vary. Typical goals include improvement in the quality of effluent combined with the production of energy (biogas), purification of manure for discharge to surface water, formulation of manure as an organic fertiliser or the conversion of manure into feedable products.

Biogas production

The anaerobic digestion process is complex both in terms of its microbiology and its biochemistry. Three main groups of bacteria are involved: the fermentative bacteria which hydrolyse and convert the biodegradable compounds to intermediate organic acids, the acetogenic bacteria which produce acetate, hydrogen and carbon dioxide, and the methanogenic bacteria which produce methane and carbon dioxide (Zehnder *et al.*, 1982; Zeikus, 1982). The overall anaerobic conversion of manure requires the synergistic action of the three groups of microorganisms involved (Iannotti *et al.*, 1982). Fortunately, anaerobic digestion works well in normal circumstances and does not need any sophisticated control systems for reliable day-to-day operation (Friman, 1984). Anaerobic digestion is usually applied to more concentrated livestock slurries and wastes from livestock processing with an optimum dry matter content of between 6 and 8%. The anaerobic digestion of piggery manure is well documented (Summers and Bousfield, 1980; Poels *et al.*, 1984, 1985; Bossier *et al.*, 1986). Typical flow diagrams are given by Hobson and Feilden (1982), Poels *et al.* (1983), Summers *et al.* (1984) and Safley *et al.* (1987).

The biogas produced consists of approximately 70% CH_4 and 30% CO_2. Generally, slurries are treated in completely mixed tanks operated at a temperature of 30° - 35°C for a period of 20-30 days (Hawkes, 1979; Hobson *et al.*, 1981). Most digesters operate satisfactorily on liquid manure without major problems at volumetric loading rates of 0.5 - 1.0 m^3 m^{-3} reactor d^{-1}. The maximal daily gas production is 0.7 - 1.2 m^3 m^{-3} reactor d^{-1}. The specific gas production from pig and cattle manure is 18 - 20 m^3 biogas m^{-3} manure (Poels *et al.*, 1983). The investment costs (> 1000 m^3) are 200 ECU m^{-3} reactor and the annual costs per m^3 digester have been calculated to be 36.6 ECU (Ten Have and Chiappini, 1993). At a production rate of 0.7 m^3 m^{-3} digester d^{-1}, the annual gas production is 256 m^3 yr^{-1}. Biogas production is therefore profitable at a price of more than 0.14 ECU m^{-3} biogas (70% methane) (Ten Have and Chiappini, 1993).

The use of farm digesters in Europe is relatively small. Farm digesters do not seem to be worthwhile unless there is, besides the biogas production, an economic benefit in improving the quality of the slurry, which is rarely the case. In most cases, individual farmers or cooperatives will install digestion facilities only when there is some form of governmental subsidy or penalty.

Discharge after biological treatment

The first plants designed to relieve farmers of their manure surpluses by allowing discharge of effluent to surface water after biological purification were installed in the mid-sixties. Their function was to concentrate and remove the solid fraction and to reduce the pollution load of the liquid fraction to a level which allowed discharge. The systems were very similar to those for the processing of sewage. However, because of the high organic matter contents and thus the high biological oxygen demand (BOD) of manure, a pretreatment was found desirable. Pig manure and cattle slurry have a BOD_5 of 10-200 g O_2 l^{-1}. Pig manure is approximately 100 times more concentrated than domestic sewage which has an average BOD_5 of 0.3 g l^{-1}. By the established waste water technologies, an acceptable purified effluent can only be obtained from the liquid fraction of manure after removal of the suspended solids and phosphorus content by filtration, sedimentation or centrifugation.

Anaerobic purification

The anaerobic purification of the liquid fraction of manure is based on the same microbiological process as biogas production. The main difference between the two technologies is that, in case of liquids, methods have to be developed to concentrate and retain the methanogenic biomass in the reactor (Switzenbaum, 1983). The upflow anaerobic sludge blanket (UASB) reactor, suited for the removal of BOD from waters with relatively low concentrations of suspended solids, can be used to purify manure from which the major part of the suspended solids have been removed. The UASB design relies on the tendency of anaerobic bacteria to form granules which are retained within the reactor by the principle of autoflocculation and gravity settling (Lettinga and Hulshoff Pol, 1986). Poels *et al.* (1981) reported laboratory experiments where 50-60% of the chemical oxygen demand (COD) of waste was removed when centrifuged pig manure (1.6% total solids) was used as feedstock. The loading rate was 30-40 kg COD m^{-3} d^{-1} and the retention time about 20 h. Schomaker *et al.* (1986) used a 19 m^3 reactor for the purification of veal calf manure. At a maximum loading rate of 5 kg COD m^{-3} d^{-1}, 70% of the COD could be removed. The effluent contained 500 mg BOD l^{-1}. As the anaerobic purification is limited to the removal of BOD or COD, a second purification stage is necessary to comply with effluent standards in terms of N, P, residual suspended solids and BOD.

Aerobic purification

A more complete purification than with anaerobic treatment is possible with the aerobic activated-sludge process. An important part of the organic material and, depending on the details of the process, also the nitrogen, is converted into CO_2 and N_2. A major benefit of aerobic treatment is that the nature and quantity of nitrogen in the treated slurry can be controlled. Depending upon operation conditions nitrogen can be conserved as ammoniacal nitrogen, lost via ammonia stripping, oxidised to nitrate and conserved, or lost via denitrification. Activated sludge organisms grow at ambient substrate concentrations of the order of 0.1 to 10 mg l^{-1}. Therefore, in the case of manure, a pretreatment is desirable before aerobic treatment. Several aerobic treatment systems have been developed and descriptions of them are available in the literature (Doyle *et al.*, 1986; Bourque *et al.*, 1987; Blouin *et al.*, 1988; Beaudet *et al.*, 1990). Treatments normally comprise of three stages: oxidation of organic matter, nitrification, and finally denitrification to remove ammonia nitrogen (Fenlon and Robinson, 1977). The last two steps are complex and difficult to achieve with pig manure (Loynachan *et al.*, 1976). Aerobic treatment systems for piggery wastes by which the manure is concentrated into sludge and a dischargeable liquid have been developed (Vanstaen *et al.*, 1976; Garraway, 1982). Besides the classical aerobic treatment, integrated aerobic-photosynthetic treatments for piggery slurry have been designed. The controlled growth of photosynthetic microalgae in the aerobically treated liquid phase of pig manure allows further removal of BOD together with removal of significant quantities of nitrogen and phosphorus (Fallowfield *et al.*, 1992; Fallowfield and Svoboda, 1993).

Manure as fertiliser

Composting. The objective of composting is to produce a stable odourless product which can be packaged, stored and used as organic fertiliser for soils. The carbon:nitrogen ratio plays an important role in the composting process. The optimum range is approximately 10-23 and may be adjusted by the addition of straw or other sources of carbon. The ratio is inversely related to the emission of ammonia. Composting of poultry manure is more difficult than pig manure due to the higher nitrogen content. Consequently, the process often results in high ammonia emissions (Kroodsma, 1986; Bonazzi *et al.*, 1988). Moisture content should be in the range of 40-60%. In the case of manure, composting is possible for relatively dry poultry manure, separated fibrous suspended solids or for liquid manure mixed with dry organic material like straw, or composted material itself (Lau and Wu, 1987; Schuchardt, 1987; Lo *et al.*, 1993). Too high a moisture content will fill the void spaces and prevent the free flow of oxygen. Temperature control is also important and usually an optimum of 55 to 60°C needs to be achieved. The temperature may be controlled by the frequency of turning when windrows are used, or by altering the flow rate of air in a system with forced aeration (Biddlestone and Gray, 1985; Finstein and Miller, 1985; Bardos and Lopez-Real, 1989). Temperature has an important influence on the evaporation of the water that is formed when microorganisms convert organic material under anaerobic conditions. The composting process itself usually takes three to four weeks, with a further two to three weeks needed for the product to cool and stabilise.

Drying. Although drying is not a "biotechnological" process, production of dried manure has received great attention, especially in the Netherlands. It is considered as an important way to transport minerals from regions with a surplus to areas with a shortage and a way to replace chemical fertiliser. A number of advantages of the production of dried manure are:
- reduction of volume and consequently a reduction in costs of transport and storage
- destruction of pathogens and weeds
- lower odour and ammonia emission
- composition can be guaranteed and adjusted by the addition of extra minerals and/or organic matter.

It is important, however, to recognise that drying of manure can lead to severe pollution of the atmosphere. As temperature increases the volatile components (volatile fatty acids, ammonia, hydrogen sulphide and carbon dioxide) are emitted. Treatment of the gases can be expensive, depending on the process and the national standards that are imposed. Evaporation and drying also are energy consuming activities. In order to minimise overall processing costs there is a tendency to install extra equipment for the recovery of evaporation heat. This often means that the bulk of the water present in the original manure is condensed and that the major part of the volatile components end up in the condensate. This condensate contains a substantial amount of BOD and N (but almost no salts or humic organic material). These components can however be removed almost completely by biological waste water treatment.

Conversion of manure into animal feed

During the last twenty years various researchers have reported efforts to produce ingredients for animal feedstuff based on manure. Many projects have been and still are aimed at the separation of protein from manure, and at the production of microbial protein (single-cell protein) or amino acids (lysine). The pellicle-forming yeast, *Candida ingens*, was found to grow on the supernatant derived from the anaerobic fermentation of piggery manure (Henry *et al.*, 1976; Henry and Thomson, 1979). More recently, Hong *et al.* (1990) reported the growth of *Schizosaccharomyces* sp. HL on the supernatant from anaerobically fermented pig waste. Both microorganisms seem to have potential value as a feed protein. Until now, however, there is little hard evidence that it is possible to produce protein of good quality and purity from animal excreta on a commercial basis.

UNIT OPERATIONS FOR AIR POLLUTION ABATEMENT

Air pollution from animal production is caused by the volatilisation of compounds from animals, their food and manure. Odours from livestock wastes are due to a mixture of a large number of volatile compounds caused by microbial degradation of plant fibre and protein (Spoelstra, 1979;1980; Hammond *et al.*, 1989). Chemical analysis of piggery wastes has resulted in the identification of some 150 volatile organic compounds (Spoelstra, 1980; Yasuhura *et al*, 1984). The problems arising from the offensiveness of these odorous compounds are well documented (Jongebreur, 1977; Johansson, 1978; Watson and Friend, 1987; O'Neil and Phillips, 1991). In general, animal odours from livestock buildings and manure stores are the cause of many complaints by the public passing within short distances of the source. Odours also emanate from the spreading of manure on to land and can be dispersed over great distances. Several methods for the measurement of odours have been developed (Carney and Dodd, 1989; Hangartner *et al.*, 1989; Van Wassenhove *et al.*, 1992).

Ammonia is one of the most important volatile compounds in manure. Ammonia and ammonium ions present in livestock wastes arise largely from the breakdown of urea. Urea is rapidly hydrolysed by the enzyme urease and converted to ammonia after excretion. The contribution of ammonia to odour concentration and intensity is less important than its effect on the environment. Ammonia, when released into the atmosphere, combines with other gases from industry and vehicles to form compounds which are deposited over wide areas on to the land and surface waters. The result is nitrogen enrichment and acidification of soils and surface waters and the pollution of ground and surface waters with nitrates (Hall, 1988). Ammonia not only has a negative effect on the environment but can adversely affect the health, performance and welfare of the animals (Drummond *et al.*, 1980; Malayer *et al.*, 1988; Donham, 1990; Robertson *et al.*, 1990) and the human attendants (Donham and Gustafason, 1982), as well as the longevity of the facility itself.

Reduction of slurry odours (biological processes)

Anaerobic digestion. Many of the compounds associated with odour emission from livestock wastes are degraded during the digestion process. Volatile fatty acids, for example, can be reduced by >90% (Summers and Bousfield, 1980). Field trials have demonstrated that, following spreading on land, odour concentration is significantly lower for digested than for undigested slurries (Pain *et al.*, 1990).

Aeration. Aeration to abate odour is applied to effluents from livestock farming processes and livestock slurries with less than 3% dry matter content. The degree of odour control depends on the treatment time. For control immediately before application to the land, aeration regimes of two days are sufficient. Storage and subsequent application to land requires a four to five day regime. For the control of ammonia emission and prevention of water pollution, at least four to five days are required to achieve nitrification of the ammonium salts (Williams *et al.*, 1986; Evans and Baines, 1986). Most efficient oxygen transfer occurs when very small bubbles of air are generated in the separated slurry or effluent. To date the most efficient aerators are sub-surface and venturi jet systems, whilst compressed-air sparge systems are more efficient in deep tanks. During continuous aeration, the air input to the aeration vessel or reactor can be controlled either by the dissolved oxygen concentration or the redox potential (Williams *et al.*, 1989).

Bioscrubbers and biofilters. The odorous chemical compounds in the air discharged from livestock buildings dissolve in water and can be utilised by microorganisms as a substrate for growth. Two main types of systems have been developed to remove the pollutants from the ventilation air from buildings i.e. bioscrubbers and biofilters. Bioscrubbers involve passing air through a film or mist of water to dissolve the pollutant in the water. The system includes a carrier, usually of plastic with a large surface area to volume ratio on which microorganisms develop and degrade the odorous compounds present in the water phase. The liquor can be recycled through the system. Monitoring has indicated that bioscrubbers can lead to a reduction of 80 to 90% in odour emission.

Biofilters are based on impeding the airflow through a porous medium colonised with microorganisms such as soil, peat or wood chippings. The medium must be kept moist to operate efficiently and this is achieved by a low rate of irrigation as required. Design principles, which have to take into account maximum airflow rates, are given by Zeisig (1987). Guidelines suggest a bed depth of approximately 1 m, a maximum load of 300 m^3 air per m^2 surface area per hour for peat and heather and 450 m^3 m^{-2} h^{-1} for compost bark. Results indicate that a reduction of 75% for odour emission and 85% for ammonia for both types of media are to be expected.

Both the biofilter and bioscrubber are dependent upon biological processes and require control. The cost of installation and operation is one of the main reasons these systems have not been generally used.

Chemical and biological additives and masking agents. The control of agricultural odours by additives and masking agents has been the subject of much debate as results obtained from farm experience have been very variable. Five main categories of additives can be considered based on the different ways to control odours:

- oxidising agents - permanganate, hypochlorite and ozone which oxidise the odorous compounds. Since slurries contain large amounts of oxidisable organic matter, large quantities of these reagents are needed
- deodorants - chemicals which react with the odorous compounds, inhibiting their release or neutralising them
- masking agents - compounds with concentrated pleasant smells
- digestive agents - usually bacterial cultures or mixtures of bacteria and enzymes in solution (Ohta and Ikeda, 1978; Ohta and Kuwada, 1988). These agents are claimed to break down the odorous compounds in the slurry
- miscellaneous chemicals - bacteriocides, disinfectants and plant extracts. These either are aimed at the destruction of the microorganisms in the slurry or at the inhibition of enzyme activity preventing the development of odorous compounds.

Odour control chemicals, enzymatic products and other digestive aids designed to alter biological pathways involved in manure decomposition are available for odour control. However, only limited data on the use of these materials is available and their efficacy in practice has proved erratic.

Decrease in ammonia concentrations

A number of options are available to achieve a reduction in the ammonia present in the animal environment. Calcium and magnesium salts added to decomposing manure can markedly reduce the amount of ammonia released (Witter and Kirchmann, 1989a). Treating

Table 3. Biotechnological processes for manure treatment.

Treatment	By-product
Total manure	
Addition of chemical or biological additives	
- Reduction of ammonia emission and/or odour reduction	
Aeration	
- Odour reduction	
Drying	
- Odour reduction	- Fertiliser with guaranteed composition
- Volume reduction	
Composting	
- Hygienization	- Stable, storable organic fertiliser
- Removal of COD/BOD	
- Odour reduction	
Anaerobic digestion	
- Hygienization	- Biogas
- Removal of COD/BOD	- Organic fertiliser
- Odour reduction	
Liquid fraction of manure	
Anaerobic purification	
- Removal of COD/BOD	- Biogas
Aerobic purification	
- Removal of COD/BOD	- Dischargeable liquid
- Removal of nitrogen	
- Removal of phosphorus	

litter with phosphoric acid and ferrous sulphate also reduces ammonia release by changing the pH. Various materials have been examined for their ability to absorb ammonia given off during aerobic decomposition of manure. In a study by Witter and Kirchmann (1989b) peat was found to be highly effective, zeolite less so, and basalt had only limited effectiveness.

Plant extracts, notably from *Yucca shidigera*, have been reported to have the ability to decrease ammonia and hydrogen sulphide emission from animals wastes. The mechanism by which this occurs is unclear. The suggestion (Mader and Brumm, 1987) that saponins in *Y. shidigera* inhibited urease appears not to be true: Headon *et al.* (1991) described a glycocomponent that bound NH_3 and suggested that this binding was for odour reductions. Little data exists at present concerning the effectiveness of these extracts.

FULL SCALE PLANTS FOR THE PROCESSING OF MANURE

The different biotechnological processes described are summarised in Table 3 according to their increasing complexity and their efficiency in dealing with the problem of a surplus of manure. As a consequence of more stringent national and international environmental legislation and in response to increasing agricultural pollution of ground and surface waters, several technologies based on one or more of the described unit operations have been developed.

Biogas plants in Denmark

Under the Danish Action Programme for Joint Large-scale Biogas Plants which commenced in 1986, nine cooperative-owned biogas facilities have been constructed (Sjahaa and Hannibal, 1990). Of these, six operate at mesophilic temperatures and three are thermophilic. The Danish programme differs from a number of other national programmes in that organic industrial and source-sorted household wastes are co-digested with animal manure. The industrial wastes are derived from slaughter houses and food processing industries and the non-manure input to the mixed feeds is not allowed to exceed 20% on a weight basis (Colleran, 1992).

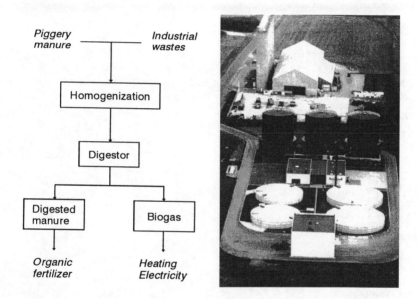

Figure 1. Schematic flow-sheet and view of the joint biogas plant at Lemvig in Denmark.

The plant of Lemvig, for example, handles the wastes of some 100 farmers in a 10 km radius from the plant. A schematic flow-sheet of the plant is given in Fig. 1. Some 440 tonnes of biomass are treated daily producing 12000 m^3 biogas. The biomass processed consists predominantly of manure supplemented with industrial biological wastes (from slaughter houses, milk factories, oil-treating factories) to a final dry matter content of 5-10%. Digestion is at 50-52°C for a period of 17 days and the production of biogas is of the order of 31 m^3 tonne^{-1}. Residual material is used as organic fertiliser by the cooperating farmers. The methane gas is used for combined heat and power production. The overall profit of the biogas plant is gathered from the sale of the methane gas to the municipality and from the tipping fees from the industrial wastes minus the total costs of hauling the biomass.

The Promest process

The Promest design converts piggery manure into a legally disposable effluent and a formulated organic fertiliser (Fig. 2). The main processes are an anaerobic digestion in two parallel digestion units in order, firstly, to produce gas, secondly, to reduce the BOD and organic material that is volatilised during heating and, thirdly, to improve the dewatering characteristics. The main part of the suspended solids is then separated and dewatered by a centrifuge. The liquid fraction is nitrified in activated sludge tanks with addition of lime for the neutralisation. The effluent, free of volatile material, is concentrated in a three stage evaporator and the distillate discharged to surface water. The centrifugation cake is dried, granulated and formulated as organic fertiliser.

The demonstration plant at Helmond, with capacity of 100,000 m^3 yr^{-1}, has been tested for more than two years and a plant with the capacity to handle 500,000 m^3 yr^{-1} manure is under construction at the same location.

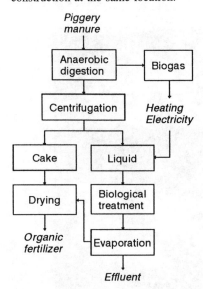

Figure. 2. Schematic flow-sheet of the Promest process.

The VerTech process

The central treatment step of the VerTech process is a chemical wet oxidation by which the organic compounds in the aqueous phase are oxidised with the formation of CO_2, ammonia, acetate and metal oxides. The VerTech technology was developed originally for the treatment of sludge (Zimmerman, 1958) but has been adapted for the processing of manure (Fig. 3). The wet oxidation of manure occurs at 270°C at a pressure of 8 MPa and results in a COD reduction of 40% (De Bekker, 1988). The COD reduction can be improved by increasing the oxygen supply. The condensate of the off-gases is, prior to discharge, purified in a conventional biological (aerobic/anaerobic) waste water treatment plant. The dry product obtained by the oxidation can be formulated as fertiliser (De Bekker, 1988).

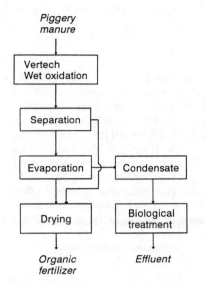

Figure 3. Schematic flow-sheet of the VerTech process.

POTENTIALS FOR PIGGERY MANURE TREATMENT

Recycling of minerals

The full scale processes described above recycle minerals within the agricultural sector and not at the level of the individual farm. The so-called Rome process (**R**ecuperative extraction of **O**ligo-elements and **M**inerals from **E**xcreta) would enable the on-farm recycling of nutrients by re-feeding the liquid fraction of manure. A central treatment step is an anaerobic thermophilic hygienization. This process results in a solid fraction with low mineral, nitrogen, phosphorus and potassium content that is fit to be spread on the land and a liquid fraction, containing essential minerals, which can be re-fed.

Solid state composting

Liquid piggery manure as such can not be composted because of its high moisture content and unfavourable carbon-to-nitrogen ratio. Tests have been carried out in which the solid fraction of manure was composted using peat and sawdust as bulking agents (Lo *et al.*, 1993). Based on measured compost characteristics and composition, the finished composts made from a manure/peat moss mixture had the best quality in terms of moisture content, nitrogen content, carbon:nitrogen ratio and the colour of the product. The liquid fraction still has to be subjected to a separate treatment.

An analogous composting process by which paper is mixed with piggery manure is under investigation. This approach has two main advantages, firstly, the composting process is carried out with the complete manure so that no liquid fraction has to be treated separately and, secondly, another waste stream (paper) is used as carbon source and bulking agent. The process results in an odourless compost that is stable and can be stored easily. Organic fertiliser is one of the possible applications of the end product.

Feed supplements

The mineral composition and odour characteristics of the manure can be influenced by the composition of the feed. Addition of phytase ensures that more of the phosphorus that is present as phytic acid in grain becomes available for the simple-stomached animal so that less phosphorous has to be formulated in the feed. Simons *et al.* (1990) reported that the addition of microbial phytase to low phosphorus diets for growing pigs increased the apparent uptake of phosphorus by 24%. Consequently, the amount of P in the faeces was 35% lower. In the case of broilers, phosphorus availability increased by 60% and the phosphorus in the droppings decreased by 50%. In both cases, the growth rate and feed conversion ratio on the low phosphorus diets containing microbial phytase were comparable to or even better than those obtained on control diets. Pen *et al.* (1993) expressed a phytase gene from *Aspergillus niger* in tobacco seeds, providing a stable and convenient packaging of the enzyme that is directly applicable in animal feed. Supplementation of broiler diets with transgenic seeds resulted in an improved growth rate, comparable to diets supplemented with fungal phytase or phosphorus, and reduced phosphorus excretion.

A new approach is the development of probiotics to control the odour formation in manure. The odour emission of manure is mainly due to the microbial degradation process during storage. Investigations are underway to formulate probiotics so that the dominating microbial populations in manure are altered towards lesser odour emissions.

CONCLUDING REMARKS

The concentration of intensive animal husbandry in certain parts of the world has led to a flux of nutrients from regions where crop production predominates (USA, Canada, S. America) to regions of intensive animal rearing (Northern Europe) where the concomitant manure surpluses cause severe environmental problems.

Biotechnology can help to abate the animal manure problems in different ways. A great deal of concern by the general public can be avoided by preventing the emission of ammonia and of malodorous compounds. Excretion of excess nutrients, particularly nitrogen, can be reduced by altering and improving nutrient capture by the animal. Technologies with the potential to recycle part of the manure, either as an organic fertiliser or as a mineral resource, are now available. Finally, by implementing processes of total conversion of the wastes, an "end-of-pipe" solution comparable to that for domestic sewage, could be provided.

The major bottleneck in the treatment of animal manure is the low economic carrying capacity of the agricultural sector. To handle and treat manure properly, increases of the order of 10-20% in the costs of animal production are to be expected. Similar increases in production prices due to environmental legislation, however, have been absorbed during the last decade by the chemical industry and, more recently, by sectors of the food industry. Such increases could be absorbed in animal husbandry, but only if legislation is enforced in an even-handed way. All farmers should be required to introduce manure treatments in situations in which more traditional methods of disposal lead to pollution. The public perception of agriculture in general, and animal husbandry in particular, is of an industry with a poor environmental record. A strategy to integrate animal husbandry in sustainable agriculture is urgently required. The world-wide imbalance in nutrients resulting from importation of animal feed argues for the development of a commerce based on products recovered from animal manure in order to redress the balance. Biotechnology can play a key role in transforming animal manure to hygienic high quality organic fertilisers. The combination of technology, international legislation and trade could transform the current problems of animal manure disposal into a positive example of how to achieve sustainable agriculture on a world-wide basis.

Acknowledgement

This work was in part supported by the IWONL (Instuut ter aanmoediging van het Wetenschappelijk Onderzoek in de Nijverheid en Landbouw). The advice of K. De Roo, M. P. Di Poorter and G. Neakermans is warmly appreciated.

REFERENCES

Bardos, R.P. and Lopez-Real, J.M.   1989.   The composting process: susceptible feedstocks, temperature, microbiology, sanitization.   In *Compost Processes in Waste Management* (W. Bidlingmaier, and P. L'Hermite, eds) pp. 179-190. E. Guyot SA, Brussels, Belgium.

Beaudet, R., Gagnon C., Bisaillon, J-G. and Ishaque, M.   1990.   Microbial aspects of aerobic themophilic treatemnt of swine waste. *Appl. Environ. Microbiol.* **56**, 971-976.

Biddlestone, A.J. and Gray, K.R.   1985.   Practical experience with farm scale systems. In *Composting of Agricultural and Other Wastes* (J.K.R. Gasser, ed.) pp. 111-134. Elsevier Applied Science Publishers, London, UK.

Blouin, M., Bisaillon, J.-G. and Beaudet, R.   1988.   Aerobic biodegradation of organic matter of swine waste. *Biol. Wastes* **25**, 127-139.

Bonazzi, G., Valli, L., and Piccinini, S.   1988.   Controlling ammonia emission from poultry manure composting plants.   In *Volatile Emissions from Livestock Farming and Sewage Operations* (V.C. Nielsen, J.H. Voorburg, and P. L'Hermite, eds) pp. 258-272. Elsevier Appied Science Publishers, London, UK.

Bossier, P., Poels, J., Van Assche, P. and Verstraete, W.   1986.   Influence of the dimensional characteristics of polyurethane foam on high rate anaerobic digestion of piggery manure. *Biotechn. Lett.* **8**, 901-906.

Bourque, D., Bisaillon, J.-G., Beaudet, R., Sylvestre, M., Ishaque, M. and Morin, A.   1987. Microbial degradation of malodorous substances of swine waste under aerobic conditions. *Appl. Environ. Microbiol.* **53**, 137-141.

Carney, P.G. and Dodd, V.A.   1989.   The measurement of agricultural malodours. *J. Agric. Eng. Res.* **43**, 197-209.

Colleran, E. 1992. Anaerobic digestion of agricultural and food-processing effluents. In *Microbial Control of Pollution* (J.C. Fry, G.M. Gadd, R.A. Herbert, C.W. Jones and I.A. Watson-Craik, eds) pp. 199-226. Cambridge University Press, Cambridge, UK.

De Bekker, P.H.A.M.J. 1988. Natte oxydatie van drijfmest op 1500 meter diepte. *Procestechniek* **43**, 38-41.

Donham, K.J.   1990.   Relationships of air quality and productivity in intensive swine housing. *J. Agri-Practice* **10**, 15-18.

Donham, K.J. and Gustafason, K.E. 1982. Human occupational hazards from swine confinement. *Ann. Am. Conf. Gov. Labs. Hyg.* **2**, 137-142.

Doyle, Y., Guay, R., de la Noue, J. and Asselin, J. 1986. Traitement aérobic du lisier de porc: aspects microbiens. *Can. J. Microbiol.* **32**, 679-686.

Drummond, J.G., Curtis, S.E., Simon, J. and Norton, H.W. 1980. Effects of aerial ammonia on growth and health of young pigs. *J. Anim. Sci.* **50**, 1085-1091.

Eurostat Regions Statistical Yearbook. 1989. Office of Official Publications of the European Community, Luxemburg.

Evans, M.R. and Baines S. 1986. Aeration and odour control by heterotrophic and autotrophic microorganisms. In *Odour Prevention and Control of Organic Sludge and Livestock Farming* (V.C. Nielsen, J.H. Voorburg, and P. L'Hermite, eds) pp. 273-287. Elsevier Applied Science Publishers, London, UK.

Fallowfield, H.J., Svoboda, I.F. and Martin, N.J. 1992. Aerobic and photosynthetic treatment of animal slurries. In *Microbial Control of Pollution* (J.C. Fry, G.M. Gadd, R.A. Herbert, C.W. Jones, and I.A. Watson-Craik, eds) pp. 171-197. Cambridge University Press, Cambridge, UK.

Fallowfield, H.J. and Svoboda, I. 1993. What can aerobic microbes do for slurry treatment? In *Proceedings of the Second Belgian Days on Pigs and Poultry, Conference organised by the Royal Flemish Society of Engineers*, Brugge 17-19 February 1993. Royal Flemish Society of Engineers, Antwerp, Belgium.

Fenlon, D.R. and Robinson, K. 1977. Denitrification of aerobically stabilised pig waste. *Water Res.* **11**, 269-273.

Finstein, M.S. and Miller, F.C. 1985. Principles of composting leading to maximization of decomposition rate, odour control and cost effectiveness. In *Composting of Agricultural and Other Wastes* (J.K.R. Gasser, ed) pp. 3-13. Elsevier Applied Science Publishers, London, UK.

Fleming, G.A. 1993. Animal waste production in the EC. In *The Production of Animal Wastes, Environment Agriculture Stock Farming in Europe* (G.A. Fleming and A. Mordenti, eds) pp. 6-10. European Conference, Mantua, Italy.

Friman, R. 1984. Monitoring anaerobic digesters on farms. *J. Agric. Eng. Res.* **29**, 357-365.

Garraway, J.L. 1982. Investigations on the aerobic treatment of pig slurry. *Agric. Wastes* **4**, 131-142.

Hall, J.E. 1988. Environmental effects of ammonia volatilisation from agriculture. In *Safe and Efficient Slurry Utilization* (H. Vetter, G. Steffens, and P. L'Hermite, eds) pp. 71-77. Commission of the European Comunities, Brussels, Belgium.

Hammond, E.G., Heppner, C. and Smith, R. 1989. Odor of swine waste lagoons. *Agric. Ecosyst. Environ.* **25**, 103-110.

Hangartner, M., Hartung, J., Paduch, M., Pain, B.F. and Voorburg, J.H. 1989. Improved recommendations on olfactometric measurements. *Environ. Techn. Lett.* **10**, 231-236.

Hawkes, D.L. 1979. Factors affecting net energy production from mesophilic anaerobic digestion. In *Anaerobic Digestion Processes* (D.A. Stafford, B.I. Wheatly and D.E. Hughes, eds) pp. 131-149. Applied Science Publishers, London, UK.

Headon, D.R., Buggle, K., Nelson, A. and Killeen, G. 1991. Glycofractions of the yucca plant and their role in ammonia control. In *Biotechnology in the Feed Industry* (T.P. Lyons, ed) pp. 95-108. Alltech, Nicholasville, Kentucky, US.

Henry, D.P., Thomson, R.H., Sizemore, D.J. and O'Leary, J.A. 1976. Study of *Candida ingens* grown on the supernatant derived from the anaerobic fermentation of monogastric animal waste. *Appl. Environ. Microbiol.* **31**, 813-818.

Henry, D.P. and Thomson R.H. 1979. Growth of *Candida ingens* on supernatant from anaerobically fermented pig waste: effect of temperature and pH. *Appl. Environ. Microbiol.* **37**, 1132-1136.

Hobson, P.N., Bousfield, S. and Summers, R. 1981. *Methane Production from Agricultural and Domestic Wastes*. Applied Science Publishers, London, UK.

Hobson, P.N. and Feilden, N.E.H. 1982. Production of biogas from agriculture wastes. *Prog. Energy Combust. Sci.* **8**, 135-158.

Hong, S.S., Pack, M.Y. and Lee, N.H. 1990. Growth of *Schizosaccharomyces* sp. HL on supernatant from anaerobically fermented pig waste: effects of VFA concentration and pH. *Biotechnol. Lett.* **12**, 309-314.

Iannotti, E.L., Fischer, J.R. and. Sievers, D.M. 1982. Characterisation of bacteria from a swine manure digester. *Appl. Environ. Microbiol.* **43**, 136-143.

Johansson, I. 1978. Determination of organic compounds in indoor air with potential reference to air quality. *Atmos. Environ.* **12**, 1371-1377.

Jongebreur, A.A. 1977. Odor problems and odor control in intensive livestock husbandry farms in the Netherlands. *Agric. Environ.* **3**, 259-265.

Kroodsma, W. 1986. Separation as a method of manure handling and odours reduction in pig buildings. In *Odour Prevention and Control of Organic Sludge and Livestock Farming* (V.C. Nielsen, J.H. Voorburg, and P. L'Hermite, eds) pp. 213-221. Elsevier Appied Science Publishers, London, UK.

Lau, D.C.W. and Wu, M.W. 1987. Manure composting as an option for utilization and management of animal waste. *Resources Conserv.* **13**, 145-156.

Lee, J. and Coulter, B. 1990. A macro view of animal manure production in the European community and implications for environment. In *Manure and Environment VIV Europe.* pp. 1-32. Misset Publishers, Utrecht, Netherlands.

Lettinga, G. and Hulshoff Pol, L.W. 1986. Advanced reactor design, operation and economy. *Water Sci. Technol.* **18**, 99-108.

Lo, K.V., Lau, A.K. and Liao, P.H. 1993. Composting of separated solid swine wastes. *J. Agric. Eng. Res.* **54**, 307-331.

Loynachan, T.E., Bartholomew, W.V. and Wollum, A.G. 1976. Nitrogen transformations in aerated swine manure slurries. *J. Environ. Qual.* **5**, 293-297.

Mader, T.L. and Brumm, M.C. 1987. Effect of feeding sarsaponin in cattle and swine diets. *J. Anim. Sci.* **65**, 9-15.

Malayer, J.R. Brandt, M.L. Green, M.L., Kelly, D.T., Sutton, A.L. and Diekman, M.A. 1988. Influence of manure gases on the onset of puberty of replacement gilts. *Anim. Prod.* **46**, 277-282.

O'Neil, D.H. and Phillips, V.R. 1991. A review of the control of odor nuisance from livestock buildings. Influence of the techniques for managing waste within the building. Part 1. *J. Agric. Eng. Res.* **50**, 1-10.

Ohta, Y. and Ikeda, M. 1978. Deodorization of pig feces by actinomycetes. *Appl. Environ. Microbiol.* **36**, 487-491.

Ohta, Y. and Kuwada, Y. 1988. Rapid deodorization of cattle feces by microorganisms. *Biol. Wastes* **24**, 227-240.

Pain, B.F., Misselbrook, T.H., Clarkson, C.R. and Rees, Y.J. 1990. Odour and ammonia emission following the spreading of anaerobically-digested pig slurry on grassland. *Biol. Wastes* **34**, 259-267.

Pen, J., Verwoerd, T.C., van Paridon, P.A., Beudeker, R.F., van den Elzen, P., Geerse, K., van der Klis, J., Versteegh, H., van Ooyen, A. and Hoekema, A. 1993. Phytase-containing transgenic seeds as a novel feed additive for improved phosphorus utilization. *Bio/Technology* **11**, 811-814.

Poels, J., Vermeiren, W. and Verstraete, W. 1981. Zuivering van voorgecentrifugeerek varhensmengmest in een anaërobe opstroomreaktor. H_2O **14**, 337-339.

Poels, J., Neukermans, G., Van Assche, P., Debruyckere M. and Verstraete, W. 1983. Performance, operation and benfits of an anaerobic digestion system on a closed piggery farm. *Agric. Wastes* **8**, 233-249.

Poels, J., Van Assche, P. and Verstraete, W. 1984. High-rate anaerobic digestion of piggery manure with polyurethane sponges on support material. *Biotechnol. Lett.* **6**, 747-752.

Poels, J., Van Assche, P. and Verstraete, W. 1985. Influence of H_2-stripping on methane production in conventional digesters. *Biotechnol. Bioeng.* **27**, 1692-1698.

Robertson, J.F., Wilson, D. and Smith, W.J. 1990. Atrophic rhinitus: the influence of the aerial environment. *Anim. Prod.* **50**, 173-182.

Safley, L.M., Vetter, R.L. and Smith, D. 1987. Operating a full-scale poultry manure anaerobic digester. *Biol. Wastes* **19**, 79-90.

Schomaker, A.H.H.M., Grootjen, D.R.J. and Lettinga G. 1986. Anaerobic treatment of calf-fattening manure using a flocculent sludge UASB reactor. In *Proceedings of the Water Treatment Conference, 'Anaerobic treatment, a grown-up technology',* Amsterdam pp. 506-513.

Schuchardt, F. 1987. Composting of liquid manure and straw. In *Proc. of 4th International Symposium of CIEC Agricultural Waste Management and Environmental Protection,* Braunschweig, pp. 271-281, Germany.

Simons, P.C., Versteegh, H., Jongbloed, A., Kemme, P., Slump, P., Bos, K.D., Wolters, G.E., Beudeker, R.F. and Verschoor, G.J. 1990. Improvement of phosphorus availability by microbial phytase in broilers and pigs. *Br. J. Nutr.* **64**, 525-540.

Sjahaa, J. and Hannibal, E. 1990. Anaerobic gasification advances. *Biocycle* **31**, 74-77.

Spoelstra, S.F. 1979. Volatile fatty acids in anaerobically stored piggery wastes. *Nether. J. Agric. Sci.* **27**, 60-66.

Spoelstra, S.F. 1980. Origin of objectionable odorous compounds in piggery wastes and the possibility of applying indicator components for studying odor development. *Agric. Environ.* **5**, 241-260.

Summers, R. and Bousfield, S. 1980. A detailed study of piggery-waste anaerobic digestion. *Agric. Wastes* **3**, 61-78.

Summers, R., Hobson, P.N., Harries, C. and Feilden, N.E.H. 1984. Anaerobic digestion on a large pig unit. *Process Biochem.* **19**, 77-78.

Switzenbaum, M.S. 1983. Anaerobic fixed film wastewater treatment. *Enz. Microb. Technol.* **5**, 242-251.

Ten Have, P.J.W. and Chiappini, U. 1993. Processing of manure surpluses. In *Environment Agricultural Stock Farming in Europe,* European Conference, Mantua, Italy, 29 pp.

Van Wassenhove, F., Vanrolleghem, P., Van Langenhove, H. and Verstraete, W. 1992. Olfactometric characterization of odour generation potential of piggery manure samples. In *Biotechniques for Air Pollution Abatement and Odour Control Policies* (A.J. Dragt and. J. Ham, eds) pp. 425-430. Elsevier, Amsterdam, Netherlands.

Vanstaen, H., Voets, J.P. and Verstraete, W. 1976. Three step treatment for piggery wastes. *Water Res.* **10**, 927-928.

Watson, R.D. and Friend, J.A.R. 1987. Pig housing and human health. In *Pig Housing and the Environment* (A.T. Smithe, and T.L.J. Lawrence, eds) pp 41-51. British Society for Animal Production.

Williams, A.G., Shaw, M., Selviah, C.M. and Cumby T.R. 1986. Oxygen requirements for controlling odours from pig slurry by aeration. In *Odour Prevention and Control of Organic Sludge and Livestock Farming* (V.C. Nielsen, J.H. Voorburg and P. L'Hermite, eds) pp. 258-272. Elsevier Applied Science Publishers, London, UK.

Williams, A.G., Shaw, M., Selviah, C.M. and Cumby T.R 1989. The oxygen requirements for deodorising and stabilising pig slurry by aerobic treatment. *Agric. Eng. Res.* **43**, 291-311.

Witter, E. and Kirchmann, H. 1989a. Peat, zeolite and basalt as absorbents of ammoniacal nitrogen during manure decomposition. *Plant Soil* **115**, 53-61.

Witter, E. and Kirchmann, H. 1989b. Effects of addition of calcium and magnesium salts on ammonia volatilization during manure decomposition. *Plant Soil* **115**, 43-52.

Yasuhura, A., Fuwa, K. and Jimbu, M. 1984. Identification of odorous compounds in fresh and rotten swine manure. *Agric. Biol. Chem.* **48**, 3001-3010.

Zehnder, A.J.B., Ingvorsen, K. and Marti, T. 1982. Microbiology of methane bacteria. In *Anaerobic Digestion 1981* (D.E. Hughes, D.A. Stattford, B.I. Wheatley, W. Baader, G. Lettinga, E.J. Nyns, W. Verstraete and R.L. Wentworth, eds) pp. 45-68. Elsevier Biomedical Press, Amsterdam, Netherlands.

Zeikus, J.G. 1982. Microbial populations in digesters. In *Anaerobic Digestion* (D.A. Stafford, B.I. Wheatley and D.E. Hughes, eds) pp. 61-85. Applied Science Publishers, London, UK.

Zeisig, M.D. 1987. Experiences with the use of biofilters to remove odours from piggeries and hen houses. In *Livestock Farming and Sewage Operations* (V.C. Nielsen, J.H. Voorburg, and P. L'Hermite, eds) pp. 209-216. Elsevier Applied Science Publishers, London, UK.

Zimmerman, F.J. 1958. New waste disposal process. *Chem. Eng.* **67**, 117-120.

17 Feed additives and other interventions for decreasing methane emissions

Christian Van Nevel and Daniel Demeyer

Department of Animal Production, University of Gent, 9090 Melle, Belgium

INTRODUCTION

Methane production in the rumen

In this chapter, only methane production and its inhibition in the rumen will be considered. Ruminant methane production is responsible for approximately 95% of total global animal and human methane emissions (Johnson *et al.*, 1991). Furthermore, 90% of ruminant methane is produced in the forestomachs, while only 10% originates from hindgut fermentation (Murray *et al.*, 1978).

During the microbial fermentation process in the rumen, carbohydrates, protein and glycerol are oxidized anaerobically to acetate, carbon dioxide and ammonia, with methane, propionate and butyrate being produced mainly as a result of electron and proton transfer reactions (hydrogen sinks). The reduction of CO_2 with H_2 via methanogenesis keeps the partial pressure of hydrogen very low, and this has an important effect on the overall fermentation: hydrogenase activity can proceed towards hydrogen production, thus avoiding the formation of lactate or ethanol as major end products and allowing more acetate to be produced (Wolin and Miller, 1988). Consequently, the ATP yield during fermentation is increased, leading to a higher microbial growth efficiency (per mole of substrate fermented) as a result of methane formation. The efficiency of microbial growth is nutritionally important, because microbial protein flowing from the rumen is the most important source of protein for the ruminant. The standard free energy change of the overall process of methane production ($CO_2 + 4H_2 \rightarrow CH_4 + 2H_2O$) is negative and allows formation of ATP, which is used by the methanogenic bacteria for maintenance and growth purposes (Russell and Wallace, 1988). Therefore, it can be argued that selective inhibition of methanogenesis in the rumen would result in a decreased bacterial protein synthesis. However, based on the fact that approximately 5 g of cells are produced per mole of methane formed (Weimer and Zeikus, 1978; Schauer and Ferry, 1980) in a cow producing 200 l of methane per day methanogens contribute only about 1% of the total microbial matter leaving the rumen.

In vitro, inhibition of methanogenesis lowered microbial growth yields only when hydrogen gas accumulated, probably because of an impairment of substrate level phosphorylation mechanisms (Van Nevel and Demeyer, 1981). It was also soon observed that inhibition of methanogenesis shifted electron transfer to propionate production as an alternative electron sink in fermentation, while acetate formation was decreased (Demeyer and Van Nevel, 1987). It can be speculated that the loss of ATP yield caused by lower acetate and methane production is compensated by an increased ATP yield from propionate formation, during which ATP is also generated (Russell and Wallace, 1988). The biochemical and bacteriological aspects of biogenic methane production have been reviewed recently (Miller, 1991; Ferry, 1992).

Finally, abundant research on rumen metabolism has shown that all reactions in the rumen are integrated parts of a series of interdependent reactions; for example, optimal fibre digestion is associated with substantial methanogenesis. This means that manipulation of the system by, for example, inhibiting one reaction will result in different interrelated effects. Inhibition of methanogenesis cannot be considered as a separate intervention, and its consequences on general rumen fermentation and animal metabolism cannot be ignored.

Negative aspects of rumen methane production

Research on rumen methanogenesis and its inhibition was initiated with the aim of increasing feed efficiency (Czerkawski, 1969). Depending on the level of feeding, composition of the diet and digestibility, 2-15% of the gross energy in the feed is lost through methane production (Johnson *et al.*, 1991; Holter and Young, 1992). By shifting electron flow from methane to propionate production, more energy and carbon are deposited in volatile fatty acids (VFA), which become available to the animal.

It has recently become clear that methane also plays an important role in global warming and in the destruction of the ozone layer, and since atmospheric methane concentrations continue to increase at 1% per annum, methanogenesis by farm animals has received renewed interest (Crutzen *et al.*, 1986; Byers and Turner, 1990; Johnson *et al.*, 1991; Tyler, 1991; Thompson *et al.*, 1992; Johnson *et al.*, in press). Total emissions of methane into the atmosphere are estimated at 400 to 600 x 10^{12} g per year, which is responsible for ca. 15% of overall global warming (Johnson *et al.*, 1991). Methane is more efficient in absorbing infrared energy than carbon dioxide, which means that, despite its very low concentration, the contribution of methane to global warming is not negligible (Tyler, 1991). Calculations in this area are inevitably of limited accuracy, but some suggest that only 2% of the global warming effect is due to methane production by domestic livestock (Johnson *et al.*, 1991). Unfortunately, in contrast with an estimated annual financial loss of approximately £15,000 million due to feed energy losses caused by methane production in ruminants (Czerkawski, 1986), the rather modest contribution of animal methane to global warming cannot be expressed in terms of striking monetary losses. It can be reasoned that inhibited methanogenesis would result in a higher production of carbon dioxide, the most important gas responsible for global warming. Stoichiometrical considerations show that this is not the case, as often confirmed in experiments *in vitro* and *in vivo* (Demeyer *et al.*, 1969; Van Nevel *et al.*, 1969; Slyter, 1979; Chalupa *et al.*, 1980; Stanier and Davies, 1981; Wakita *et al.*, 1986; Kone *et al.*, 1989).

INHIBITION OF METHANOGENESIS IN THE RUMEN

Intervention at the dietary level by ration manipulation

Methane production (kJ per 100 kJ in feed) was found to be negatively related to the level of intake, while at a maintenance level of feeding, increases in digestibility resulted in higher methane production (Blaxter and Clapperton, 1965). The rate of fermentation is also important: substrates which are fermented at a slower rate, such as structural carbohydrates, yield more methane per unit substrate fermented than highly fermentable food components (Czerkawski, 1969; Holter and Young, 1992). This was illustrated clearly in experiments with cows receiving rations varying in hay to concentrate ratio from 100:0 to 20:80 (Ørskov *et al.*, 1968). Methane production was gradually decreased with increasing amounts of concentrates, the 20:80 type ration giving half the methane production of the 100% hay diet. High amounts of concentrates decrease rumen pH and it is known that methanogenic bacteria are inhibited at lower pH values (Demeyer and Henderickx, 1967b). Molar proportions of propionic acid increased from 17 to 31%, in agreement with the inverse relationship between methane and propionate production in rumen fermentation (Van Nevel *et al.*, 1974). Based on this relationship, it can be predicted that any intervention at the dietary level (composition, quantity) which causes a shift in VFA proportions in the rumen will also result in changes in methane production: a decreased acetate:propionate (A/P) ratio will result in lower methane production. A great number of factors affect the A/P ratio in the rumen, and numerous papers in the literature deal with this subject. Some interventions which can lower the A/P ratio are:

- increasing the amount of highly fermentable carbohydrates and decreasing proportions of roughage in the diet (Ørskov *et al.*, 1968; Thomas and Rook, 1977; Broster *et al.*, 1979; Sutton, 1986; Ilian *et al.*, 1986; Oshio *et al.*, 1987; Cecava *et al.*, 1990)
- physical treatment of the ration: grinding and pelleting of roughages and heat treatment (steam flaking, micronization) of grain (Thomson, 1972; Thomas and Clapperton, 1972; Aimone and Wagner, 1977; Zinn, 1987; Moore *et al.*, 1992)
- sodium hydroxide treatment of straw (Hvelplund *et al.*, 1978)
- feeding frequency: low frequencies tend to increase molar proportions of propionate (Roth and Kirschgessner, 1976; Jensen and Wolstrup, 1977; Sutton *et al.*, 1986)
- increasing the level of feeding with hay-concentrate based diets (Thomas and Rook, 1977; Broster *et al.*, 1979; Norgaard, 1987)
- feeding buffers and other types of dietary manipulation (Harrison *et al.*, 1975,1976; Hodgson *et al.*, 1976; Thomson *et al.*, 1978; Rogers and Davis, 1982; Hadjipanayiotou *et al.*, 1982; Estell and Galyean, 1985).

Effect of additives fed with the ration

Halogenated methane analogues and other compounds. Inhibition of methanogenesis by diversion of electrons from the reduction of CO_2 to other acceptors was found in *in vitro* experiments with the addition of methylene blue, riboflavin, NAD, nitrate, sulfate, sulfite, methyl- and benzyl viologen. Sometimes hydrogen gas accumulated in the system (McNeill, 1957; Wolin *et al.*, 1964). In addition to its action as alternative electron acceptor, sulfite also had a direct toxic effect on methanogenic bacteria (Van Nevel *et al.*, 1970a). A daily dose of 10 g of Na_2SO_3 infused in the rumen of a sheep resulted in a 65% inhibition of methane production. However, the effect was transient and 5 h after addition methane production was almost completely restored, due to reduction and/or absorption of the added compound (Van Nevel *et al.*, 1970a). The decrease in methane was accompanied by an altered VFA pattern in the rumen: acetate decreased in favour of propionate and butyrate. From all these experiments, it seemed that the effect of most alternative electron acceptors was not very specific, rendering practical application of any of the compounds unlikely.

Direct inhibition of methanogenesis has been found with halogenated methane analogues and some other compounds. Small quantities of chloroform, carbon tetrachloride and methylene chloride were accidentally found to be potent inhibitors of methane production in incubations of mixed rumen bacteria metabolizing formate or CO_2/H_2 (Bauchop, 1967). Further research showed methane-inhibitory properties for a series of halogenated compounds, including chloral hydrate (Van Nevel *et al.*, 1969), methylene bromide (Van Nevel *et al.*, 1970), di-and trichloroacetamide (Trei *et al.*, 1971; Slyter, 1979), nitrapyrin (2-chloro-6-(trichloromethyl)-pyridine) (Salvas and Taylor, 1980), bromochloromethane (Johnson *et al.*, 1972), hemi-acetal of chloral and starch (HCS) (Johnson, 1972), trichloroethyl adipate and -pivalate (Czerkawski and Breckenridge, 1975) and chloro-substituted benzo-1,3-dioxins (Stanier and Davies, 1981) (Table 1). Chloral hydrate is converted in the rumen to chloroform, either enzymically or chemically (Prins, 1965; Quaghebeur and Oyaert, 1971). Methane production by pure strains of methanogens was inhibited by chloroform, carbon tetrachloride and chloral hydrate (Prins *et al.*, 1972). 2-Bromoethanesulfonic acid (BES) is a bromine analogue of coenzyme-M and interferes with methanogenesis by inhibiting the methyl coenzyme-M reductase in methanogenic bacteria (Balch and Wolfe, 1979). In the pathway of methane formation, coenzyme-M is a carrier of C_1 units at the methanol level of oxidation (McBride and Wolfe, 1971). BES is a potent methane inhibitor (Table 1), yet even huge amounts of the compound, much higher than needed for inhibition of methane production, had only a small inhibitory effect on substrate degradation as shown by VFA production (Table 2). The VFA pattern was altered: molar proportions of propionate and butyrate were increased at the expense of acetate production, while hydrogen gas accumulated (Table 2). Growth studies with a wide range of microbes, including eubacteria, archaebacteria and yeast, have shown that BES inhibited growth only of methanogens (Sparling and Daniels, 1987). Similar specificity was also reported by Sauer and Teather (1987).

In an experiment in our laboratory to investigate the effects of BES *in vivo* (I. Immig *et al.*, manuscript in preparation) a pulse dose of 2 g of BES, followed by continuous infusion of 2 g per day into the rumen of a sheep decreased the proportion of methane in rumen gases from 40 to 0.4% after 7 h. However, after three days the methane content increased to 26%, clearly showing that adaptation of the methanogenic population occurred.

The exact mechanism of action of halogenated methane analogues on methanogenesis remains uncertain. They form complexes with corrinoid compounds, thus inhibiting cobamide dependent methyl transfer (Wood *et al.*, 1968). However, in extracts of *Methanobacterium* M.o.H. no cobamide-containing proteins could be detected (Wolfe, 1971). Pyromellitic diimide, a by-product formed during the conversion of natural gas to petrol, was found to be a very potent methane inhibitor but unfortunately it was inactivated in the rumen within 24 h (Martin and Macy, 1985; Eijssen *et al.*, 1990). Dimethyldiphenyliodonium chloride (DDIC) was used in rumen manipulation as a deaminase inhibitor, but methane production also decreased (Table 1). Its mechanism of action on methane formation or methanogens is unknown (Chalupa, 1980). Inhibition of methane production by the dietary addition of compounds mentioned above can eventually be accompanied by a series of phenomena not always favourable for the animal or production system:

- hydrogen accumulation in the rumen, still representing an energy loss (Demeyer and Van Nevel, 1975)
- lowered substrate utilization and depressed microbial protein yields *in vitro* (Marty and Demeyer, 1973; Chalupa *et al.*, 1980; Russell and Martin, 1984), although this is not always confirmed *in vivo* (Mathers and Miller, 1982)
- inhibition of amino acid degradation (Chalupa *et al.*, 1980; Russell and Martin, 1984)
- depressed feed intake and better feed efficiency (Chalupa, 1980). Favourable effects can only be expected with high roughage diets giving appreciable amounts of methane in the rumen (Demeyer and Van Nevel, 1987)

Table 1. Inhibition of ruminal methane production by halogenated compounds.

Compound[1]	In vitro			In vivo				
	Concn	Inhibition (%)	Ref.	Compound	Amount	Inhibition (%)	Animal	Ref.
TCA	13 ppm	95	1	TCE-P	120 mg d^{-1}	21-53	Sheep	12
CHCl$_3$	0.04 mM	100	2		240 mg d^{-1}	53-57		
CCl$_4$	0.04 mM	100	2	TCE-A	150 mg d^{-1}	6-25	Sheep	12
CH$_2$Br$_2$	0.05 mM	100	2					
Chloral hydrate	0.1 mM	66	3	BCM	300 mg d^{-1}	28-87		
DCA	32 mg d^{-1}	100	4		5.5 g d^{-1}	100	Steers	13
ICI 111075	1 mg l^{-1}	68	5		108 mg d	84	Sheep	14
	2 mg l^{-1}	91		HCS	213 mg d^{-1}	85	Sheep	14
Nitrapyrin	0.005 mM	99	6		2.2 g d^{-1}	50-82	Sheep	15
					3.2 g d^{-1}	54	Sheep	16
Pyromellitic diimide	10 ppm	97	7	TCA	0.3%[3]	34	Cattle	17
					120 mg d^{-1}	94	Sheep	1
BES	0.03 mM	76	7		170 mg d^{-1}	43	Sheep	18
	0.05 mM	86	8	Chloral hydrate	4 g d^{-1}	100	Sheep	3
HCS	20 ppm	87	9		1-4 g d^{-1}	96	Sheep	19
	40 ppm	92		ICI 13409	1 mg kg^{-1} BW[4]	67	Sheep	20
DDIC	8 ppm (starch)[2]	28	10		6 mg kg^{-1} BW	90	Cattle	
	8 ppm (hay)[2]	65		CHCl$_3$	140 mg d^{-1}	89	Sheep	18
	5 ppm	76	11					

[1] TCA - trichloroacetamide; DCA - dichloroacetamide; ICI 111075 - 2-trichloromethyl-4-dichloro-methylene benzo [1,3] dioxin-6-carboxylic acid; Nitrapyrin - 2-chloro-6-(trichloromethyl)pyridine; BES - bromoethanesulfonic acid; HCS - hemiacetal of chloral and starch; DDIC - dimethyldiphenyliodonium chloride; TCE-P - trichloroethylpivalate; TCE-A - trichloroethyladipate; BCM - bromochloromethane; ICI 13409 - 2,4-bis(trichloromethyl)-benzo[1,3]dioxin-6-carboxylic acid.

[2] Substrate.

[3] In ration.

[4] Bodyweight.

References: 1, Trei et al., 1971; 2, Van Nevel et al., 1970b; 3, Van Nevel et al., 1969; 4, Slyter, 1979; 5, Stanier and Davies, 1981; 6, Salvas and Taylor, 1980; 7, Martin and Macy, 1985; 8, Sauer and Teather, 1987; 9, Chalupa, 1980; 10, Van Nevel and Demeyer, 1992; 11, Chalupa, 1980; 12, Czerkawski and Breckenridge, 1975; 13, Johnson et al., 1972; 14, Sawyer et al., 1974; 15, Johnson, 1972; 16, Trei et al., 1972; 17, Cole and McCroskey, 1975; 18, Clapperton, 1974; 19, Mathers and Miller, 1982; 20, Davies et al., 1982.

Table 2. Effect of 2-bromoethanesulfonic acid (BES) on incubations of rumen contents from slaughtered cattle.

Incubation[1]	Fermentation products (μmol per incubation)					
	Acetate	Propionate	Butyrate	Total VFA	CH$_4$	H$_2$
Control	885	299	369	1553	444	1
BES (0.1 mM)	676	342	396	1414	166	102
Control	786	201	356	1343	445	1
BES (20 mM)	551	247	420	1218	0	439

From De Graeve *et al.* (1990).
[1] 10 ml of strained rumen fluid were incubated at 37°C with 0.5 g of grass hay and 40 ml of Burrough's solution (1 g NH$_4$HCO$_3$ l^{-1}; pH 6.8) for 24 h under CO$_2$.

- the effect of the drugs on methane production is often transient because the inhibitor is broken down to a non-toxic product or because the bacterial population adapts to become more resistant to the drug (Johnson, 1972; Johnson *et al.*, 1972; Clapperton, 1974; Cole and McCroskey, 1975). Only chloroform and the chloro-substituted benzo-1,3-dioxins had a very persistent long-term effect (Clapperton, 1974; Davies *et al.*, 1982)
- toxicity of the inhibitor. For example, chlorinated methane analogues are hepatotoxic (Lanigan *et al.*, 1978).

Direct comparison of the potency of the additives given in Table 1 is not possible due to differences in experimental animals (cattle or sheep), ration type and dose administered. However, it is clear that halogenated compounds are potent inhibitors.

Antibiotics. For many years, antibacterial substances have been used widely in animal production as growth promoting substances. Antibiotics are mixed in the ration at very low, non-therapeutic doses. In order to explain favourable effects on growth and fattening, their influence on digestion has often been studied.

About four decades ago, it was found that methane production in *in vitro* incubations with rumen contents from steers fed chlortetracycline (ca. 11 ppm in feed) was lower (9-22%) than control animals (Hungate *et al.*, 1955). The authors suggested that the inhibition was not the result of a direct effect of the antibiotic on methanogenic bacteria, but due to inhibition of the microbes producing hydrogen and formate, both intermediate precursors of methane. During the last two decades, many reports have been published describing the effects of antibiotics, especially ionophores and glycopeptides, on rumen and post-ruminal digestion (Goodrich *et al.*, 1984; Schelling, 1984; Parker and Armstrong, 1987; Van Nevel and Demeyer, 1988; Van Nevel, 1991; Russell and Strobel, 1989). Optimization or manipulation of digestive processes, especially rumen fermentation, with the aim of increasing production was again the ultimate goal with these compounds. However, many of the antibiotics and ionophores used in ruminant feeding as growth promoters or against lactic acidosis (Van Nevel and Demeyer, 1990) also affect methane production (Table 3). Their effect on methane production is rather inconsistent, as decreases, increases or no effect at all was observed. However, it is clear that avoparcin, a glycopeptide, and ionophores, both of which are known to act on Gram-positive bacteria, inhibit methanogenesis, simultaneously shifting the VFA pattern to a higher propionate production at the expense of acetate and butyrate (Van Nevel and Demeyer, 1992).

Bacitracin, a polypeptide antibiotic which also affects Gram-positive bacteria, also lowered methane production, but its action was less potent than ionophores (Table 3; Russell and Strobel, 1988). Two other glycopeptide antibiotics which inhibit methane production are actaplanin and aridicin, the latter of which inhibited methane production by about 16% *in vitro* (Barao *et al.*, 1985; Lindsey *et al.*, 1985). It is interesting to note that some compounds stimulated methanogenesis, and in agreement with stoichiometry acetate formation increased while propionate decreased (Van Nevel and Demeyer, 1992). Higher acetate production is linked to increases in formate or hydrogen production, both of which are precursors of methane. Such incubations are only a first phase in the evaluation of additives, and should be followed by *in vivo* trials, lasting long enough to reveal eventual adaptation of the microbes to the drugs.

Table 3. Effect of antibiotics on methane production in incubations of mixed rumen microbes metabolizing hay or starch.

Compound (8 ppm)	CH_4 production (% of control)[1]	
	Hay[2]	Starch[2]
Control	100.0	100.0
Non ionophores		
Avoparcin	66.4*	74.7*
Capreomycin	109.8	109.1
Flavomycin	114.3	101.8
Thiopeptin	95.8	70.8*
Novobiocin	165.7*	115.5
Virginiamycin	172.3*	109.9
Terramycin	177.0*	154.6*
Aureomycin	162.9*	154.9*
Bacitracin	87.8[3]	81.3[3]
Ionophores		
Lasalocid	54.5*	73.3*
Monensin	78.8	57.9*
Salinomycin	83.1	55.6*

From Van Nevel and Demeyer (1992).
[1] Methane production was calculated as mmol per 100 mmol of volatile fatty acids produced, thus correcting for inhibition of substrate degradation.
[2] Detergent washed hay; soluble starch.
[3] No statistics.
* Significantly different from control ($P < 0.05$).

Monensin, an ionophore used widely in beef fattening, inhibits methane production *in vivo* by an average of about 25% (Table 4). Yet, when animals were fed hourly, no effect at all was observed (O'Kelly and Spiers, 1992). From *in vitro* research, Van Nevel and Demeyer (1977) concluded that monensin was not directly toxic to rumen methanogens, but inhibited organisms converting formate to carbon dioxide and hydrogen by formate lyase, the most important substrate for methane bacteria. This confirmed the suggestion made by Hungate *et al.* (1955). Pure strains of *Methanobacterium ruminantium* were not or were only slightly inhibited by monensin or lasalocid. Some other methanogens showed a delayed growth response,

Table 4. Effect of monensin on methane production *in vivo*.

Ration	Animal	Dose	Inhibition (%)	Reference
Cracked corn and silage	Steers	3 mg d^{-1} kg MW$^-$	26	Wedegaertner and Johnson (1983)
Low roughage	Steers	200 mg d^{-1}	16	Thornton and Owens (1981)
High roughage	Steers	200 mg d^{-1}	24	Thornton and Owens (1981)
Lucerne hay *ad libitum*	Steers	33 mg (kg feed)$^{-1}$	26	O'Kelly and Spiers (1992)
Lucerne hay (250 g h^{-1})	Steers	33 mg (kg feed)$^{-1}$	0	O'Kelly and Spiers (1992)
Lucerne hay and concentrates (50:50)	Lambs	10 ppm 20 ppm	26 31	Joyner *et al.* (1979)

MW - metabolic weight.

but complete growth inhibition was never observed. At the same dose of inhibitor, growth of some other bacteria (e.g. ruminococci) ceased completely (Chen and Wolin, 1977; Henderson *et al.*, 1981). Besides its inhibition of methane production, monensin altered rumen VFA pattern in the same way as described above for other antibiotics. Many other ionophores change fermentation pattern in a similar way, including lasalocid, salinomycin, lysocellin, tetronasin, gramicidin, narasin, and cationomycin (see also Chapter 9; Bartley *et al.*, 1979; Webb *et al.*, 1980; Barao *et al.*, 1985; Jarrell and Hamilton, 1985; Wakita *et al.*, 1986; Bartle *et al.*, 1988; Newbold *et al.*, 1988; Bogaert *et al.*, 1989; Gates *et al.*, 1989; Spears *et al.*, 1989; Kung *et al.*, 1992). Weight gain of beef cattle is not always increased by ionophores, but a lower feed intake usually results in an improved efficiency of feed conversion.

In their review, Russell and Strobel (1989) explained the effect of ionophores on rumen fermentation. The sensitivity of different species of microbes to the compounds is different, while ion selectivity (affinity for mono- or divalent cations) of the drug is also important. Altered ion fluxes through the cell membrane are part of the mechanism of action. Experiments with different pure strains of rumen bacteria and monensin and lasalocid indicated that the overall effect on rumen fermentation is probably due to shifts in the microbial population towards ionophore-resistant organisms, which tend to produce more propionate (Chen and Wolin, 1977; Henderson *et al.*, 1981).

Unfortunately, some long-term *in vivo* trials have shown that inhibition of methanogenesis by monensin and lasalocid did not persist. Control values were restored after ca. two weeks (Rumpler *et al.*, 1986; Johnson *et al.*, 1991). From a stoichiometric point of view, this conflicts with the altered rumen VFA patterns with ionophores which persist during and at the end of long-term growth trials (Richardson *et al.*, 1976). The effect of salinomycin on methane production seemed to be somewhat more persistent (Wakita *et al.*, 1986).

The effect of ionophores on methanogenesis may not be restricted to their effects on rumen bacteria. Ionophores may also affect the fermentation in the lower gut. Incubations of caecal contents with monensin *in vitro* resulted in inhibition of methane production (Marounek *et al.*, 1990). Since a substantial proportion of monensin passes through the digestive tract intact, post-ruminal effects may be significant (Marounek *et al.*, 1990). O'Kelly and Spiers (1992), when feeding monensin to steers, calculated that 55% of the reduction in methane production could be accounted for by the depressed feed intake, leaving 45% due to specific effects on rumen fermentation.

The use of ionophores is limited to fattening cattle for the most part. Their effects on milk yield and composition have been variable (Sprott *et al.*, 1988), but in any case ionophores are not used in the ration of dairy cows. An exception is New Zealand, where monensin boluses are used to control pasture bloat in dairy animals. In contrast, the use of avoparcin in dairy cow feeding has recently been approved in the EC.

Methane inhibition by lipid supplements. Some twenty five years ago, it was found that long-chain fatty acids (LCFA) inhibited methane production in the rumen *in vitro* and *in vivo*, while propionic acid production was increased (Czerkawski *et al.*, 1966; Demeyer and Henderickx, 1967a; Demeyer *et al.*, 1969). Some data are summarized in Table 5. The inhibitory effect on methanogenesis depends on the nature and amount of lipid supplement, free fatty acids being more potent than triacylglycerols, while sheep seem to be more sensitive than cattle (Van Nevel, 1991). *In vitro* studies confirmed that, for inhibition of methane production, a free carboxyl group was necessary and a greater effect was found with unsaturated fatty acids (Van Nevel and Demeyer, 1988). The latter are hydrogenated by rumen bacteria, but the amount of metabolic hydrogen used in this process cannot account for the inhibited methane production. The effect of triacylglycerols in the diet on rumen fermentation will be dependent on the rate of lipolysis. High proportions of concentrates, causing low pH values in the rumen, seem to lower this rate (Demeyer, 1973). Experiments with pure strains of rumen bacteria indicated that fatty acids inhibited growth of methanogenic bacteria, oleic acid being the most potent. Several Gram negative bacteria, contributing to propionate production, remained unaffected (Prins *et al.*, 1972; Henderson, 1973). This may explain the change in fermentation pattern when lipid supplements were fed: molar proportions of propionate increased, and this was accompanied by a corresponding decrease in acetate and butyrate production. Under these conditions, considerable decreases in numbers of ciliate protozoa have often been observed (Czerkawski *et al.*, 1975; Broudiscou *et al.*, 1990a). As soybean oil hydrolysate had similar effects on methane production and the fermentation pattern in the rumen of both normal faunated and protozoa-free sheep, it is clear that the decrease in protozoal numbers is not entirely responsible for the effects observed (Broudiscou *et al.*, 1990a,b). Attachment of methanogenic bacteria to ciliate protozoa has been observed, and it has been assumed that both types of organism benefit from interspecies hydrogen transfer as a result of this association (Stumm *et al.*, 1982). The experiment with protozoa-free sheep however also indicated that methane inhibition cannot be accounted for completely by elimination of the methanogens associated with protozoa (Van der Honing and Tamminga, 1986). The toxic effect of fatty acids is thought to be due to adsorption on to the microbial cell wall, thus interfering with passage of essential nutrients (Galbraith *et al.*, 1971; Henderson, 1973).

Lipids are not specific inhibitors of methane production. Decreases in organic matter and crude fibre degradation in the rumen occurred after feeding diets rich (>5%) in fat, an effect

Table 5. Inhibition of methane production in ruminants as a result of feeding lipid supplements.

Animal	Ration type	Lipid	Amount (g d^{-1})	CH$_4$ inhibition (%)	Reference
Sheep	Hay	Oleic acid	30	3	Czerkawski *et al.*, (1966)
			50	31	
			73	39	
		Linoleic acid	28	10	
			59	24	
			75	43	
		Linolenic acid	44	12	
			60	38	
			87	47	
			124	62	
Sheep	Concentr/hay	Linseed oil hydrolysate	30	67	Demeyer *et al.* (1969)
Sheep	Concentr/hay	Beef tallow	56	17	Van der Honing *et al.* (1983)
			96	33	
Cow	Concentr/hay	Beef tallow	650	7	Van der Honing *et al.* (1981)
			910	5	
		Soybean oil	650	14	
Steers	Concentr/hay	Yellow grease and blended animal fat	226	14	Zinn (1989)
			452	23	

seen mainly in sheep and less frequently in cows (Kowalczyk *et al.*, 1977; Ørskov *et al.*, 1978; Rohr *et al.*, 1978; Zinn, 1989). As total tract digestibility of these fractions was influenced by lipids much less than rumen digestibility, a shift in digestion from rumen to hindgut must have taken place. Such a shift would also decrease methane production, as the production of methane (mol per mol of substrate) from fibre or soluble sugars in the hindgut is only 0.45 of the rumen value (Demeyer and de Graeve, 1991).

Feeding lipid supplements to dairy cows influences milk composition: protein concentration is depressed as a consequence of lower uptake of amino acids by the mammary gland (Casper and Schingoethe, 1989) while, particularly with unsaturated LCFA, milk fat content can be depressed severely (Sutton and Morant, 1989).

BIOTECHNOLOGICAL INTERVENTIONS

Effect of microbial feed additives on methane production

General aspects of microbial feed additives for ruminants have been treated extensively in Chapter 13. Therefore, their effect on methane production in the rumen will be mentioned only briefly here. The most widely used preparations (live cells and growth medium) are based on *Saccharomyces cerevisiae* (SC) and *Aspergillus oryzae* (AO), and their effect on rumen fermentation and animal productivity has been reviewed recently by several authors (Williams, 1988; Williams and Newbold, 1990; Martin and Nisbet, 1992; Newbold, 1992).

Papers reporting effects on methane production are scarce, and all of these experiments were done *in vitro* (in batch culture or in the rumen simulation technique, Rusitec). In two experiments, SC and AO stimulated methane production (50-60%) in incubations without substrate, while no effect at all was seen when starch, Trypticase or bermuda grass were incubated (Martin *et al.*, 1989; Martin and Nisbet, 1990). More consistent results were obtained by Frumholtz *et al.* (1989) and Mutsvangwa *et al.* (1992). The first group added 250 mg AO daily to Rusitec and the percentage of methane in the headspace gas decreased to approximately 50% of the control value. The A/P ratio remained unchanged but the production of butyrate and valerate was increased in line with stoichiometry. Protozoal numbers were reduced by 45%. Because of the close association between methanogens and ciliates, and between ciliates and other members of the bacterial population, the microbial additives could therefore change the composition of the microbial flora and decrease methane inhibition indirectly by altering the balance of the population. Mutsvangwa *et al.* (1992) fed SC (1.5 kg per tonne of feed) to bulls and measured methane production from rumen fluid *in vitro*. After 12 h incubation, a 10% decrease, compared with control incubations, was observed, but after 24 h no difference was found. Until now, the available data relating microbial feed additives and methane production are not convincing and much more research is needed before it can be concluded that yeast cultures or *A. oryzae* extracts decrease methane production *in vivo*.

Defaunation of the rumen

Although the presence of protozoa in the rumen is not essential for the host, it is now certain that they play an important role in overall rumen digestion. A negative aspect is the turnover of microbial protein in the rumen, thus lowering the efficiency and amount of microbial protein synthesis. This is largely due to the predatory activity of protozoa towards bacteria, but also to the fact that protozoa are retained selectively in the rumen. In order to unravel the role of protozoa in the digestion of different feed components and in other processes in the rumen such as microbial growth yield, fermentation pattern, and the kinetics of digesta flow, a one-shot intervention called defaunation, whereby protozoa are eliminated from the rumen, has often been used. Several reviews of the subject have been published (Kreuzer, 1986; Veira, 1986; Jouany *et al.*, 1988; Ushida *et al.*, 1991; Williams and Coleman, 1992).

In almost every experiment, defaunation of the rumen of cattle, sheep and goats has resulted in considerable (20-50%) decreases in methane production compared with the normal faunated state (Kreuzer *et al.*, 1986; Williams and Coleman, 1992). Reviewing the literature, Kreuzer (1986) calculated that defaunation decreased energy losses through methanogenesis from 7.87 to 5.49% of gross energy intake. In some *in vivo* experiments, the effect on methane production was dependent on the composition of the diet: with a semi-synthetic diet based on cellulose or steam-flaked starch, defaunation lowered methane production in sheep, but not when native starch was fed (Kreuzer *et al.*, 1986). With goats, the intervention had no effect with an all-hay ration, but inhibition was noted when concentrates were fed with hay (Itabashi *et al.*, 1984). However, in both experiments methane production was already lower during the control periods (faunated) with the native starch and all-hay diets.

Decreased methanogenesis in defaunated animals can be explained by the following:
- lower rumen digestibility of the crude fibre fraction of the ration

- an altered VFA pattern in the rumen, with an increased proportion of propionate, due to changes in the composition of the microflora. However, the effect of defaunation on the VFA pattern is not consistent (Williams and Coleman, 1992)
- loss of methanogens attached to ciliates
- loss of protozoa which produce hydrogen or formate, which in turn are precursors of methane.

It is clear that defaunation, like other forms of manipulation, has a series of interrelated effects on overall rumen fermentation, as summarized by Jouany *et al.* (1988). The influence on animal performance has been reviewed extensively by Williams and Coleman (1992). Increases, decreases or no effect at all on liveweight gain and food conversion have been observed. Only wool growth was improved in all experiments. Defaunation usually increased protein flow to the small intestine, but this positive effect will only improve performance of animals when protein supply limits growth.

Defaunation on a large practical scale however is seriously limited by the fact that no satisfactory method has yet been described for eliminating protozoa from the rumen. The following requirements must be fulfilled for a method of defaunation to be acceptable: it must be selective, effective and persistent, easy to administer, and not harmful to the animal. In some defaunation studies, death of animals has been reported and severe anorexia may occur, causing serious weight losses during the defaunation process. Many different methods have been described for the experimental defaunation of ruminants (Kreuzer, 1986; Jouany *et al.*, 1988; Jouany, 1991). Chemical defaunating agents include copper sulfate, dioctylsodium sulfosuccinate, nonylphenoletoxylates, sodium lauryldietoxysulfate, calcium peroxide, and large amounts of fatty acids. Emptying the rumen and washing with formaldehyde is also effective, and isolating newborn animals from their dams and rearing in isolation also gives ciliate-free animals. Nutritional defaunation can be carried out by feeding pelleted concentrates *ad libitum* or large amounts of milk has also been effective, but the rumen of these animals was only checked for the absence of protozoa for at most seven days after treatment (Kreuzer and Kirchgessner, 1987). Only after three weeks' absence of ciliates can it be assumed that the procedure was successful. Defaunated animals must be kept separated from conventional ruminants to avoid spontaneous recontamination. The lower methane production in the rumen of chemically defaunated animals is not the result of toxic effects of the defaunating agent on bacteria as a same effect was found in animals raised ciliate-free from birth (Kreuzer *et al.*, 1986).

Introduction of reductive acetogenesis in the rumen

In the hindgut of mammals and termites, acetogenic bacteria produce acetic acid by the reduction of carbon dioxide with hydrogen

$$2CO_2 + 8H \rightarrow CH_3COOH + 2H_2O$$

(Ljungdahl, 1986). This process, referred to as hydrogenotrophic or reductive acetogenesis, does not occur in the rumen, but acts as an important hydrogen sink in the hindgut fermentation (Demeyer and de Graeve, 1991; Lajoie *et al.*, 1988). Although hydrogen- and CO_2-utilizing acetogenic bacteria have been isolated from the rumen of sheep and cattle, under normal conditions they grow fermentatively on organic substrates (Genthner *et al.*, 1981; Leedle and Greening, 1988; Greening and Leedle, 1989). It was speculated that methane production in the rumen might be inhibited by changing the metabolism of the indigenous reductive acetogens from an organotrophic mode to hydrogen-oxidizing, carbon dioxide-reducing acetate production or by introducing allochtonous species (Wolin and Miller, 1988). Descriptions of species able to grow on $H_2 + CO_2$, together with the metabolic pathways involved can be found in the review by Ljungdahl (1986). Before introduction can be achieved successfully, it must be known under what conditions these bacteria can compete successfully with methanogens for available H_2 in the rumen. During the inoculation process, competition by methanogens might be inhibited by an inhibitor of methane production such as BES, thus facilitating the establishment and growth of acetogens. Although the effect of BES would only be temporary, the transient inhibition of methanogens might permit an acetogenic population to become active in reductive acetogenesis.

The differences in fermentation between rumen and hindgut may be related to differences in physicochemical characteristics of the environment or the substrates available. In the hindgut, sloughed epithelial cells, bile and pancreatic secretions and glycoproteins from mucins are available to the bacteria (Cummings *et al.*, 1989).

CONCLUSIONS

Extensive research has revealed that methanogenesis is a rather sensitive process, very susceptible to instantaneous inhibition. Several methods for inhibiting methane production have been described, but none of them seems to be unequivocally effective. Inhibitors of methanogenesis often cause a series of interrelated effects in the animal which sometimes impair productive performance, for example fibre digestion may be inhibited. The ideal inhibitor must be very specific and persistent in its action, not toxic for the animal in the dosage used and completely safe concerning residues in edible tissue or milk. Ecological aspects are also important because additives inevitably may be secreted into the environment. It is rather doubtful that further research will show that halogenated methane inhibitors, being the most potent agents, will ever comply with all the requirements mentioned above. Ionophores are widely used but their ability to prevent methane production is rather modest. The biotechnological interventions presented here are unconvincing (yeasts), not applicable on a practical scale (defaunation) or speculative (reductive acetogenesis). Finally, feeding high concentrate diets and/or fats to dairy cattle, causing a low-methane, high-propionate stoichiometry in the rumen, has to take into account the milkfat depressing properties of such diets.

ACKNOWLEDGEMENT

Much of the research done in the University of Gent and described in this Chapter was sponsored by IWONL and FWO, Brussels.

REFERENCES

Aimone, J.C. and Wagner, D.G. 1977. Micronized wheat. I. Influence on feedlot performance, digestibility, VFA and lactate levels in cattle. *J. Anim. Sci.* **44**, 1088-1095.
Balch, W.E. and Wolfe, R.S. 1979. Transport of coenzyme M (2-mercaptoethanesulfonic acid) in *Methanobrevibacterium ruminantium*. *J. Bacteriol.* **137**, 264-273.

Barao, S.M., Bergen, W.G. and Hawkins, D.R. 1985. Effect of narasin and actaplanin alone or in combination on feedlot performance and carcass characteristics of finishing steers. *J. Anim. Sci.* **61** (Suppl. 1), 471. (Abstract).

Bartle, S.J., Preston, R.L. and Bailie, J.H. 1988. Dose-response relationship of the ionophore tetronasin in growing-finishing cattle. *J. Anim. Sci.* **66**, 1502-1507.

Bartley, E.E., Herod, E.L., Bechtle, R.M., Sapienza, D.A. and Brent, B.E. 1979. Effect of monensin or lasalocid, with and without niacin or amicloral, on rumen fermentation and feed efficiency. *J. Anim. Sci.* **49**, 1066-1075.

Bauchop, T. 1967. Inhibition of rumen methanogenesis by methane analogues. *J. Bacteriol.* **94**, 171-175.

Blaxter, K.L. and Clapperton, J.L. 1965. Prediction of the amount of methane produced by ruminants. *Br. J. Nutr.* **19**, 511-522.

Bogaert, C., Gomez, L., Jouany, J.P. and Jeminet, G. 1989. Effects of the ionophore antibiotics lasalocid and cationomycin on ruminal fermentation in vitro (Rusitec). *Anim. Feed Sci. Technol.* **27**, 1-15.

Broster, W.H., Sutton, J.D. and Bines, J.A. 1979. Concentrate:forage ratios for high-yielding dairy cows. In *Recent Advances in Animal Nutrition* (W. Haresign and D. Lewis, eds) pp. 99-126. Butterworths, London, UK.

Broudiscou, L., Van Nevel, C.J. and Demeyer, D.I. 1990a. Effect of soya oil hydrolysate on rumen digestion in defaunated and refaunated sheep. *Anim. Feed Sci. Technol.* **30**, 51-67.

Broudiscou, L., Van Nevel, C.J. and Demeyer, D.I. 1990b. Incorporation of soya oil hydrolysate in the diet of defaunated or refaunated sheep - effect on rumen fermentation in vitro. *Arch. Anim. Nutr.* **40**, 329-337.

Byers, F.M. and Turner, N.D. 1990. The role of methane from beef cattle in global warming. In *Beef Cattle Research in Texas* (J.W. Turner, J.S. Oman and R.L. Crum, eds) pp. 69-74. Texas Agric. Expt. Station, College Station, Texas, US.

Casper, D.P. and Schingoethe, D.J. 1989. Model to describe and alleviate milk protein depression in early lactation dairy cows fed a high fat diet. *J. Dairy Sci.* **72**, 3327-3335.

Cecava, M.J., Merchen, N.R., Berger, L.L. and Nelson, D.R. 1990. Effect of energy level and feeding frequency on site of digestion and postruminal nutrient flows in steers. *J. Dairy Sci.* **73**, 2470-2479.

Chalupa, W. 1980. Chemical control of rumen microbial metabolism. In *Digestive Physiology and Metabolism in Ruminants* (Y. Ruckebusch and P. Thivend, eds) pp. 325-347. MTP Press, Falcon House, Lancaster, UK.

Chalupa, W., Corbett, W. and Brethour, J.R. 1980. Effects of monensin and amicloral on rumen fermentation. *J. Anim. Sci.* **51**, 170-179.

Chen, M. and Wolin, M.J. 1979. Effect of monensin and lasalocid-sodium on the growth of methanogenic and rumen saccharolytic bacteria. *Appl. Environ. Microbiol.* **38**, 72-77.

Clapperton, J.L. 1974. The effect of trichloroacetamide, chloroform and linseed oil given into the rumen of sheep on some of the end-products of rumen digestion. *Br. J. Nutr.* **32**, 155-161.

Cole, N.A. and McCroskey, J.E. 1975. Effects of hemiacetal of chloral and starch on the performance of beef steers. *J. Anim. Sci.* **41**, 1735-1741.

Crutzen, P.J., Aselmann, I. and Seiler, W. 1986. Methane production by domestic animals, wild ruminants, other herbivorous fauna, and humans. *Tellus* **38B**, 271-284.

Cummings, J.H., Gibson, G.R., and Macfarlane, G.T. 1989. Quantitative estimates of fermentation in the hind gut of man. *Acta Vet. Scand.* **86**, 76-82 (Suppl.).

Czerkawski, J.W. 1969. Methane production in the rumen and its significance. *World Rev. Nutr. Diet.* **11**, 240-282.

Czerkawski, J.W. 1986. *An Introduction to Rumen Studies.* Pergamon Press, Oxford, UK.

Czerkawski, J.W. and Breckenridge, G. 1975. New inhibitors of methane production by rumen micro-organisms. Experiments with animals and other practical possibilities. *Br. J. Nutr.* **34**, 447-457.

Czerkawski, J.W., Blaxter, K.L. and Wainman, F.W. 1966. The metabolism of oleic, linoleic and linolenic acids by sheep with reference to their effects on methane production. *Br. J. Nutr.* **20**, 349-362.

Czerkawski, J.W., Christie, W.W., Breckenridge, G. and Hunter, M.L. 1975. Changes in rumen metabolism of sheep given increasing amounts of linseed oil in their diet. *Br. J. Nutr.* **34**, 25-44.

Davies, A., Nwaonu, H.N., Stanier, G. and Boyle, F.T. 1982. Properties of a novel series of inhibitors of rumen methanogenesis; in vitro and in vivo experiments including growth trials on 2,4-bis(trichloromethyl)-benzo[1,3]dioxin-6-carboxylic acid. *Br. J. Nutr.* **47**, 565-576.

De Graeve, K.G., Grivet, J.P., Durand, M. and Demeyer, D. 1990. Effect van een methaanremmer, 2-broomethaansulfonzuur, op de fermentatie door dikkedarmbacterien, pp. 11-12. 15^e Studiedag Ned. Voedingsonderzoekers, Utrecht, The Netherlands.

Demeyer, D. 1973. Lipidstoffwechsel im Pansen. In *Biologie und Biochemie der Mikrobiellen Verdauung* (D. Giesecke und H. Henderickx, eds) pp. 209-234. BLV Verlaggesellschaft, München, Germany.

Demeyer, D.I. and De Graeve, K. 1991. Differences in stoichiometry between rumen and hindgut fermentation. *J. Anim. Physiol. Anim. Nutr.* **22**, 50-61.

Demeyer, D.I. and Henderickx, H.K. 1967a. The effect of C_{10} unsaturated fatty acids on methane production in vitro by mixed rumen bacteria. *Biochim. Biophys. Acta* **137**, 484-497.

Demeyer, D.I. and Henderickx, H.K. 1967b. Methane production *in vitro* by mixed rumen bacteria. *Biochem. J.* **105**, 271-277.

Demeyer, D.I. and Van Nevel, C.J. 1975. Methanogenesis, an integrated part of carbohydrate fermentation, and its control. In *Digestion and Metabolism in the Ruminant* (I.W. McDonald and A.C.I. Warner, eds) pp. 366-382. The University of New England Publishing Unit. Armidale, N.S.W., Australia.

Demeyer, D.I. and Van Nevel, C.J. 1987. Chemical manipulation of rumen metabolism. In *Physiological and Pharmacological Aspects of the Reticulo-Rumen* (L.A.A. Ooms, A.D. Degryse and A.S.J.P.A.M. van Miert, eds) pp. 227-251. M. Nijhoff Publishers, Dordrecht, Netherlands.

Demeyer, D.I., Van Nevel, C.J., Henderickx, H.K. and Martin, J. 1969. The effect of unsaturated fatty acids upon methane and propionic acid in the rumen. In *Energy Metabolism of Farm Animals* (K.L. Blaxter, J. Kielanowski and G. Thorbek, eds) pp. 139-147. Oriel Press, Newcastle upon Tyne, UK.

Estell, R.E. and Galyean, M.L. 1985. Relationship of rumen fluid dilution rate to rumen fermentation and dietary characteristics of beef steers. *J. Anim. Sci.* **60**, 1061-1071.

Eijssen, A.F.M.M., Barry, T.N. and Brookes, I.M. 1990. The effect of pyromellitic diimide upon the rumen fermentation of sheep fed a forage diet. *Anim. Feed Sci. Technol.* **28**, 145-153.

Ferry, J.G. 1992. Biochemistry of methanogenesis. *Crit. Rev. Biochem. Mol. Biol.* **27**, 473-503.

Frumholtz, P.P., Newbold, C.J. and Wallace, R.J. 1989. Influence of *Aspergillus oryzae* fermentation extract on the fermentation of a basal ration in the rumen simulation technique (Rusitec). *J. Agric. Sci., Camb.* **113**, 169-172.

Galbraith, H., Miller, T.B., Paton, A. and Thompson, J.K. 1971. Antibacterial activity of long chain fatty acids and the reversal with calcium, magnesium, ergocalciferol and cholesterol. *J. Appl. Bacteriol.* **34**, 803-813.

Gates, R.N., Roland, L.T., Wyatt, W.E., Hembry, F.G. and Bailie, J.H. 1989. Dose-response relationship of tetronasin administered to grazing steers. *J. Anim. Sci.* **67**, 3419-3424.

Genthner, B.R.S., Davis, C.L. and Bryant, M.P. 1981. Features of rumen and sewage sludge strains of *Eubacterium limosum,* a methanol and H_2-CO_2 using species. *Appl. Environ. Microbiol.* **42**, 12-19.

Goodrich, R.D., Garrett, J.E., Gast, D.R., Kirick, M.A., Larson, D.A. and Meiske, J.C. 1984. Influence of monensin on the performance of cattle. *J. Anim. Sci.* **58**, 1484-1498.

Greening, R.C. and Leedle, J.A.Z. 1989. Enrichment and isolation of *Acetitomaculum ruminis*, gen. nov., sp. nov. - acetogenic bacteria from the bovine rumen. *Arch. Microbiol.* **151**, 399-406.

Hadjipanayiotou, M., Harrison, D.G. and Armstrong, D.G. 1982. The effects upon digestion in sheep of the dietary inclusion of additional salivary salts. *J. Sci. Food Agric.* **33**, 1057-1062.

Harrison, D.G. Beever, D.E., Thomson, D.J. and Osbourn, D.F. 1975. Manipulation of rumen fermentation in sheep by increasing the rate of flow of water from the rumen. *J. Agric. Sci., Camb.* **85**, 93-101.

Harrison, D.G., Beever, D.E., Thomson, D.J. and Osbourn, D.F. 1976. Manipulation of fermentation in the rumen. *J. Sci. Food Agric.* **27**, 617-620.

Henderson, C. 1973. The effects of fatty acids on pure cultures of rumen bacteria. *J. Agric. Sci., Camb.* **81**, 107-112.

Henderson, C., Stewart, C.S. and Nekrep, F.V. 1981. The effect of monensin on pure and mixed cultures of rumen bacteria. *J. Appl. Bacteriol.* **51**, 159-169.

Hodgson, J.C., Thomas, P.C. and Wilson, A.G. 1976. Influence of the level of feeding on fermentation in the rumen of sheep receiving a diet of ground barley, ground hay and flaked maize. *J. Agric. Sci., Camb.* **87**, 297-302.

Holter, J.B. and Young, A.J. 1992. Methane production in dry and lactating Holstein cows. *J. Dairy Sci.* **75**, 2165-2175.

Hungate, R.E., Fletcher, D.W. and Dyer, I.A. 1955. Effects of chlortetracycline feeding on bovine rumen microorganisms. *J. Anim. Sci.* **14**, 997-1002.

Hvelplund, T., Stigsen, P., Møller, P.D. and Jensen, K. 1978. Propionic acid production rate in the bovine rumen after feeding untreated and sodium hydroxide-treated straw. *Zeitschr. Tierphys. Tierernähr. Futtermittelkde* **40**, 183-190.

Ilian, M.A., Razzaque, M.A., Suleiman, A.R, Salman, A.J. and Salman, A.R. 1986. Sheep diets with various roughage to concentrate ratios. 1. Effects on performance and rumen characteristics. *Nutr. Rep. Int.* **33**, 353-361.

Itabashi, H., Kobayashi, T. and Matsumoto, M. 1984. The effects of rumen ciliate protozoa on energy metabolism and some constituents in rumen fluid and blood plasma of goats. *Jap. J. Zootech. Sci.* **55**, 248-256.

Jarrell, K.F. and Hamilton, E.A. 1985. Effect of gramicidin on methanogenesis by various methanogenic bacteria. *Appl. Environ. Microbiol.* **50**, 179-182.

Jensen, K. and Wolstrup, J. 1977. Effect of feeding frequency on fermentation pattern and microbial activity in the bovine rumen. *Acta Vet. Scand.* **18**, 108-121.

Johnson, E.D., Wood, A.S., Stone, J.B. and Moran, E.T., Jr. 1972. Some effects of methane inhibition in ruminants (steers). *Can. J. Anim. Sci.* **52**, 703-712.

Johnson, D.E. 1972. Effects of a hemiacetal of chloral and starch on methane production and energy balance of sheep fed a pelleted diet. *J. Anim. Sci.* **35**, 1064-1068.

Johnson, D.E., Hill, T.M. Carmean, B.R. Lodman, D.W. and Ward, G.M. 1991. New perspectives on ruminant methane emissions. In *Energy Metabolism of Farm Animals* (C. Wenk and M. Boessinger, eds) pp. 376-379. ETH, Zürich, Switzerland.

Johnson, D.E., Hill, T.M., Ward, G.M., Johnson, K.A., Branine, M.E., Carmean, B.R. and Lodman, D.W. The global methane budget. In *Atmospheric Methane* (M.A.K. Khalil, ed.) Springer Verlag, New York, US (in press).

Jouany, J.P. 1991. Defaunation of the rumen. In *Rumen Microbial Metabolism and Ruminant Digestion* (J.P. Jouany, ed.) pp. 239-261. INRA, Paris, France.

Jouany, J.P., Demeyer, D.I. and Grain, J. 1988. Effect of defaunating the rumen. *Anim. Feed Sci. Technol.* **21**, 229-265.

Joyner, A.E., Brown, L.J., Fogg, T.J., and Rossi, R.T. 1979. Effect of monensin on growth, feed efficiency and energy metabolism of lambs. *J. Anim. Sci.* **48**, 1065-1069.

Kone, P., Machado, P.F. and Cook, R.M. 1989. Effect of the combination of monensin and isoacids on rumen fermentation in vitro. *J. Dairy Sci.* **72**, 2767-2771.

Kowalczyk, J., Ørskov, E.R., Robinson, J.J. and Stewart, C.S. 1977. Effect of fat supplementation on voluntary food intake and rumen metabolism in sheep. *Br. J. Nutr.* **37**, 251-257.

Kreuzer, M. 1986. Methods and application of defaunation in the growing ruminant. *J. Vet. Med.* **A 33**, 721-745.

Kreuzer, M. and Kirchgessner, M. 1987. Investigations on the nutritive defaunation of the rumen of ruminants. *Arch. Anim. Nutr.* **37**, 489-503.

Kreuzer, M., Kirchgessner, M. and Müller, H.L. 1986. Effect of defaunation on the loss of energy in wethers fed different quantities of cellulose and normal or steamflaked maize starch. *Anim. Feed Sci. Technol.* **16**, 233-241.

Kung, L., Tung, R.S. and Slyter, L.L. 1992. In vitro effects of the ionophore lysocellin on ruminal fermentation and microbial populations. *J. Anim. Sci.* **70**, 281-288.

Lajoie, S.F., Bank, S., Miller, T.L. and Wolin, M.J. 1988. Acetate production from hydrogen and [C-13] carbon dioxide by the microflora of human feces. *Appl. Environ. Microbiol.* **54**, 2723-2727.

Lanigan, G.W., Payne, A.L. and Peterson, J.E. 1978. Antimethanogenic drugs and *Heliotropum europeum* poisoning in penned sheep. *Aust. J. Agric. Res.* **29**, 1281-1292.

Leedle, J.A.Z. and Greening, R.C. 1988. Postprandial changes in methanogenic and acidogenic bacteria in the rumens of steers fed high-forage or low-forage diets once daily. *Appl. Environ. Microbiol.* **54**, 502-506.

Lindsey, T.O., Hedde, R.D., Sokolek, J.A., Quach, R. and Morgenthien, E.A. 1985. *In vitro* characterization of aricidin activity in the rumen. *J. Anim. Sci.* **61** (Suppl. 1), 464. (Abstract).

Ljungdahl, L.G. 1986. The autotrophic pathway of acetate synthesis in acetogenic bacteria. *Annu. Rev. Microbiol.* **40**, 415-450.

Marounek, M., Petr, O. and Machanova, L. 1990. Effect of monensin on in vitro fermentation of maize starch by hindgut contents of cattle. *J. Agric. Sci., Camb.* **115**, 389-392.

Martin, S.A. and Macy, J.M. 1985. Effects of monensin, pyromellitic diimide and 2-bromoethanesulfonic acid on rumen fermentation in vitro. *J. Anim. Sci.* **60**, 544-550.

Martin, S.A. and Nisbet, D.J. 1990. Effects of *Aspergillus oryzae* fermentation extract on fermentation of amino acids, bermudagrass and starch by mixed ruminal microorganisms in vitro. *J. Anim. Sci.* **68**, 2142-2149.

Martin, S.A. and Nisbet, D.J. 1992. Effects of direct-fed microbials on rumen microbial fermentation. *J. Dairy Sci.* **75**, 1736-1744.

Martin, S.A., Nisbet, D.J. and Dean, R.G. 1989. Influence of a commercial yeast supplement on the in vitro ruminal fermentation. *Nutr. Rep. Int.* **40**, 395-403.

Marty, R.J. and Demeyer, D.I. 1973. The effect of inhibitors of methane production on fermentation pattern and stoichiometry in vitro using rumen contents from sheep given molasses. *Br. J. Nutr.* **30**, 369-376.

Mathers, J.C. and Miller, E.L. 1982. Some effects of chloral hydrate on rumen fermentation and digestion in sheep. *J. Agric. Sci., Camb.* **99**, 215- 224.

McBride, B.C. and Wolfe, R.S. 1971. A new coenzyme of methyl transfer, coenzyme M. *Biochemistry* **10**, 2317-2324.

McNeill, J.J. 1957. Methane formation and the hydrogen metabolism of bovine rumen bacteria. Ph.D. Thesis, Univ. Maryland, US.

Miller, T.L. 1991. Biogenic sources of methane. In *Microbial Production and Consumption of Greenhouse Gases: Methane, Nitrogen Oxides, and Halomethanes* (J.E. Rogers and W.B. Whitman, eds) pp. 175-187. Am. Soc. Microbiol., Washington D.C., US.

Moore, J.A., Poore, M.H., Eck, T.P., Swingle, R.S., Huber, J.T. and Arana, M.J. 1992. Sorghum grain processing and buffer addition for early lactation cows. *J. Dairy Sci.* **75**, 3465-3472.

Murray, R.M., Bryant, A.M. and Leng, R.A. 1978. Methane production in the rumen and lower gut of sheep given lucerne chaff: effect of level of intake. *Br. J. Nutr.* **39**, 337-345.

Mutsvangwa, T., Edwards, I.E., Topps, J.H. and Paterson, G.F.M. 1992. The effect of dietary inclusion of yeast culture (Yea-sacc) on patterns of rumen fermentation, food intake and growth of intensively fed bulls. *Anim. Prod.* **55**, 35-40.

Newbold, C.J. 1992. Probiotics - a new generation of rumen modifiers? *Med. Fac. Landbouww. Univ. Gent* **57/4b**, 1925-1933.

Newbold, C.J., Wallace, R.J., Watt, N.D. and A.J. Richardson. 1988. Effect of the novel ionophore tetronasin (ICI 139603) on ruminal microorganisms. *Appl. Environ. Microbiol.* **54**, 544-547.

Nørgaard, P. 1987. The influence of level of feeding and physical form of the feed in the-reticulo-rumen fermentation in dairy cows fed 12 times daily. *Acta Agric. Scand.* **37**, 353-365.

O'Kelly, J.C. and Spiers, W.G. 1992. Effect of monensin on methane and heat productions of steers fed lucerne hay. *Aust. J. Agric. Res.* **43**, 1789-1793.

Ørskov, E.R., Flatt, W.P. and Moe. P.W. 1968. Fermentation balance approach to estimate extent of fermentation and efficiency of volatile fatty acid formation in ruminants. *J. Dairy Sci.* **51**, 1429-1435.

Ørskov, E.R., Hine, R.S. and Grubb, D.A. 1978. The effect of urea on digestion and voluntary intake by sheep of diets supplemented with fat. *Anim. Prod.* **27**, 241-245.

Oshio, S., Tahata, I. and Minato, H. 1987. Effect of diets differing in ratios of roughage to concentrate on microflora in the rumen of heifers. *J. Gen. Appl. Microbiol.* **33**, 99-111.

Parker, D.S. and Armstrong, D.G. 1987. Antibiotic feed additives and animal production. *Proc. Nutr. Soc.* **46**, 415-421.

Prins, R.A. 1965. Action of chloral hydrate on rumen microorganisms in vitro. *J. Dairy Sci.* **48**, 991-993.

Prins, R.A., Van Nevel, C.J. and Demeyer, D.I. 1972. Pure culture studies of inhibitors for methanogenic bacteria. *Ant. van Leeuwen.* **38**, 281-287.

Quaghebeur, D. and Oyaert, W. 1971. Effect of chloral hydrate and related compounds on the activity of several enzymes in extracts of rumen microorganisms. *Zentrabl. Veterinaer Med.* A **18**, 417-427.

Richardson, L.F., Raun, A.P., Potter, E.L., Cooley, C.O. and Rathmacher, R.P. 1976. Effect of monensin on rumen fermentation in vitro and in vivo. *J. Anim. Sci.* **43**, 657-664.

Rogers, J.A. and Davis, C.L. 1982. Effects of intraruminal infusions of mineral salts on volatile fatty acid production in steers fed high-grain and high-roughage diets. *J. Dairy Sci.* **65**, 953-962.

Rohr, K., Daenicke, R. and Oslage, H.J. 1978. Untersuchungen über den Einfluss verschiedner Fettbeimischungen zum Futter auf Stoffwechsel und Leistung von Milchkühen. *Landbauforsch. Völkenrode* **28**, 139-150.

Roth, F.X. and Kirchgessner, M. 1976. Nahrstoffverdaulichkeit und N-Umsatz beim Schaf bei unterscheidlicher Futterungsfrequenz mit Kraftfutter. *Zeitschr. Tierphys. Tierernähr. Futtermittelkde* **37**, 322-329.

Rumpler, W.V. Johnson, D.E. and Bates, D.B. 1986. The effect of high dietary cation concentration on methanogenesis by steers fed diets with and without ionophores. *J. Anim. Sci.* **62**, 1737-1741.

Russell, J.B. and Martin, S.A. 1984. Effect of various methane inhibitors on the fermentation of amino acids by mixed rumen microorganisms in vitro. *J. Anim. Sci.* **59**, 1329-1338.

Russell, J.B. and Strobel, H.J. 1988. Effects of additives on in vitro ruminal fermentation: a comparison of monensin and bacitracin, another Gram-positive antibiotic. *J. Anim. Sci.* **66**, 552-558.

Russell, J.B. and Strobel, H.J. 1989. The effect of ionophores on ruminal fermentation. *Appl. Environ. Microbiol.* **55**, 1-6.

Russell, J.B. and Wallace, R.J. 1988. Energy yielding and consuming reactions. In *The Rumen Microbial Ecosystem* (P.N. Hobson, ed.) pp. 185-215. Elsevier Applied Science, London, UK.

Salvas, P.L. and Taylor, B.F. 1980. Blockage of methanogenesis in marine sediments by the nitrification inhibitor 2-chloro-6-(trichloromethyl)pyridine (nitrapyrin or N-serve). *Curr. Microbiol.* **4**, 305-308.

Sauer, F.D. and Teather, R.M. 1987. Changes in oxidation-reduction potentials and volatile fatty acid production by rumen bacteria when methane synthesis is inhibited. *J. Dairy Sci.* **70**, 1835-1840.

Sawyer, M.S., Hoover, W.H. and Sniffen, C.J. 1974. Effects of a ruminal methane inhibitor on growth and energy metabolism in the ovine. *J. Anim. Sci.* **38**, 908-914.

Schauer, N.L. and Ferry, J.G. 1980. Metabolism of formate in *Methanobacterium formicicum*. *J. Bacteriol.* **142**, 800-807.

Schelling, G.T. 1984. Monensin mode of action in the rumen. *J. Anim. Sci.* **58**, 1518-1527.

Slyter, L.L. 1979. Monensin and dichloroacetamide influences on methane and volatile fatty acid production by rumen bacteria *in vitro* continuous rumen fermentations. *Appl. Environ. Microbiol.* **37**, 283-288.

Sparling, R. and Daniels, L. 1987. The specificity of growth inhibition of methanogenic bacteria by bromoethanesulfonate. *Can. J. Microbiol.* **33**, 1132-1136.

Spears, J.W., Burns, J.C. and Wolfrom, G.W. 1989. Lysocellin effects on growth performance, ruminal fermentation, nutrient digestibility and nitrogen metabolism in steers fed forage diets. *J. Anim. Sci.* **67**, 547-556.

Sprott, L.R., Goehring, T.B., Beverly, J.R. and Corah, L.R. 1988. Effects of ionophores on cow herd production: a review. *J. Anim. Sci.* **66**, 1340-1346.

Stanier, G. and Davies, A. 1981. Effects of the antibiotic monensin and an inhibitor of methanogenesis on *in vitro* continuous rumen fermentations. *Br. J. Nutr.* **45**, 567-578.

Stumm, C.K., Gijzen, H.J. and Vogels, G.D. 1982. Association of methanogenic bacteria with ovine rumen ciliates. *Br. J. Nutr.* **47**, 95-99.

Sutton, J.D. 1986. Rumen fermentation and gastro-intestinal absorption of protein. In *New Developments and Future Perspectives in Research on Rumen Function* (A. Neimann-Sørensen, ed.) pp. 21-38. C.E.C., Brussels, Belgium.

Sutton, J.D. and Morant. S.V. 1989. A review of the potential of nutrition to modify milk fat and protein. *Livest. Prod. Sci.* **23**, 219- 237.

Sutton, J.D., Hart, I.C., Broster, W.H., Elliott, R.J. and Schuller, E. 1986. Feeding frequency for lactating cows: effects on rumen fermentation and blood metabolites and hormones. *Br. J. Nutr.* **56**, 181-192.

Thomas, P.C. and Clapperton, J.L. 1972. Significance to the host of changes in fermentation activity. *Proc. Nutr. Soc.* **31**, 165-170.

Thomas, P.C. and Rook, J.A.F. 1977. Manipulation of rumen fermentation. In *Recent Advances in Animal Nutrition* (W. Haresign and D.J.A. Cole, eds) pp. 157-183. Butterworths, London, UK.

Thompson, A.M., Hogan, K.B. and Hoffman, J.S. 1992. Methane reductions - implications for global warming and atmospheric chemical change. *Atm. Environm.* **26A**, 2665-2668.

Thomson, D.J. 1972. Physical form of the diet in relation to rumen fermentation. *Proc. Nutr. Soc.* **31**, 127-139.

Thomson, D.J., Beever, D.E., Latham, M.J., Sharpe, M.E. and Terry, R.A. 1978. The effect of the inclusion of mineral salts in the diet on dilution rate, the pattern of rumen fermentation and the composition of the rumen microflora. *J. Agric. Sci., Camb.* **91**, 1-7.

Thornton, J.H. and Owens, F.N. 1981. Monensin supplementation and in vivo methane production by steers. *J. Anim. Sci.* **52**, 628-634.

Trei, J.E., Parish, R.C., Singh, Y.K. and Scott, G.C. 1971. Effect of methane inhibitors on rumen metabolism and feedlot performance of sheep. *J. Dairy Sci.* **54**, 536-540.

Trei, J.E., Scott, G.C. and Parish, R.C. 1972. Influence of methane inhibition on energetic efficiency of lambs. *J. Anim. Sci.* **34**, 510-515.

Tyler S.C. 1991. The global methane budget. In *Microbial Production and Consumption of Greenhouse Gases: Methane, Nitrogen Oxides, and Halomethanes* (J.E. Rogers and W.B. Whiteman, eds) pp. 7-38. Am. Soc. Microbiol., Washington D.C., US.

Ushida, K., Jouany, J.P. and Demeyer, D. 1991. Effects of presence or absence of rumen protozoa on the efficiency of utilization of concentrate and fibrous feeds. In *Physiological Aspects of Digestion and Metabolism in Ruminants* (T. Tsuda, Y. Sasaki and R. Kawashima, eds) pp. 625-654. Academic Press, San Diego, US.

Van der Honing, Y. and Tamminga, S. 1986. Effect of fat on rumen fermentation and gastrointestinal absorption. In *New Developments and Future Perspectives in Research on Rumen Function* (A. Neimann-Sϕrensen, ed.) pp. 55-68. C.E.C., Brussels, Belgium.

Van der Honing, Y. , Wieman, B.J., Steg, A. and van Donselaar, B. 1981. The effect of fat supplementation of concentrates on digestion and utilization of energy by productive dairy cows. *Neth. J. Agric. Sci.* **29**, 79-92.

Van der Honing, Y., Tamminga, S., Wieman, B.J., Steg, A., van Donselaar, B. and van Gils, L.G.M. 1983. Further studies on the effects of fat supplementation of concentrates fed to lactating dairy cows. 2. Total digestion and energy utilization. *Neth. J. Agric. Sci.* **31**, 27-36.

Van Nevel, C.J. 1991. Modification of rumen fermentation by the use of additives. In *Rumen Microbial Metabolism and Ruminant Digestion.* (J.-P. Jouany, ed.) pp. 263-280. INRA, Paris, France.

Van Nevel, C.J. and Demeyer, D.I. 1977. Effect of monensin on rumen metabolism *in vitro*. *Appl. Environ. Microbiol.* **34**, 251-257.

Van Nevel, C.J. and Demeyer, D.I. 1981. Effect of methane inhibitors on the metabolism of rumen microbes *in vitro*. *Arch. Tierernährung* **31**, 141-151.

Van Nevel, C.J. and Demeyer, D.I. 1988. Manipulation of rumen fermentation. In *The Rumen Microbial Ecosystem* (P.N. Hobson, ed.) pp. 387-443. Elsevier Applied Science, London, UK.

Van Nevel, C.J. and Demeyer, D.I. 1990. Effect of antibiotics, a deaminase inhibitor and sarsaponin on nitrogen metabolism of rumen contents *in vitro*. *Anim. Feed Sci. Technol.* **31**, 323-348.

Van Nevel, C.J. and Demeyer, D.I. 1992. Influence of antibiotics and a deaminase inhibitor on volatile fatty acids and methane production from detergent washed hay and soluble starch by rumen microbes *in vitro*. *Anim. Feed Sci. Technol.* **37**, 21-31.

Van Nevel, C.J., Henderickx, H.K., Demeyer, D.I. and J. Martin. 1969. Effect of chloral hydrate on methane and propionic acid in the rumen. *Appl. Microbiol.* **17**, 695-700.

Van Nevel, C.J., Demeyer, D.I., Cottyn, B.G. and Henderickx, H.K. 1970a. Effect of sodium sulphite on methane and propionate in the rumen. *Zeitschr. Tierphys. Tierernähr. Futtermittelkde.* **26**, 91-100.

Van Nevel, C., Demeyer, D. and Henderickx, H.K. 1970b. Effect of chlorinated methane analogues on methane and propionic acid production in the rumen in vitro. *Med. Fac. Landbouww. Univ. Gent* **25**, 145-152.

Van Nevel, C.J., Prins, R.A. and Demeyer, D.I 1974. Observations on the inverse relationship between methane and propionate in the rumen. *Zeitschr. Tierphys. Tierernähr. Futtermittelkde* **33**, 121-125.

Veira, D.M. 1986. The role of ciliate protozoa in nutrition of the ruminant. *J. Anim. Sci.* **63**, 1547-1560.

Wakita, M., Masuda, T. and Hoshino, S. 1986. Effects of salinomycin on the gas production by sheep rumen contents in vitro. *J. Anim. Phys. Anim. Nutr.* **56**, 243-251.

Webb, K.E., Fontenot, J.P. and Lucas, D.M. 1980. Metabolism studies in steers fed different levels of salinomycin. *J. Anim. Sci.* **51** (Suppl.), 407. (Abstract).

Wedegaertner, T.C. and Johnson, D.E. 1983. Monensin effects on digestibility, methanogenesis and heat increment of a cracked corn silage diet fed to steers. *J. Anim. Sci.* **57**, 168-177.

Weimer. P.J. and Zeikus, J.G. 1978. One carbon metabolism in methanogenic bacteria. Cellular characterization and growth of *Methanosarcina barkeri.* *Arch. Microbiol.* **119,** 49-57.

Williams, A.G. and Coleman, G.S. 1992. *The Rumen Protozoa.* Springer-Verlag, New York, US.

Williams, P.E.V. 1988. Understanding the biochemical mode of action of yeast culture. In *Biotechnology in the Feed Industry* (T.P. Lyons, ed), pp. 79-99. Alltech Techn. Public., Nicholasville, Kentucky, US.

Williams, P.E.V. and Newbold, C.J. 1990. Rumen probiosis: the effects of novel microorganisms on rumen fermentation and ruminant productivity. In *Recent Advances in Animal Nutrition* (W. Haresign and D.J.A. Cole, eds) pp. 211-227. Butterworths, London, UK.

Wolfe, R.S. 1971. Microbial formation of methane. *Adv. Microb. Physiol.* **6**, 107-146.

Wolin, E.A., Wolfe, R.S. and Wolin, M.J. 1964. Microbial formation of methane. *J. Bacteriol.* **87,** 993-998.

Wolin, M.J. and Miller, T.L. 1988. Microbe-microbe interactions. In *The Rumen Microbial Ecosystem* (P.N. Hobson, ed.) pp. 343-359. Elsevier Applied Science, London, UK.

Wood, J.M., Kennedy, F.S. and Wolfe, R.S. 1968. The reaction of multihalogenated hydrocarbons with free and bound reduced vitamin B_{12}. *Biochemistry* **7**, 1707-1719.

Zinn, R.A. 1987. Influence of lasalocid and monensin plus tylosin on comparative feeding value of steam-flaked versus dry-rolled corn in diets for feedlot cattle. *J. Anim. Sci.* **65**, 256-266.

Zinn, R.A. 1989. Influence on level and source of dietary fat on its comparative feeding value in finishing diets for feedlot steers. *J. Anim. Sci.* **67**, 1038-1049.

Index

Acetogenesis, relation to methane production
340-341
Acetyl CoA carboxylase 288
Acidification of milk replacer 254
Acidosis
– *Fusobacterium necrophorum* infection 193
– prevention by ionophores and antibiotics
180, 194
Acute pulmonary edema and emphysema, pre-
vention by monensin 180
ADP glucose pyrophosphorylase 285, 286
Aerobic phase of silage preservation 37
Aerobic purification of animal wastes 314
Agricultural production growth 1-2
Agrobacterium tumefaciens in transformation
of plant cells 73-74
Albumins
– Brazil nut methionine-rich 75
– plant 71
Amino acids
– availability 86-87, 95
– biosynthetic pathways 82*ff*
– chelates 110
– composition, animal products 117
– composition, rumen microorganisms 116-
118
– D-amino acids 93
– digestibility in poultry 109
– dispensable and indispensable 97
– essential, for ruminants 115
– extraction 105
– formulation of diets to balance 100-102,
107-110
– imbalances, metabolic effects 99
– intestinal digesta 119-120
– limiting, for ruminants 127-128
– modification of profile in plant seed proteins
74*ff*
– nonruminants 93*ff*
– products registered for feeding 104
– requirements for pigs and poultry 99, 106
– structure 93-94
– UDP for ruminants 118-119
Ammonia
– formation in the intestine 98
– from animal wastes 312, 316, 317-318
– treatment of silage 46
Amylase 36, 37, 296, 298
Anaerobic purification of animal wastes 314
Antibacterials see Antibiotics
Antibiotics
– combination with copper 161, 162, 164,
165, 166
– economics of use 145-147, 150, 151-153
– effects on feed intake 153-155
– growth promoters 9, 173
– growth promotion in ruminants 187*ff*
– inhibition of methanogenesis 334*ff*
– interactions with probiotics 218-210
– modes of action in non-ruminants 144, 146
– mode of action in ruminants 191-192
– non-ruminant nutrition 143*ff*
– poultry nutrition 147, 148, 151
– pig nutrition 147, 148, 151
– posology 151
– rotation 166
– variables in determining responses 149
– variations in response 144, 148
Antisense RNA 279, 283
Arabidopsis 2S albumin gene 81
Arabinosidase 296
Arabinoxylanase 298, 301
Arabinoxylans 297, 298, 301
Arginine bioavailability, 95
Arsenilic acid, 144
Aspartate family of amino acids
– biosynthetic pathways 82-83
– deregulation by aspartate kinase mutation
82-84
– deregulation by dihydropicolinate synthase
mutation 84-85
Aspergillus oryzae

– in pre-ruminants   252, 253
– post-ruminal effects   263-264
– probiotic for ruminants   259*ff*, 307, 338-339
Aureomycin   335
Avilamycin   144, 165
Avoparcin   144, 145, 153, 156, 158, 161, 187-190, 191, 192, 195, 196, 197, 334, 335
Bacillus spp.
– as probiotics   208, 214, 215, 216, 217, 218, 247, 251, 252
– as rumen inoculants   253
Bacitracin   144, 145, 148, 151, 156, 158, 159, 160, 161, 162, 165, 187-189, 193, 195, 196, 216, 335
Bacteriocins   211, 249
Barley
– composition   297
– feeding to pigs   301, 302, 323
– feeding to poultry   301, 322-323
Bacteroides
– as probiotic   208, 214
– stimulation by oligosaccharides   239
Beans, heat and enzyme treatments   305-306
Bifidobacterium spp.
– as probiotics   208, 212, 214, 215, 217, 220, 247, 252
– stimulation by oligosaccharides   239
Biogas   312, 313
– large-scale plants   318*ff*
Bioscrubbers and biofilters   317
Bloat prevention by ionophores and antibiotics   180, 194
Broilers
– effects of antibacterials on mortality   153
– effects of enzyme supplementation   299, 304
– production effects of antibacterials   155-158
– variation in response to antibacterials   148
2-Bromoethanesulfonic acid   331, 332, 333, 334
Brown midrib (*bmr*) mutants of lignin biosynthesis   282
By-products
– avoidance of pollution   6
– solid state fermentation   55-70
Capreomycin   335
Carbadox   144, 145, 153, 163

Carnosine bioavailability   96
Cellulase   36, 48, 295, 296
Chickens
– response to dietary enzymes   298, 299
– response to dietary oligosaccharides   237-238
Chlortetracycline   144, 145, 148, 151, 153, 158, 159, 160, 161, 162, 164, 165, 188, 189, 190, 192, 193, 194, 195, 196, 197, 334
Cinnamate 4-hydroxylase   281, 282
Cinnamoyl-CoA reductase   281, 282
Cinnamyl alcohol dehydrogenase   281, 282, 283
Citrulline bioavailability   95
Clostridium spp.
– probiotics   208, 248
Clostridium butyricum   208
Clostridium difficile   206
Clostridium perfringens   146, 248, 249, 250
Coccidiosis, prevention by ionophores   174, 186-187
Competitive exclusion   206, 211, 250
Composting of animal wastes   314-315
Conglycinins   72, 79
Consumer awareness   4
Conservation of feeds   1314
Coprinus fimetarius   55-56
Cutin   307
Cyadox   145
Cysteine and cystine bioavailability   95
Cysteine-rich proteins in plants   80-81
Defaunation of the rumen   339-340
Digesters for animal waste processing   312*ff*
Digestibility estimation in pigs   98
Dimethyldiphenyliodonium   bromide   332, 333
Direct-fed microbials, see Probiotics
– definition   207
Ducks, antibacterials in   161
Egg production
– influence of antibiotics   159-160
– influence of probiotics   217
– variation in response to antibiotics   144
Energy content of feedstuffs   297
Escherichia coli   146, 206, 211, 212, 213, 215, 248, 249, 250, 255
Enterococcus spp.
– as probiotics   208, 212, 214, 247, 252

Enterococcus faecalis
- as silage inoculant 39
- in chick intestinal tract 206
- in probiotics 208, 250
Enterococcus faecium
- antagonism towards other bacteria 250
- as silage inoculant 39
- in probiotics 208, 213, 215, 216, 220, 249
Enzymes
- applications as feed additives 11-12, 295*ff*
- barley diets supplementation 302-303
- digestive 296
- effect on viscosity of gut contents 298
- effects with various feedstuffs 305-307
- for ruminants 307
- in place of heat treatment 305-306
- properties required as feed additives 11
- silage additives 47-48
- wheat diets supplementation 303-305
Epiphytic bacteria of crops, influence on silage
    fermentation 46-47
Esterases of *Aspergillus oryzae* 268
Fat for suppressing methane production 337-
    338
Feed additives 2-4
- see Antibiotics, Enzymes, Oligosaccharides,
    Probiotics
Feedout phase of silage making 40
Fermentation, solid state 55-70
Fermentation phase of silage preservation 37-
    38
Ferulate O-methyl transferase 281, 282, 283
Flavomycin 156, 158, 187-189, 190, 335
Flavophospholipol 145, 159, 160, 161, 162
Formaldehyde treatment of proteins for rumi-
    nants 123-125, 126
Formic acid as silage preservative 43, 124
Fructan biosynthesis 287
Fructooligosaccharides 219, 233-234, 237,
    239, 254
Fructosyltransferase 233, 234
Fungi
- as feed additives for ruminants 259*ff*
- solid state fermentation of by-products 55-
    70
Fusobacterium necrophorum 193
a-Galactooligosaccharides 235, 238
Geese, antibacterials in 161

Genetic engineering
- advantages over conventional plant breeding
    280
- forage crops 88
- ligninolytic microorganisms 59-60
- plants 73*ff*, 279*ff*
- rumen microorganisms 270-271
b-Glucanase 296, 301, 304
b-Glucans 295, 297, 301
a-Glucooligosaccharides 234-235, 237, 238,
    239, 240
b-Glucooligosaccharides 236
Glutamic acid, biotechnological production
    102
Glutaraldehyde, use of to protect proteins for
    ruminants 125
Glycinins 72, 79
- hypervariable regions for genetic modifica-
    tion 80
Grass silage
- production effects of yeast 261, 263, 270
Growth in agricultural production 1-2
Guinea fowl, antibacterials in 161-162
Halogenated methane analogues 331
Heat treatment of proteins 121-123, 126-127,
    305-306
Histidine bioavailability 96
Homocysteine, bioavailability 95
Hydrogen peroxide 249
Ideal protein 101-102
Immune response
- effect of probiotics 212-213
- effect of oligosaccharides 241
Intestinal microflora
- composition 206
- role in animal health 206-207
Ionophores 173-197
- acidosis prevention 180, 194
- acute pulmonary edema and emphysema
    prevention 180
- antimicrobial effects 181-185
- bloat prevention 180
- calf growth promotion 186
- dairy cows 337
- dietary fat interactions 185-186
- effects on ionic homeostasis 183-184
- effects on mineral uptake 185
- effects on rumen protein metabolism 179

– inhibition of methanogenesis   334
– modes of action   174, 175, 177*ff*
– post-ruminal effects   185, 186
– responses with beef cattle   175, 176, 336
– ruminal effects   177-181
Irpex lacteus, enzymes as feed additive   12
Isoleucine bioavailability   96
Klebsiella spp.   255
Lactitol   216
Lactobacillus spp.
– adhesion to chicken crop and piglet gut   209
– as silage inoculant   39, 41, 42, 43
– influence of numbers on silage   44, 45
– probiotics   208, 210, 213*ff*, 247*ff*
– stimulation by oligosaccharides   239
Lactobacillus acidophilus   205, 208, 210, 220, 241, 247, 250
Lactococcus lactis
– as silage inoculant   39
– as probiotic   208, 211
Lactulose   216, 239
Laidlomycin   174, 175
Lanthionine bioavailability   95
Lasalocid   174, 175, 177, 335, 336
Legislation governing feed additives
– Australia   17-20
– Canada   20-22
– Europe   22-26
– Japan   26-28
– Unites States   28-31
Leucine bioavailability   96
Leuconostoc mesenteroides
– as silage inoculant   39
– synthesis of a-glucooligosaccharides   235
Lignin
– *bmr* mutants of biosynthesis   282-283
– effect on digestibility   280-281, 307
– ferulic acid cross-links   281
– manipulation of biosynthesis   281
– peroxidase mutants   284
Lignin degradation   55-57
– anaerobic   56-57
– effects of alkali treatment   281
– genetic manipulation of ligninolytic micro-organisms   59-60
– in lignified by-products   57-61
– selection of fungi for   57-59
Limiting amino acids for ruminants   127-128

Lincomycin   145, 158, 219
Lipid supplements for suppressing methane production   337-338
Liver abscesses in ruminants   193
Listeria monocytogenes
– inhibition by *Enterococcus faecium* extract   250
– inhibition by hydrogen peroxide   249
– proliferation in silages exposed to O_2 39
Lysine
– antagonism by arginine   99
– bioavailability of D- and L-isomers   95
– encapsulation with polymers   133-134
– diet formulation   100
– industrial production   103, 105
– loss on heating protein supplements   121-123
– methods for protection   110, 128-134
– plant biosynthetic pathways   82-83, 84
– regulation of synthesis   82*ff*
– requirement of pigs   106
– ruminant digesta   130
– threonine/lysine ratio   106-107
Lysine supplementation
– costs   72
– need in ruminants   128, 129, 130
– responses in pigs   106,107
– responses in ruminants   134-135
Lysocellin   174, 175
Maize
– *bmr* mutants of lignin biosynthesis   283
– composition   297
– effects of increasing lignin content   280
– improved cell wall digestibility   280
– increasing oil content   287-288
– methionine content   76
– starch mutants   286
– starch synthesis   285
– sucrose phosphate synthase   286
– transformation   74
Malic acid in probiotics for ruminants   265
Mannan-oligosaccharide   255, 256
Mannose-specific lectins   254
Manure
– aerobic treatment   314
– anaerobic treatment   314
– biogas production   313
– biotechnological treatments   311-326, 318

– composting 314-315
– conversion to animal feed 315
– disposal problem 311-312
– drying 315
– processing plants 318*ff*
– production in Europe 312
Metchnikoff 205, 247
Methane
– antibiotics for inhibiting 334*ff*
– ATP formation 329
– defaunation of the rumen for decreasing 339-340
– dietary interventions for decreasing 330*ff*
– environmental damage 330
– from animal wastes 313
– inhibition by ionophores in ruminants 177-178
– inhibitors 331-334
– lipid supplements for decreasing 337-338
– mechanism of formation 329
– relation to propionate production 329, 331, 332, 334, 340
– relation to reductive acetogenesis 340-341
Methionine
– bioavailability 95
– derivatives tested in ruminants 131
– encapsulation with lipids 132
– encapsulation with polymers 133-134
– in plants 74*ff*
– industrial production 103
– methods for protection 110, 128-134
– requirement for protected methionine in ruminants 128, 129
– responses in ruminants 134-135
– ruminant digesta 130
Methionine hydroxy analogue 129, 132
Methionine-rich proteins 74*ff*
– Brazil nut albumin 75-77
– chimeric genes 75-77
– soybean 10.8 kDa protein 78
– zein 15 kDa protein 78
Milk production
– response to microbial feed additives 259-262
Minerals, extraction from manure 321
Monensin
– discovery 174

– inhibition of methane production 177-178, 335-337
– influence on rumen N metabolism 178-179
– mode of action 175
– performance responses in ruminants 174-175
– stimulation of propionate formation 177-178
Narasin 175
Neomycin 187-189, 195, 196
Nitrovin 145, 153, 158, 161
Nonprotein nitrogen
– as silage additive 48-50
Novobiocin 335
Nurmi concept 211
Nystose 234
Oats
– as broiler feed 7-8
– enzyme supplementation 298
Odours
– control of air pollution 316*ff*
– from animal manure 312
Oilseeds
– increasing oil content 287-288
Olaquindox 144, 145
Oligosaccharides
– as enzyme inducers 240
– commercially available 12-13
– feed additives 233*ff*
– human milk 241
– immune response 241
– interaction with probiotics 219
– in calves 237, 238
– in cows 238
– in humans 239
– in piglets 237
– in poultry 219
– in rabbits 237, 238
– interactions with cell surfaces 241
– manufacture 233-237
– mechanism of action 238*ff*
– stimulation of specific bacteria 239, 240
Ornithine bioavailability 95
Oxo-amino acids bioavailability 96
Oxytetracycline 144, 145, 158, 161, 162, 165, 188, 189, 190, 191, 193, 195, 196
Peas composition 297
Pediococcus spp.

– as silage inoculant   39, 41, 42, 43
– probiotics   208, 217
Penicillin   160, 161
Phanerochaete chrysosporium   60, 61
Phaseolin
– increased methionine content   79, 80
Phaseolin-Brazil nut albumin chimeric gene
   75-77
Phenolic acids   281
Phenylalanine ammonia-lyase   281
Phenylalanine bioavailability   96
Phytase   322
Pigs
– amino acid requirements   99, 106-107
– dietary enzymes for   301*ff*
– fructooligosaccharides in piglet diet   237
– nutritional response to antibacterials   162-
   165
– probiotics for   205*ff*
– reproductive performance   217-218
– variation in response to antibiotics   146
Polygalacturonidase   296
Polyporus versicor   57
Population growth   1
Poultry
– amino acid requirements   99
– amino acid digestibility   109
– antibacterials for   143*ff*
– probiotics for   205*ff*
Probiotics   10, 165
– colonisation of gut   251
– composition   208
– definition   207
– effects on digestion   218
– effects on gut microflora of poultry   214
– effects on gut microflora of pre-ruminants
   248-249
– effects on gut microflora of young pigs
   213-214
– effects on growth rate of pigs   215-216
– effects on growth rate of poultry   216-217
– effects on reproductive performance   217-
   218
– for pigs and poultry   205*ff*
– for pre-ruminants   247*ff*
– housing and hygiene effects   220, 221
– immune response effects   212-213, 251-252

– interactions with other feed additives   218-
   220
– mode of action   210*ff*, 250*ff*
– neonate health   252
– post-ruminal effects   262-263
– quality control   221
– selection of organisms   208-209
– stability   210, 221
– standardization   221-222
– stimulation of rumen development   252*ff*
– yeast for ruminants   259*ff*
Product registration
– Australia   17-20
– Canada   20-22
– Europe   22-26
– Japan   26-28
– Unites States   28-31
Promest process   320
Promoter sequences
– regulation of plant gene expression   279,
   280
Protease   36, 296
Protected proteins for ruminants
– formaldehyde use   123-125, 126
– methods for making   120-127
– requirement   120
Protein breakdown in the rumen
– influence of monensin   179
Protein digestion in nonruminants   98
Protein supplements
– essential amino acid composition   117
– heating, protection for ruminants   121-123
– ideal   101-102
Protein turnover   98
Pullets, influence of antibacterials   158-159
Quail, antibacterials in   162
Raffinose   235, 236, 307
Rapeseed   8, 76, 297
Recombinant DNA techniques   10
– modification of plants   73*ff*, 279*ff*
– rumen microorganisms   270-271
Registration of biotechnology products
– Australia   17-20
– Canada   20-22
– Europe   22-26
– Japan   26-28
– Unites States   28-31
Rumen inoculants   253

Rumen microorganisms
- amino acid composition 116-118
- development of population 248
- effects of ionophores 181-184, 195, 196
- methane production 329
- nutritive value 116-118
- sensitivity to antibiotics 194-197
- stimulation by yeast and fungi 263-264
Rumen protected proteins 120
Saccharomyces cerevisiae
- effects on poultry 217
- post-ruminal effects 262-263
- probiotic for ruminants 259*ff*, 338-339
- probiotic for pre-ruminants 247, 252
Salinomycin 165, 175, 336
Salmonella 206, 208, 210, 211, 212, 214, 220, 221, 237, 240, 255
Seed storage proteins
- biosynthesis and assembly 72-73
- cloning 73
Selenium-enriched yeast 6
Shigella sonnei 212
Silage additives 33-54
- acids and acid salts 50-51
- bacterial inoculants 36, 40-47
- enzymes 47-48
- fermentation inhibitors 34
- fermentation stimulants 35
- nonprotein N 48-50
- nutrient sources 36, 48-50
Silage making
- aerobic phase 37
- factors affecting quality 34, 35
- feedout phase 40
- fermentation phase 37
- nutritive value of silage 44-47
- stable phase 38-39
Solid state fermentation 55-70, 321-322
Sorghum
- *bmr* mutants of lignin biosynthesis 283
Soybean
- composition 297
- enzyme supplementation 306
- glycinin genes 80
- methionine content 76
- phaseolin-Brazil nut albumin gene insertion 76, 77, 87
- proteins 72

- transformation 74
Spiramycin 188, 189
Stable phase of silage making 38-39
Stachyose 235, 236
Staphylococcus aureus 249, 250
Starch synthesis
- branching enzymes 285
- control 285
- target for genetic modification 284-286
- "waxy_ gene 285
Storage carbohydrates in plants 284
Straw breakdown
- influence of probiotics 267-269
Streptococcus agalactiae 249, 250
Streptococcus bovis 250
Streptomycin 161
Sucrose accumulation in plants 286
Sulfanilamides 205
Tannins, for protection of proteins for ruminants 126
Terramycin 335
Tetracyclines 187
Tetronasin 174, 175, 179, 336
Thiopeptin 335
Threonine
- bioavailability 95
- industrial production 103, 105
Tobacco as model genetic system 74, 78, 81, 84, 85, 283, 284, 287
Transformation
- by *Agrobacterium tumefaciens* 74
- of crop plants 73-74
Transgenic plants
- agronomic properties 86
- expression of chimeric genes 88
- for improved protein quality 71-92
- for improved energy characteristics 279-293
- fructan biosynthesis 287
- lignin biosynthesis 281-283
- safety 87
- strategies for trait manipulation 279
- sucrose accumulation 286-287
Tryptophan
- bioavailability 95
- industrial production 103
- use as serotonin precursor 109, 110
Turkeys

– antibiotics in nutrition   155-156
– probiotics effects   217
Tylosin   144, 145, 148, 151, 158, 161, 162, 163, 164, 165, 188, 189, 193, 194, 195, 196, 197, 216
Tyrosine/phenylalanine bioavailability   96
Valine bioavailability   96
Variable regions in plant genes suitable for modification   80, 81
VerTech process   320
Viability
– storage effects in probiotics   210
Viscosity of gut contents, effect of enzymes 298, 300-301
Virginiamycin   144, 145, 148, 151, 156, 158, 159, 160, 161, 162, 165, 188, 189, 190, 193, 216, 335
Wheat
– composition   297
– feeding to pigs   301, 302, 304-305

– feeding to poultry   300, 301, 303-304
White-rot fungi
– digestion of lignified by-products   57-59
Xylanase   36, 48, 296, 298, 299, 306
b-Xylooligosaccharides   237
Yeast, see *Saccharomyces cerevisiae*
– mannan-oligosaccharide   255, 256
– oxygen scavenging in rumen   266-267
– post-ruminal effects   262-263
– probiotic for pre-ruminants   247
– probiotic for ruminants   259*ff*
– selenium-enriched   6
– stimulation of lactate uptake   253, 265
Yogurt   205, 247
Yucca shidigera   318
Zeins   72
– insertion of lysine into genes   81
Zinc bacitracin, see Bacitracin
Zinc sulfate, protein protection for ruminants 127